Algorithmic Diagnosis
of Symptoms and Signs:
A Cost-Effective Approach
THIRD EDITION

Algorithmic Diagnosis of Symptoms and Signs:
A Cost-Effective Approach

THIRD EDITION

R. Douglas Collins, M.D., F.A.C.P.

Former Associate Professor of Medicine
Medical University of South Carolina
Former Associate Clinical Professor of Medicine
University of Florida School of Medicine
Chatsworth, CA

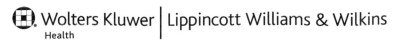

. Wolters Kluwer | Lippincott Williams & Wilkins
Health

Philadelphia · Baltimore · New York · London
Buenos Aires · Hong Kong · Sydney · Tokyo

Senior Acquisitions Editor: Sonya Seigafuse
Senior Product Manager: Kerry Barrett
Vendor Manager: Bridgett Dougherty
Senior Manufacturing Manager: Benjamin Rivera
Senior Marketing Manager: Kim Schonberger
Design Coordinator: Steve Druding
Production Service: Aptara, Inc.

© 2013 by LIPPINCOTT WILLIAMS & WILKINS, a WOLTERS KLUWER business
Two Commerce Square
2001 Market Street
Philadelphia, PA 19103 USA
LWW.com

Printed in China

Library of Congress Cataloging-in-Publication Data
Collins, R. Douglas.
  Algorithmic diagnosis of symptoms and signs : a cost-effective
approach / R. Douglas Collins. — 3rd ed.
      p. ; cm.
  Includes bibliographical references and index.
  ISBN 978-1-4511-7343-7 (alk. paper) — ISBN 1-4511-7343-1 (alk. paper)
  I. Title.
  [DNLM: 1. Diagnosis—Handbooks.   2. Signs and Symptoms—Handbooks.
3. Algorithms—Handbooks.   4. Cost Savings—Handbooks. WB 39]

  616.07'5—dc23

                                           2012016937

To purchase additional copies of this book, call our customer service department at (800)
638-3030 or fax orders to (301) 223-2320. International customers should call (301) 223-
2300.

Visit Lippincott Williams & Wilkins on the Internet: at LWW.com. Lippincott Williams &
Wilkins customer service representatives are available from 8:30 AM to 6 PM, EST.

I am delighted to be asked to write a third edition of this text!

How can the third edition be more useful to students, primary care providers and physicians in practice? Because I have added the algorithmic diagnosis of several more useful laboratory tests. Furthermore, I have provided the reader with actual case histories to illustrate how to utilize the algorithms in clinical practice. Finally, I have added an appendix with an extensive list of diagnostic tests to be ordered when faced with the most common symptoms.

I would like to acknowledge my wife, Norie Collins, for performing the tedious job of typing the manuscript for this edition. It is my hope that this edition will continue to serve as a useful tool to the clinician on the front lines of medical practice.

R. Douglas Collins, M.D., F.A.C.P.

The average textbook of medicine is not very useful to the busy practicing physician because all of the information in these texts is catalogued according to specific diseases. Until the physician has a diagnosis, he cannot look up diagnostic tests or treatment that would address the patient's problem.

This book applies algorithms to the clinical diagnosis of symptoms and signs. It is aimed at organizing the approach to diagnosis and reducing the cost of a diagnostic workup. To facilitate this procedure, the symptoms and signs are arranged alphabetically. Once the physician turns to a certain symptom or sign, he will find not just a list of diseases, but the diseases are arranged in an algorithm. At a glance he will be able to find what other historical and clinical data he needs to look for, to pin down the diagnosis. Then in the accompanying text he will find the tests to order for a diagnostic workup.

A highlight of this book is a discussion on when to refer to the appropriate specialist. Once a specific diagnosis has been established, the clinician can move on to treatment. I have written this book to provide primary care physicians and specialists with a useful tool in the rapid diagnosis of symptoms and signs that they can use in their offices, in the emergency room, or in the hospital wards.

R. Douglas Collins, M.D., F.A.C.P.

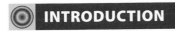

HOW TO USE THESE ALGORITHMS

The algorithms presented in these pages are, at the very least, a list of the most common disorders that may cause a given symptom or sign. As such, however, they are not all inclusive. Rare or unusual conditions are excluded. The reader is referred to other treatises of differential diagnosis, such as *French's Index of Differential Diagnosis,* edited by I.A.D. Bouchier, H. Ellis, and P.R. Fleming, *and Handbook of Difficult Diagnosis,* edited by A.A. Louis, for a more complete list of diagnostic possibilities.

The list of diagnostic possibilities is broken down by the presence or absence of additional symptoms and signs. The reader should be aware that any specific patient may not present with an additional symptom necessary for this analysis, and, therefore, the entire list of possibilities must still be entertained. Alternatively, the patient may present with the additional symptom but still have one of the other disorders on the diagnostic tree; therefore, at all times, the clinician should maintain an index of suspicion that the patient could have any one of the disorders listed on the page and not exclude any of the possibilities completely until a positive laboratory, x-ray, or tissue diagnosis is ready. For example:

A 47-year-old white female reported progressive numbness and tingling and weakness of the lower extremities. Examination showed loss of vibratory and position sense in the lower extremities and positive Babinski's sign. A tentative diagnosis of pernicious anemia was made. However, tests for serum B_{12} and folic acid were normal. Magnetic resonance imaging (MRI) of the thoracic spine showed a neurofibroma at the T6-7 level.

From this example, one can see that, had the clinician not kept an open mind about the entire list of diagnostic possibilities, he or she would not have ordered MRI of the thoracic spine and would have missed the diagnosis.

Finally, the text accompanying each algorithm contains valuable information on how to approach the patient with each presenting symptom and sign and how to proceed with the diagnostic workup. For example:

A 35-year-old white female presents to the emergency room with acute abdominal pain and diffuse tenderness and rebound.

The text on acute abdominal pain shows that the routine diagnostic tests are a flat and upright plate of the abdomen, a complete blood cell count, urinalysis, amylase, and chemistry panel. Most clinicians would remember to order these tests without referring to this handbook. However, some clinicians might forget to order a chest x-ray or electrocardiogram and pregnancy test. Furthermore, there are additional tests to order in case the routine tests are unrevealing. The clinician is reminded to order x-ray contrast studies and ultrasound of the gallbladder and pelvis, and he or she is reminded to do a peritoneal tap to diagnose a ruptured ectopic pregnancy.

Most of the time, this little handbook is not presenting anything new to the experienced diagnostician. However, the materials presented here will jog the memory and help the diagnostician proceed with a thorough workup.

CONTENTS

CASE HISTORY

A 67-year-old white female presents to the emergency department with generalized abdominal pain that began this morning. Following the algorithm, you check her for cough, shortness of breath, and an unusual odor to her breath, and find none of these signs. She is not aware of being bitten by a spider and you do not find any bite-like lesions on her body. Her blood pressure is 95/60 and her pulse is 110 per minute so you keep in mind the possibility of an inferior wall myocardial infarct.

Examination of the abdomen reveals generalized rebound tenderness and guarding and hypoactive bowel sounds. You perform a rectal examination and find bloody stools. You suspect a mesenteric thrombosis and you would be correct.

ASK THE FOLLOWING QUESTIONS:

1. **Where is the pain located?** If it is diffuse, one should consider pancreatitis, mesenteric artery occlusion, or ruptured peptic ulcer. In addition, another viscus may be perforated, such as a ruptured ectopic, and there may be peritonitis. Pain out of proportion to the objective findings suggests mesenteric artery occlusion. If it is focal, we need to know what quadrant it is in. For example, acute cholecystitis is in the right upper quadrant, whereas diverticulitis is usually in the left lower quadrant.
2. **What is the nature of the pain?** Colicky abdominal pain suggests intestinal obstruction, renal calculus, and cholelithiasis or common duct stone, whereas constant pain is typical of pancreatitis, a ruptured peptic ulcer, appendicitis, diverticulitis, and a ruptured ectopic pregnancy.
3. **Does the pain radiate?** The pain of acute cholecystitis typically radiates to the right scapula or right shoulder. The pain of a ruptured peptic ulcer may also radiate to the shoulder. The pain of acute renal calculus may radiate to the testicle.
4. **What are the associated signs and symptoms?** Shock with generalized tenderness and rebound and diminished or absent bowel sounds should suggest a ruptured peptic ulcer or acute pancreatitis. However, acute right upper quadrant pain with nausea and vomiting should suggest acute cholecystitis. On the other hand, appendicitis is more insidious in onset and is associated with anorexia and nausea, rarely vomiting, as well as constipation. Renal colic presents with hematuria.
5. **Could this patient's abdominal pain be due to an extra-abdominal condition?** Remember, lobar pneumonia, myocardial infarction, diabetic acidosis, and porphyria may be responsible for acute abdominal pain. There are numerous other conditions that need to be considered.
6. **If the patient is an infant, is there projectile vomiting or current jelly stools?** Projectile vomiting suggests pyloric stenosis, whereas bloody stools would suggest intussusception.

DIAGNOSTIC WORKUP

It is wise to consult a general surgeon at the outset. All patients with acute abdominal pain should have a stat, flat, and upright plate of the abdomen; a chest x-ray to rule out pneumonia; an electrocardiogram (EKG) to rule out myocardial infarction; and a complete blood count (CBC), urinalysis, amylase, lipase, lactic acid, and chemistry panel. Sometimes lateral decubitus films of the abdomen are necessary to show the step ladder pattern of intestinal obstruction. A pregnancy test is ordered when age and sex dictate it!

When these tests fail to confirm the clinical diagnosis, x-ray contrast studies or ultrasound may be necessary. For example, a computed tomography (CT) scan of the abdomen can be done for a suspected renal calculus. Serial cardiac enzymes may confirm a myocardial infarction. Gallbladder ultrasound can be done to confirm cholecystitis and cholelithiasis. A nuclear scan of the gallbladder with iminodiacetic acid derivatives is very accurate in detecting acute cholecystitis. An angiogram is done for suspected mesenteric thrombosis. Ultrasonography may also help diagnose impending rupture of an abdominal aneurysm, appendicitis, or ectopic pregnancy. A peritoneal tap may diagnose a ruptured ectopic pregnancy. Laparoscopy should also be considered. A urine porphobilinogen helps exclude porphyria. A double enema may help diagnose intestinal obstruction. Magnetic resonance imaging (MRI) can be done when the diagnosis remains obscure, but it is cheaper to consult a general surgeon first.

If the diagnosis remains in doubt, an exploratory laparotomy must be done before the patient's condition deteriorates. The only case where this might be risky is acute pancreatitis. If this is suspected and the serum amylase is repeatedly normal, a quantitative urine amylase or peritoneal tap may confirm the diagnosis. Endoscopy may need to be done to diagnose a peptic ulcer, gastritis, gastric tumor, or reflux esophagitis. In obscure cases of appendicitis and diverticulitis, a contrast barium enema may help confirm the diagnosis. Angiography can diagnose an aneurysm or mesenteric infarction.

ABDOMINAL PAIN, ACUTE

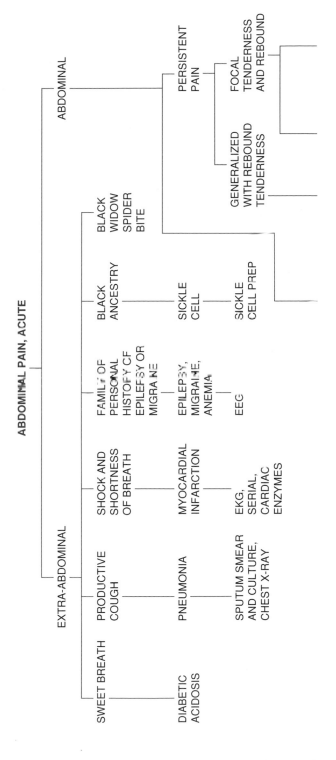

(continued)

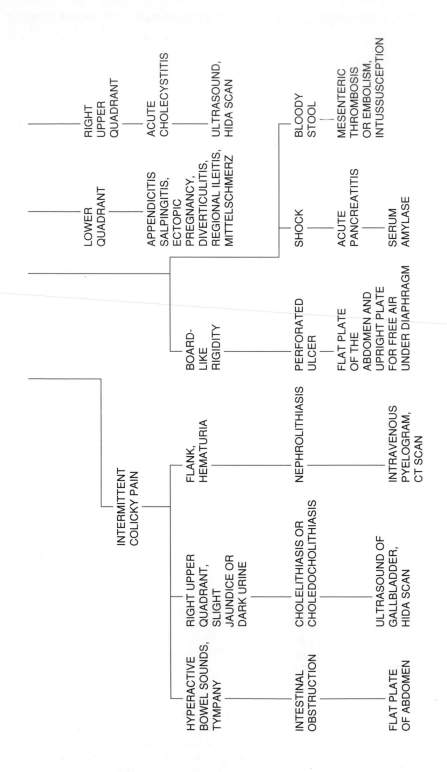

ASK THE FOLLOWING QUESTIONS:

1. **Is there a family history of migraine or epilepsy?** Migraine and epilepsy both present with abdominal pain.
2. **Is the pain colicky or persistent?** Chronic colicky abdominal pain may be due to chronic cholecystitis, cholelithiasis, renal calculus, or partial intestinal obstruction.
3. **What is the location of the pain?** If the pain is located in the upper abdomen, then one should consider peptic ulcer disease, pancreatitis, cholecystitis, and cholelithiasis. If the pain is located in the flanks, one should consider renal calculus and pyelonephritis. If the pain is located in the lower abdomen, one should consider diverticulitis, salpingitis, endometritis, and chronic appendicitis. Regional ileitis also may be located in the lower abdomen, particularly in the right lower quadrant.
4. **What is the relationship to meals?** Abdominal pain relieved by food may be due to a peptic ulcer. Abdominal pain brought on by food may be due to abdominal angina. If the pain comes on 2 to 3 hr after a meal, it may be due to a peptic ulcer. On the other hand, pain that comes on 1 to 2 hr after meals, especially if it's a fatty meal, may be related to cholecystitis and cholelithiasis.
5. **Is there fever associated with the abdominal pain?** Fever and abdominal pain may be due to pyelonephritis, diverticulitis, or appendicitis.
6. **Is there a history of chronic alcoholism?** The history of chronic alcoholism suggests acute and chronic pancreatitis.
7. **Is there blood in the stool?** The presence of blood in the stool would, of course, suggest peptic ulcer disease and diverticulitis.
8. **Is there an abdominal mass?** The presence of an abdominal mass, particularly in the midepigastrium, suggests a pancreatic cyst related to chronic pancreatitis. A mass in the right lower quadrant might be related to regional ileitis or salpingitis. A mass in the left lower quadrant may be related to diverticulitis and salpingitis.

DIAGNOSTIC WORKUP

Routine laboratory tests include a CBC, sedimentation rate, urinalysis, urine culture, sensitivity, colony count, chemistry panel, serum amylase and lipase, pregnancy test, stool for occult blood, and stools for ovum and parasites. A chest x-ray, EKG, and flat plate of the abdomen should also be done. A urine porphobilinogen will help exclude porphyria.

If these tests are negative, then an upper gastrointestinal (GI) series, esophagogram, and gallbladder ultrasound would be done for upper abdominal pain; an intravenous pyelogram (IVP) or CT scan would be done for flank pain; and a barium enema and sigmoidoscopy would be performed for lower abdominal pain. At this point a trial of H_2 antagonists or PPI's may be appropriate.

If these studies are inconclusive, a gastroenterologist should be consulted for endoscopic procedures. If there is upper abdominal pain, esophagoscopy, gastroscopy, and duodenoscopy would be performed. Endoscopic retrograde cholangiopancreatography (ERCP) may be required to diagnose cholangitis or common duct stones. If there is lower abdominal pain, colonoscopy would be performed. A CT scan of the abdomen and pelvis is a useful diagnostic tool also. Gallium scans may detect a diverticular abscess or other localized area of chronic inflammation. Ultrasonography is useful in diagnosing a mesenteric artery occlusion. Pelvic ultrasound may be useful in lower abdominal pain, especially in females. Aortography and angiography will be useful in abdominal angina. Lymphangiography can be helpful in discovering retroperitoneal tumors. Ultimately, exploratory laparotomy may still be necessary in some cases.

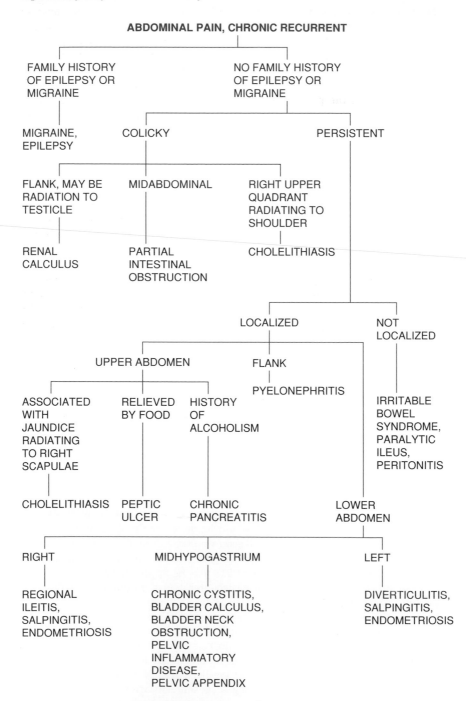

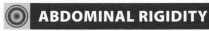

ASK THE FOLLOWING QUESTIONS:

1. **Is there tenderness and rebound tenderness?** If this is absent, consider voluntary rigidity. If this is present, the finding must be considered serious.
2. **Is there a history of trauma?** A history of trauma brings to mind the possibility of a ruptured spleen or other abdominal organ rupture or laceration.
3. **Is there a history of recurrent abdominal pain?** This finding should make one think of a ruptured peptic ulcer or diverticulum or a perforated gallbladder, although appendicitis may occasionally be preceded by bouts of abdominal pain. If there is no history of trauma or abdominal pain, consider ruptured appendix, pelvic inflammatory disease (PID), ruptured ectopic pregnancy, peritonitis, pancreatitis, mesenteric, thrombosis, and ruptured abdominal aneurysm.

DIAGNOSTIC WORKUP

A stat CBC, urinalysis, chemistry panel, amylase and lipase, and flat plate and upright film of the abdomen should be done. Immediate consult with a general surgeon is in order. If surgery is to be delayed or when the exact cause of the rigidity is in doubt, consider ordering a chest x-ray to rule out pneumonia and a peritoneal tap to exclude ruptured ectopic pregnancy, generalized peritonitis, and laparoscopy. Blood cultures, abdominal ultrasound, and CT scans of the abdomen may be necessary to diagnose cholecystitis, diverticulitis, aortic aneurysm, and various neoplasms associated with rupture. Exploratory laparotomy must be considered in any case of unexplained tenderness and rigidity when the diagnosis is in doubt.

ABDOMINAL RIGIDITY

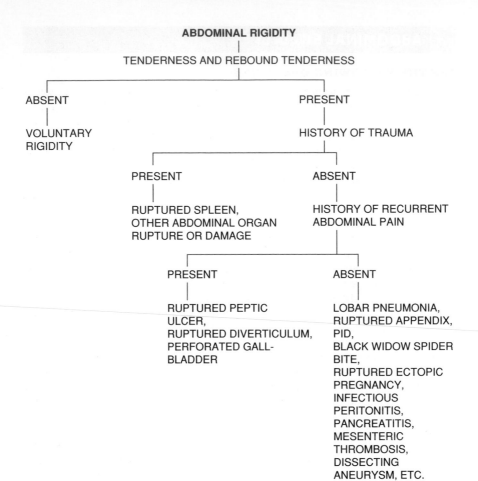

TENDERNESS AND REBOUND TENDERNESS

ABSENT

VOLUNTARY
RIGIDITY

PRESENT

HISTORY OF TRAUMA

PRESENT

RUPTURED SPLEEN,
OTHER ABDOMINAL ORGAN
RUPTURE OR DAMAGE

ABSENT

HISTORY OF RECURRENT
ABDOMINAL PAIN

PRESENT

RUPTURED PEPTIC
ULCER,
RUPTURED DIVERTICULUM,
PERFORATED GALL-
BLADDER

ABSENT

LOBAR PNEUMONIA,
RUPTURED APPENDIX,
PID,
BLACK WIDOW SPIDER
BITE,
RUPTURED ECTOPIC
PREGNANCY,
INFECTIOUS
PERITONITIS,
PANCREATITIS,
MESENTERIC
THROMBOSIS,
DISSECTING
ANEURYSM, ETC.

ASK THE FOLLOWING QUESTIONS:

1. **Is it in the right upper quadrant?** A mass in the right upper quadrant is most often an enlarged liver. However, the liver may be pushed down by a subphrenic abscess, and there may be an enlarged gallbladder due to cholecystitis or bile duct obstruction. There may be perinephric abscesses, tumors of the colon, renal tumors, adrenal tumors, hydrops of the gallbladder, fecal impaction, or an abdominal wall hematoma.

2. **Is it in the epigastrium?** A mass in the epigastrium also may be an enlarged liver, but other types of masses must be considered, including an omental hernia, pancreatic tumor, pancreatic cyst, gastric carcinoma, pyloric stenosis, aortic aneurysm, and retroperitoneal sarcoma.

3. **Is it in the left upper quadrant?** Left upper quadrant masses are often a splenomegaly, but abdominal wall hematomas occur in this area, as well as pancreatic tumors, pancreatic cysts, gastric tumors, colon tumors, kidney tumors or enlargement, and fecal impaction.

4. **Is it in the right lower quadrant?** A mass in the right lower quadrant is frequently a carcinoma of the colon, appendiceal abscess, psoas abscess, pyosalpinx, regional ileitis, intussusception, or an ovarian tumor.

5. **Is it in the hypogastrium?** A mass in the hypogastrium may be bladder, pregnant uterus, uterine fibroids, regional ileitis, urachal cyst, omental cyst, and, rarely, endometrial carcinoma.

6. **Is it in the left lower quadrant?** A left lower quadrant mass is most often a palpable sigmoid colon, but pathologic conditions such as diverticulitis with abscess, carcinoma of the colon, and ovarian tumors may be present

7. **Is the mass tender?** The presence of a tender mass in the right upper quadrant often means congestive heart failure, a tender liver from hepatitis, or a tender gallbladder from cholecystitis, subphrenic abscess, perinephric abscess, or an abdominal wall hematoma. A tender mass in the epigastrium may be a pancreatic cyst. A tender mass in the left upper quadrant may be an abdominal wall hematoma or a perinephric abscess. A tender mass in the right lower quadrant may be appendiceal abscess, psoas abscess, pyosalpinx, regional ileitis, or intussusception. A tender mass in the left lower quadrant may be a diverticulitis or pyosalpinx.

8. **Is there blood in the urine or stool?** The presence of blood in the urine, of course, would suggest a tumor of the kidney such as hypernephroma or Wilms' tumor. The presence of blood in the GI tract would suggest either a gastric carcinoma or colon carcinoma but may also be seen in intussusception, diverticulitis, and regional ileitis. Occasionally, it is seen in carcinoma of the ampulla of Vater.

9. **Is there fever?** The presence of fever would suggest that the mass is an abscess such as subphrenic abscess, perinephric abscess, diverticular abscess, appendiceal abscess, or pyosalpinx. Fever also suggests hepatitis, cholecystitis, or cholangitis.

DIAGNOSTIC WORKUP

Routine diagnostic tests include a CBC, sedimentation rate, urinalysis, chemistry panel with electrolytes, amylase and lipase, stool for occult blood, EKG, chest x-rays, and a flat plate of the abdomen. A carcinoembryonic antigen (CEA) test may diagnose colon cancer. Alpha-1-fetoprotein may diagnose carcinoma of the liver. If there are chills and fever, blood cultures ought to be done. Next in line are contrast radiographic studies such as upper GI series, barium enema, small bowel series, IVP, or cholecystogram.

At this point, before ordering more expensive tests, a surgeon or gastroenterologist should be consulted. An abdominal ultrasound will be helpful in differentiating cholecystitis and other cystic masses of the pancreas, kidneys, and reproductive organs.

Endoscopic procedures will help diagnose carcinoma of the stomach and colon and diverticulitis. ERCP is useful in diagnosing carcinoma of the pancreas and bile ducts.

Lymphangiography will help differentiate retroperitoneal tumors. CT scans of the abdomen and pelvis are useful in differentiating all types of masses. Gallium scans will help uncover subdiaphragmatic, perinephric, diverticular, and pelvic abscesses. Peritoneal taps will help differentiate ascites, pancreatitis, and peritoneal bleeding. Needle biopsy of the liver or any mass lesion under laparoscopic guidance may be diagnostic. A laparoscopy is useful in differentiating many types of masses also. Ultimately, exploratory laparotomy is still an excellent way of establishing a diagnosis.

ABDOMINAL SWELLING, FOCAL

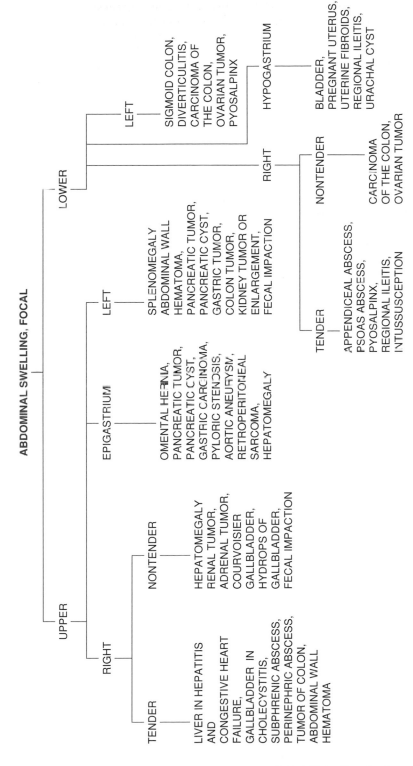

UPPER

RIGHT

TENDER

LIVER IN HEPATITIS AND CONGESTIVE HEART FAILURE, GALLBLADDER IN CHOLECYSTITIS, SUBPHRENIC ABSCESS, PERINEPHRIC ABSCESS, TUMOR OF COLON, ABDOMINAL WALL HEMATOMA

NONTENDER

HEPATOMEGALY RENAL TUMOR, ADRENAL TUMOR, COURVOISIER GALLBLADDER, HYDROPS OF GALLBLADDER, FECAL IMPACTION

EPIGASTRIUM

OMENTAL HERNIA, PANCREATIC TUMOR, PANCREATIC CYST, GASTRIC CARCINOMA, PYLORIC STENOSIS, AORTIC ANEURYSM, RETROPERITONEAL SARCOMA, HEPATOMEGALY

LEFT

SPLENOMEGALY ABDOMINAL WALL HEMATOMA, PANCREATIC TUMOR, PANCREATIC CYST, GASTRIC TUMOR, COLON TUMOR, KIDNEY TUMOR OR ENLARGEMENT, FECAL IMPACTION

LOWER

LEFT

SIGMOID COLON, DIVERTICULITIS, CARCINOMA OF THE COLON, OVARIAN TUMOR, PYOSALPINX

HYPOGASTRIUM

BLADDER, PREGNANT UTERUS, UTERINE FIBROIDS, REGIONAL ILEITIS, URACHAL CYST

RIGHT

NONTENDER

CARCINOMA OF THE COLON, OVARIAN TUMOR

TENDER

APPENDICEAL ABSCESS, PSOAS ABSCESS, PYOSALPINX, REGIONAL ILEITIS, INTUSSUSCEPTION

ABDOMINAL SWELLING, GENERALIZED

ASK THE FOLLOWING QUESTIONS:

1. **Is there hepatomegaly?** If there is hepatomegaly, one should suspect congestive heart failure, emphysema, constrictive pericarditis, hepatic vein thrombosis, and cirrhosis of the liver.
2. **Is there dyspnea or cardiomegaly?** If there is dyspnea or cardiomegaly, one should suspect congestive heart failure or emphysema.
3. **Is there hypertension or proteinuria?** The presence of hypertension or proteinuria should arouse suspicion of nephritis or nephrosis.
4. **Is there diffuse abdominal tenderness and rebound?** These findings are suggestive of tuberculous peritonitis, ruptured viscus, pancreatic cyst, advanced intestinal obstruction, mesenteric thrombosis or embolism, acute pancreatitis, and ruptured ectopic pregnancy.

DIAGNOSTIC WORKUP

Routine diagnostic tests include a CBC, sedimentation rate, urinalysis, microscopic examination of the urine sediment, chemistry panel, amylase and lipase, tuberculin test, stool for occult blood, chest x-ray, EKG, and flat plate of the abdomen with lateral decubiti. In women of child-bearing age, a pregnancy test should be done.

The presence of ascites or smaller amounts of fluid can be established by ultrasonography or CT scan. If peritoneal fluid is established, a peritoneal tap is done and the fluid analyzed and cultured. Cultures should be done for both routine and acid-fast bacilli (AFB). The fluid may be spun down and a Papanicolaou (Pap) smear made or cell block study done. Contrast radiographic studies may identify a primary neoplasm or primary source for infection. Gallium scans may be utilized to identify a source of infection. Laparoscopy or exploratory laparotomy is useful in establishing the diagnosis. A general surgeon or gastroenterologist should be consulted early in the diagnostic evaluation.

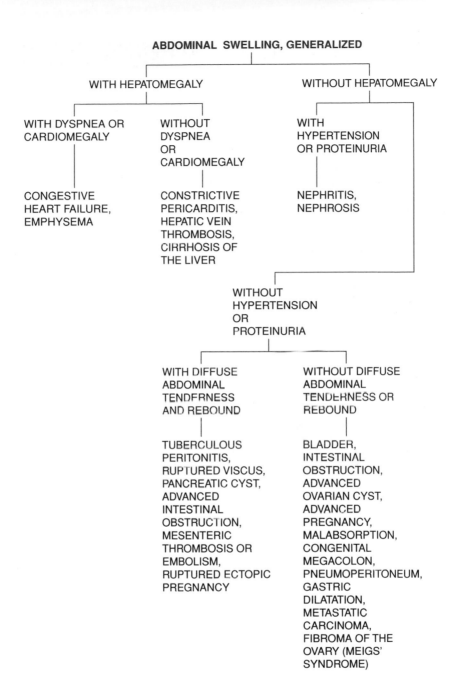

ABDOMINAL SWELLING, GENERALIZED

WITH HEPATOMEGALY

WITHOUT HEPATOMEGALY

WITH DYSPNEA OR CARDIOMEGALY

CONGESTIVE HEART FAILURE, EMPHYSEMA

WITHOUT DYSPNEA OR CARDIOMEGALY

CONSTRICTIVE PERICARDITIS, HEPATIC VEIN THROMBOSIS, CIRRHOSIS OF THE LIVER

WITH HYPERTENSION OR PROTEINURIA

NEPHRITIS, NEPHROSIS

WITHOUT HYPERTENSION OR PROTEINURIA

WITH DIFFUSE ABDOMINAL TENDERNESS AND REBOUND

TUBERCULOUS PERITONITIS, RUPTURED VISCUS, PANCREATIC CYST, ADVANCED INTESTINAL OBSTRUCTION, MESENTERIC THROMBOSIS OR EMBOLISM, RUPTURED ECTOPIC PREGNANCY

WITHOUT DIFFUSE ABDOMINAL TENDERNESS OR REBOUND

BLADDER, INTESTINAL OBSTRUCTION, ADVANCED OVARIAN CYST, ADVANCED PREGNANCY, MALABSORPTION, CONGENITAL MEGACOLON, PNEUMOPERITONEUM, GASTRIC DILATATION, METASTATIC CARCINOMA, FIBROMA OF THE OVARY (MEIGS' SYNDROME)

CASE HISTORY

A 62-year-old white man complained of pain, numbness, and tingling in both lower extremities which is increased by walking more than one-half a block for the past 6 months. He also complains of erectile dysfunction. On physical examination, his blood pressure is 110/80, but he demonstrates weak dorsalis pedis, tibialis, popliteal, and femoral pulses in both lower extremities. There was a loud bruit over both femoral arteries. Following the algorithm, you suspect a Leriche syndrome and you would be correct.

ASK THE FOLLOWING QUESTIONS:

1. **Is it in the upper or lower extremities?** Diminished pulse in the upper extremities should suggest dissecting aneurysm, embolism, fracture, arteriovenous fistula, coarctation of the aorta, aortic aneurysm, thoracic outlet syndrome, and subclavian steal syndrome. Diminished pulse in the lower extremities should suggest embolism, fracture, arteriovenous fistula, peripheral arteriosclerosis, Leriche's syndrome, and coarctation of the aorta, as well as dissecting aneurysm. Diminished pulses in all four extremities would suggest shock or constrictive pericarditis.

2. **Is it unilateral or bilateral?** The presence of unilateral absent or diminished pulse should suggest dissecting aneurysm, embolism, fracture, arteriovenous fistula, some cases of coarctation of the aorta, aortic aneurysm, thoracic outlet syndrome, and subclavian steal if it is in the upper extremity. In the lower extremities, unilateral decrease in the pulse may be due to arteriosclerosis or arterial embolism. Bilateral diminished pulses would suggest Leriche's syndrome, saddle embolism, dissecting aneurysm, and coarctation of the aorta if it is in the lower extremity; and if it is in the upper extremity, it may also be related to a dissecting aneurysm and rarely arteriosclerosis.

3. **Is it sudden in onset?** The presence of a sudden onset in diminished pulse should suggest an embolism or dissecting aneurysm regardless of where the diminished or absent pulse may be. However, if it is just the lower extremities, it could be Leriche's syndrome as well. If all four extremities are involved, of course, it could be shock.

DIAGNOSTIC WORKUP

Routine tests include a CBC, sedimentation rate, urinalysis, chemistry panel, VDRL test, EKG, and chest x-ray. If there is a history of trauma, x-rays of the involved extremity or extremities should be done. If it is acute onset with fever, a blood culture should be done to rule out bacterial endocarditis. Because an acute onset suggests an embolism, a search for the embolic source should be undertaken. This would include serial EKGs and cardiac enzymes to rule out myocardial infarction, echocardiography to rule out a thrombus in the atrium or ventricle, and 24-hr Holter monitoring to rule out auricular fibrillation of the paroxysmal variety. A cardiologist should be consulted for further guidance in determining if there is an embolic source.

If there are transient ischemic attacks, four-vessel angiography should be done to determine if there is a subclavian steal. If a dissecting aneurysm is suspected, a CT scan of the chest or angiography is the diagnostic procedure of choice, and this must be done without delay. Doppler studies are of assistance in diagnosing the peripheral arteriosclerosis regardless of where it is, but angiography will ultimately need to be done to determine the exact location of the blockage and whether surgery could be effective in alleviating the condition.

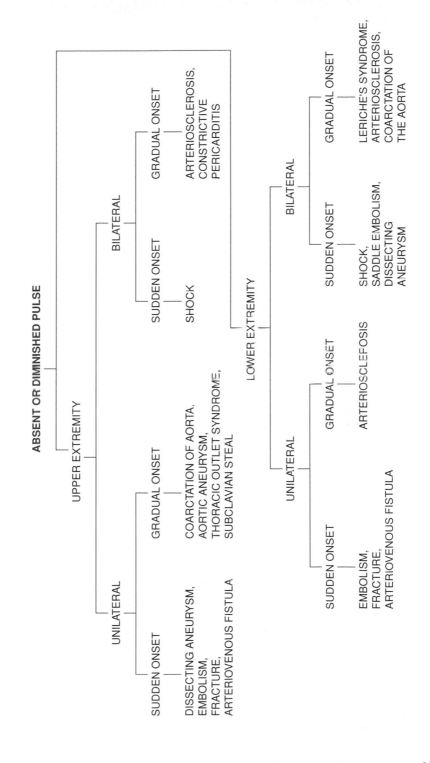

ABSENT OR DIMINISHED PULSE

UPPER EXTREMITY

UNILATERAL

SUDDEN ONSET

DISSECTING ANEURYSM,
EMBOLISM,
FRACTURE,
ARTERIOVENOUS FISTULA

GRADUAL ONSET

COARCTATION OF AORTA,
AORTIC ANEURYSM,
THORACIC OUTLET SYNDROME,
SUBCLAVIAN STEAL

BILATERAL

SUDDEN ONSET

SHOCK

GRADUAL ONSET

ARTERIOSCLEROSIS,
CONSTRICTIVE
PERICARDITIS

LOWER EXTREMITY

UNILATERAL

SUDDEN ONSET

EMBOLISM,
FRACTURE,
ARTERIOVENOUS FISTULA

GRADUAL ONSET

ARTERIOSCLEFOSIS

BILATERAL

SUDDEN ONSET

SHOCK,
SADDLE EMBOLISM,
DISSECTING
ANEURYSM

GRADUAL ONSET

LERICHE'S SYNDROME,
ARTERIOSCLEROSIS,
COARCTATION OF
THE AORTA

ACID PHOSPHATASE ELEVATION

ASK THE FOLLOWING QUESTIONS:

1. **Is there a prostatic mass or prostate-specific antigen (PSA) elevation?** These findings point to a diagnosis of prostatic carcinoma. If there is also an elevated alkaline phosphatase, there may be bony metastasis. If there is no prostatic mass or elevated PSA, one should look for Gaucher's disease, liver disease, Niemann–Pick disease, or various hematologic disorders.

2. **Is the alkaline phosphatase elevated?** As stated previously, an elevated alkaline phosphatase with a prostatic mass or elevated PSA points to prostatic carcinoma with bony metastasis. If both the alkaline phosphatase and acid phosphatase are elevated in the absence of a prostatic mass or elevated PSA, one should suspect Paget's disease, osteogenic sarcoma, and advanced Gaucher's disease.

3. **Is there no prostatic mass, no elevation of PSA, and no elevation of the alkaline phosphatase?** This picture may occur in liver disease, early Gaucher's disease, and multiple myeloma.

DIAGNOSTIC WORKUP

Initially, this may include a prostatic examination, a CBC, PSA, chemistry panel, protein electrophoresis, liver profile, skeletal survey, and bone scan. If the diagnosis is in doubt at this point, a urologist should be consulted. The urologist may order ultrasonography of the prostate, CT scan of the abdomen and pelvis, and a biopsy of the prostate.

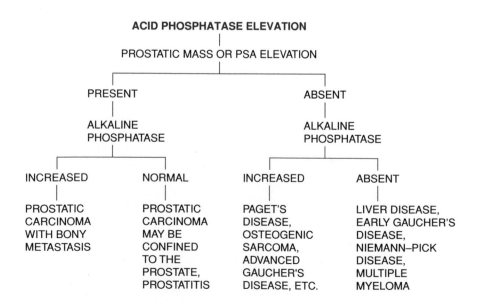

ASK THE FOLLOWING QUESTIONS:

1. **What is the blood glucose and serum acetone level?** If these are increased, consider diabetic acidosis. If these are normal, consider other causes of acidosis.
2. **What is the bicarbonate level?** An increased bicarbonate level points to respiratory acidosis, whereas a decreased bicarbonate level points to renal disease, diarrhea, and the use of certain diuretics.

DIAGNOSTIC WORKUP

This should include a CBC, chemistry panel, electrolytes, arterial blood gas analysis, serum and urine ketones, lactic acid, pulmonary function tests, EKG, and consultation with a pulmonologist or nephrologist.

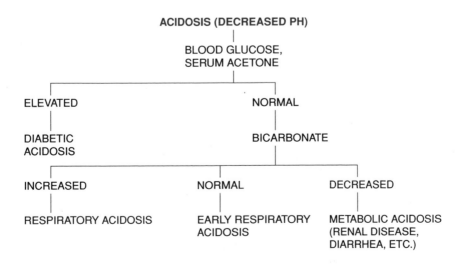

ACIDOSIS (DECREASED PH)
|
BLOOD GLUCOSE, SERUM ACETONE

ELEVATED → DIABETIC ACIDOSIS

NORMAL → BICARBONATE
- INCREASED → RESPIRATORY ACIDOSIS
- NORMAL → EARLY RESPIRATORY ACIDOSIS
- DECREASED → METABOLIC ACIDOSIS (RENAL DISEASE, DIARRHEA, ETC.)

ALKALINE PHOSPHATASE ELEVATION

ASK THE FOLLOWING QUESTIONS:

1. **What is the calcium level?** If this is increased, one should look for primary hyperparathyroidism and bone metastasis. These two findings can be further differentiated with parathyroid hormone (PTH) assay. If calcium is decreased, the patient may have vitamin D deficiency, malabsorption syndrome, Fanconi's syndrome, or other renal diseases.

2. **Are there abnormalities of liver function tests?** If the calcium is normal but liver function tests are abnormal, think of liver disease, obstructive jaundice, and liver metastasis. If the patient is not pregnant, sepsis, Paget's disease, osteogenic sarcoma, gynecologic malignancies, and liver and bone metastasis may be considered.

3. **What is the phosphate level?** In the face of a low calcium level, a low phosphatelevel will help distinguish vitamin D deficiency, malabsorption syndrome, and Fanconi's syndrome from other renal diseases in which the phosphate level will be high.

4. **Is there a high 5'-nucleotidase or γ-glutamyltransferase level?** This will help distinguish liver disease from Paget's disease, metastatic bone disease, and osteogenic sarcoma.

DIAGNOSTIC WORKUP

The workup should include a CBC, sedimentation rate, urinalysis, chemistry panel, protein electrophoresis, liver profile, PTH assay, skeletal survey, bone scan, CT scan of the abdomen, alkaline phosphatase isoenzymes, acid phosphatase, and a PSA to rule out prostatic carcinoma.

ALKALINE PHOSPHATASE ELEVATION

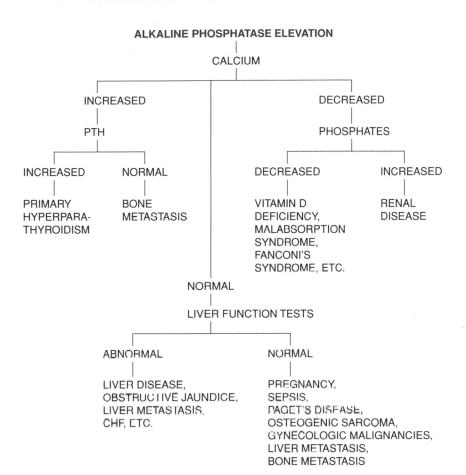

CALCIUM

INCREASED   DECREASED

PTH   PHOSPHATES

INCREASED   NORMAL   DECREASED   INCREASED

PRIMARY
HYPERPARA-
THYROIDISM

BONE
METASTASIS

VITAMIN D
DEFICIENCY,
MALABSORPTION
SYNDROME,
FANCONI'S
SYNDROME, ETC.

RENAL
DISEASE

NORMAL

LIVER FUNCTION TESTS

ABNORMAL   NORMAL

LIVER DISEASE,
OBSTRUCTIVE JAUNDICE,
LIVER METASTASIS,
CHF, ETC.

PREGNANCY,
SEPSIS,
PAGET'S DISEASE,
OSTEOGENIC SARCOMA,
GYNECOLOGIC MALIGNANCIES,
LIVER METASTASIS,
BONE METASTASIS

ALKALOSIS (INCREASED PH)

ASK THE FOLLOWING QUESTIONS:

1. **What is the bicarbonate level?** If this is elevated, the patient has a metabolic alkalosis. If this is decreased, the patient has a respiratory alkalosis associated with salicylate intoxication or hyperventilation syndrome.
2. **Has the patient been vomiting?** If so, look for gastric outlet obstruction, intestinal obstruction, and other causes of vomiting. If there is no history of vomiting, the alkalosis may be due to diuretics, Cushing's disease, or chronic antacid use.

DIAGNOSTIC WORKUP

The workup of alkalosis should include a CBC, chemistry panel, urinalysis, electrolytes, arterial blood gas analysis, flat plate of the abdomen, chest x-ray, and consultation with an endocrinologist.

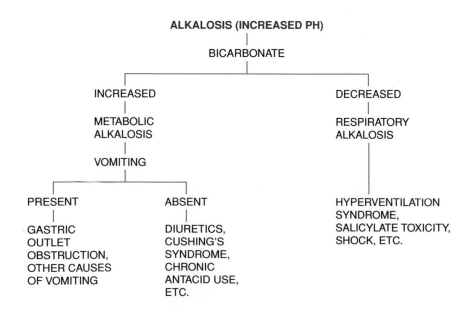

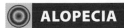

The clinician faced with a patient with hair loss must decide whether it is focal or diffuse. If it is focal, one should determine whether there is a rash in the area of hair loss. If there is a rash, one should consider conditions such as tinea capitis, lupus erythematosus, psoriasis, and seborrheic dermatitis. If there is no rash, one should consider alopecia areata, syphilis, burns, and other injuries to the skin.

If the area of hair loss is diffuse, one must consider that it might be male pattern baldness, as well as female pattern baldness in later years. If it is not typically a male pattern baldness, then one must consider that it might be due to a systemic disease myxedema, hyperpituitarism, hyperthyroidism, anticoagulant drug therapy, or cancer chemotherapy.

DIAGNOSTIC WORKUP

If you are looking for pyoderma or a fungal infection, then a smear and culture of the scrapings for bacteria and fungi should be done. If these are negative, a skin biopsy should be performed. The skin biopsy will help identify lupus erythematosus, psoriasis, and alopecia areata. Systemic disorders may need to be ruled out with thyroid function tests, antinuclear antibody (ANA) assay, VDRL test, CBC, and serum iron and ferritin. A dermatologist should be consulted in difficult cases.

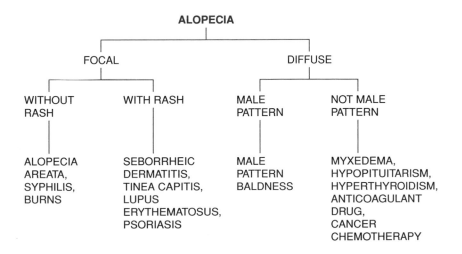

ALTERATIONS IN SERUM IRON

INCREASED

ASK THE FOLLOWING QUESTION:

1. **What is the red cell count?** If it is decreased, think of aplastic anemia and hemolytic anemia. If it is normal, look for hemochromatosis or a side effect from pyridoxine (B_6) therapy.

DECREASED

ASK THE FOLLOWING QUESTION:

1. **What is the serum ferritin?** If it is increased, look for chronic infection or malignancy. If it is decreased, then iron deficiency anemia is confirmed.

DIAGNOSTIC WORKUP

Aplastic anemia will be confirmed by a bone marrow examination as well as iron deficiency anemia and malignancy. Hemachromatosis is best confirmed by a liver biopsy. Hemolytic anemia will show elevated serum haptoglobins and reticulocyte count.

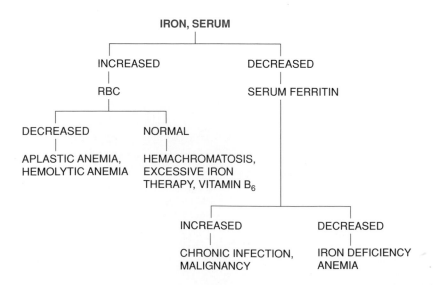

INCREASED

ASK THE FOLLOWING QUESTIONS:

1. **Is the patient an infant or child?** If so, the patient may have Lesch–Nyhan syndrome or Down's syndrome.
2. **Is the blood urea nitrogen (BUN) increased?** Under these circumstances, look for renal failure obstructive uropathy or multiple myeloma.
3. **Is there associated increase of the white or red cell count?** This would indicate leukemia or polycythemia.
4. If none of the foregoing questions can be answered positively, the patient probably has gout. Other conditions to be considered are drugs (thiazides, cytotoxics, and ethambutol) and various hematologic conditions (lymphoma, megaloblastic anemia, etc.).

DECREASED

A decreased uric acid is found in renal tubular acidosis and associated with diuretics and other drugs.

DIAGNOSTIC WORKUP

Order a CBC to diagnose leukemia and polycythemia. An arthrocentesis may be indicated to diagnose gout, although a therapeutic trial of Colchicine will be useful if there are significant arthritic symptoms. A chemistry panel and urinalysis will help pin down a diagnosis of renal disease. Serum protein electrophoresis should be ordered in cases of suspected multiple myeloma. A hematologist or nephrologist should be consulted if the diagnosis is still in doubt.

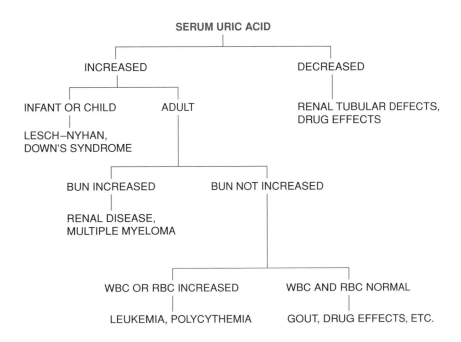

ASK THE FOLLOWING QUESTIONS:

1. **Is there galactorrhea?** Of course, the most common cause of galactorrhea would be the galactorrhea following pregnancy and delivery. However, if there is galactorrhea, one should consider the possibility that the patient is taking drugs, including contraceptive pills and marijuana. Also, one should consider pituitary tumors and hypothalamic tumors.

2. **Are there abnormal or absent secondary sex characteristics?** If there is masculinization, then an adrenal or ovarian tumor or polycystic ovaries should be considered. If there is simply absence of female secondary sex characteristics, one should consider Turner's syndrome or Simmonds' disease and other pituitary disorders.

3. **Are there abnormal findings on the vaginal examination?** The amenorrhea may be due to an imperforate hymen, an imperforate vagina, absence of the vagina, a cervical stenosis with hematometra, and absence of a uterus, as in testicular dysgenesis. If there are normal female secondary sex characteristics and a normal vaginal examination and no galactorrhea, then some systemic disease such as anemia, leukemia, or Hodgkin's disease must be considered as well as psychogenic causes. Perhaps the amenorrhea is secondary to a neurologic disorder.

DIAGNOSTIC WORKUP

The first thing to do is a pregnancy test, as pregnancy is the most common cause of secondary amenorrhea. If the pregnancy test is negative, referral to a gynecologist may be done at this time. If a specialist is not handy, one may proceed with the workup. A trial of medroxyprogesterone acetate (Provera®) may be done by intramuscular injection or by mouth. If bleeding occurs on withdrawal of the progesterone, then it is established that the uterus is functional. It also establishes that the cervix and vagina are patent. If bleeding does not occur, uterine pathology is likely, and referral to a gynecologist is necessary.

If there is no galactorrhea, a normal response to progesterone, and the patient is a teenager, one may simply discontinue studies at this point and observe for the normal onset of the menstrual cycle.

If the patient with primary amenorrhea has already reached her 20s or if there is definite secondary amenorrhea, then further diagnostic studies should be done. If there is galactorrhea, a serum for prolactin should be done. If that is elevated, a CT scan or MRI of the brain should be done to look for a pituitary tumor or hypothalamic tumor. If there is no galactorrhea, one should still order a prolactin, but also order tests for follicle-stimulating hormone (FSH), luteinizing hormone (LH), and serum estradiol. If the FSH and LH are elevated and the estradiol is decreased, primary ovarian failure must be considered. A buccal smear for sex chromogens should be done to rule out Turner's syndrome. Other causes of primary ovarian failure are ovarian agenesis and polycystic ovary syndrome. An elevated free testosterone will support the diagnosis of polycystic ovary syndrome (Stein–Leventhal syndrome).

If the FSH, LH, and estradiol are all decreased, then hypopituitarism should be considered, as well as hypothalamic disorders. Referral to an endocrinologist is wise at this point. When an adrenocortical tumor is suspected, a serum cortisol and cortisol suppression test should be done.

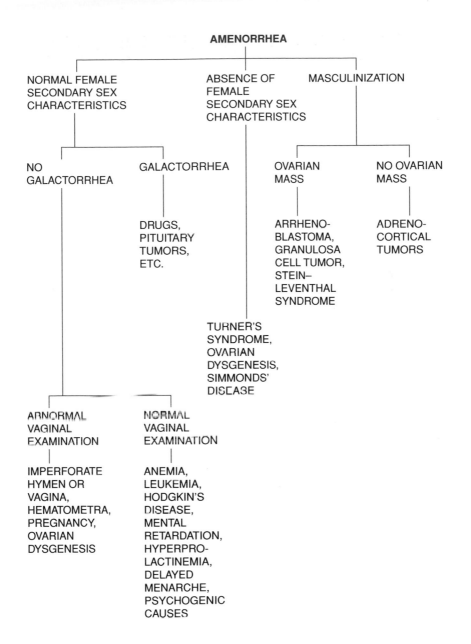

ASK THE FOLLOWING QUESTIONS:

1. **Is the amnesia transient or persistent?** If it is transient, one should look for evidence of a head injury. If there is no evidence of a head injury, then one should consider epilepsy, transient ischemic attacks, and migraine. If there is evidence of a head injury, one would consider concussion and some of the other more serious conditions of the brain that occur with a head injury.

2. **Is there a fever?** If the amnesia is persistent and there is a fever, one needs to consider encephalitis, meningoencephalitis, cerebral abscesses, and encephalomyelitis. If there is no fever, one must ask if there is a reduction of memory for recent events. If there is reduction of memory for recent events, one should consider some of the more serious diseases of the brain, such as cerebral tumors, chronic drug or alcohol use, Alzheimer's disease, cerebral arterial sclerosis, and neurosyphilis. If there is no reduction of memory for recent events, then a psychiatric disorder such as hysteria, dissociated reaction, or schizophrenia must be considered.

DIAGNOSTIC WORKUP

All patients with a history of amnesia deserve a CT scan or MRI. The CT scan would be more cost-effective and would be the diagnostic test of choice because it also helps detect acute brain hemorrhages. Patients with fever should have a spinal tap as well as CBC, urinalysis, and chemistry panel. These patients also probably should have a blood culture. An electroencephalogram (EEG) should be ordered to rule out epilepsy and toxic, metabolic, and inflammatory diseases of the brain.

If all these studies are negative and an organic cause is still considered, then referral to a neurosurgeon or neurologist is in order. If these studies are negative and a psychiatric disorder is suspected, a psychiatrist should be consulted.

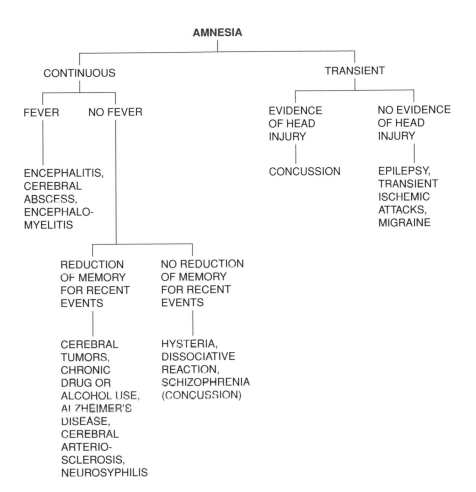

CASE HISTORY

A 59-year-old white male complains of difficulty with his memory and tingling of his hands and feet for the past year. His physical examination reveals a slight decrease in vibratory sense below the knees and a smooth tongue. His hemoglobin in your office is 13.1 g. While this is not striking, you know that this is below the normal of 14 to 17 for males.

Following the algorithm, you find he denies alcohol abuse and has not noted bloody or tarry stools in the past year. He is not jaundiced. You order a CBC and find among other things that his white count is low. You suspect pernicious anemia and further studies confirm your diagnosis.

ASK THE FOLLOWING QUESTIONS:

1. **Is there a history of chronic blood loss?** A history of peptic ulcer, ulcerative colitis, or other causes of chronic GI bleeding would indicate the anemia is most likely due to iron deficiency. Likewise, chronic hypermenorrhea or metror-rhagia in women of child-bearing age may lead to iron deficiency anemia.
2. **Are there neurologic signs?** Paresthesias, loss of vibratory sense, ataxia, and mild dementia should lead one to suspect pernicious anemia.
3. **Is there jaundice?** Clinical jaundice should arouse the suspicion of a hemo-lytic anemia, but mild clinical jaundice may be seen in pernicious anemia also. Chronic liver disease, such as alcoholic cirrhosis, is often associated with folate deficiency or sideroblastic anemia.
4. **What is the white count?** A decreased white count should alert one to the possibility of aplastic anemia, myelofibrosis, or infiltrative diseases of the bone marrow, such as carcinomatosis, Gaucher's disease, or lymphoma. It may also be related to pernicious anemia. An increased white count would suggest leukemia, chronic infections, anemia, or bacteremia.
5. **Is the tourniquet test positive?** This would suggest disseminated intravascular coagulation (DIC) or thrombocytopenia purpura of various etiologies.

DIAGNOSTIC WORKUP

The most important thing to do initially is to examine a blood smear for red cell morphology. If the anemia is microcytic, one would consider iron deficiency or chronic blood loss. If it is macrocytic, consideration should be given to pernicious anemia or folate deficiency. If there are schistiocytes, look for DIC. Further workup should include a chemistry panel, sickle cell prep, Hb electrophoresis, stool for occult blood, liver function tests, reticulocyte count, serum iron and iron-binding capacity, serum B_{12} and folic acid, serum haptoglobin, and platelet count. A urine test for methyl-malonic acid will help diagnose pernicious anemia. A positive stool for occult blood would prompt a GI workup. If these studies are inconclusive, a hematologist should be consulted. A hematologist will perform a bone marrow examination for a more definitive diagnosis. Perhaps a liver–spleen scan, CT scan of the abdomen, or therapeutic trial of iron, B_{12}, or folic acid is indicated.

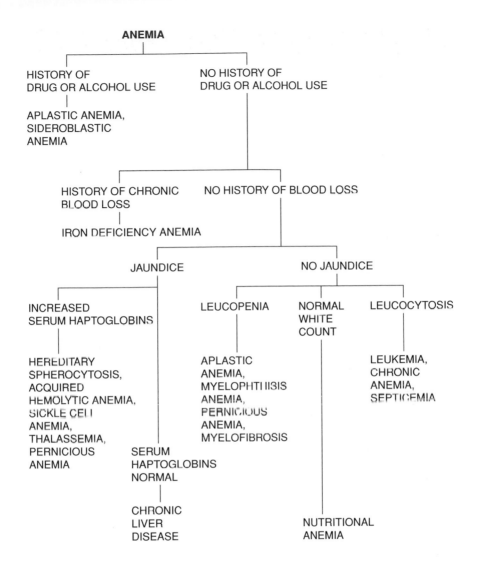

ANEMIA

HISTORY OF
DRUG OR ALCOHOL USE

APLASTIC ANEMIA,
SIDEROBLASTIC
ANEMIA

NO HISTORY OF
DRUG OR ALCOHOL USE

HISTORY OF CHRONIC
BLOOD LOSS

IRON DEFICIENCY ANEMIA

NO HISTORY OF BLOOD LOSS

JAUNDICE

NO JAUNDICE

INCREASED
SERUM HAPTOGLOBINS

HEREDITARY
SPHEROCYTOSIS,
ACQUIRED
HEMOLYTIC ANEMIA,
SICKLE CELL
ANEMIA,
THALASSEMIA,
PERNICIOUS
ANEMIA

SERUM
HAPTOGLOBINS
NORMAL

CHRONIC
LIVER
DISEASE

LEUCOPENIA

APLASTIC
ANEMIA,
MYELOPHTHISIS
ANEMIA,
PERNICIOUS
ANEMIA,
MYELOFIBROSIS

NORMAL
WHITE
COUNT

NUTRITIONAL
ANEMIA

LEUCOCYTOSIS

LEUKEMIA,
CHRONIC
ANEMIA,
SEPTICEMIA

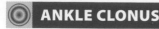

ANKLE CLONUS

ASK THE FOLLOWING QUESTIONS:

1. **What other symptoms and signs are present?** Ankle clonus rarely occurs by itself. Usually, there are pathologic reflexes such as a Babinski's sign on the lower extremities. The patient usually will also complain of weakness and may be found to have weakness when the muscles are tested. If the ankle clonus is long-standing, there will be atrophy. There will also frequently be sensory findings, as well as sensory complaints. Finally, with bilateral ankle clonus there will often be hyperactive reflexes throughout the lower extremities and sometimes in the upper extremities.

2. **Is the ankle clonus unilateral or bilateral?** If it is unilateral, then it is a sign of either hemiparesis or monoplegia; and if it is hemiplegia or hemiparesis, one should consider the possibility of a cerebral disorder. If there is headache and papilledema, that disorder is most likely a space-occupying lesion of the brain such as a brain tumor, abscess, or hematoma. If there is hemiparesis and it is acute in onset, there is most likely an occlusion of one of the cerebral arteries, whereas if the hemiparesis is gradual in onset, one should consider multiple sclerosis and, once again, a brain tumor. Ankle clonus associated with monoplegia is more likely related to a spinal cord tumor, but a parasagittal tumor could also be present. Bilateral ankle clonus is more likely due to a disorder of the spinal cord such as a spinal cord tumor, amyotrophic lateral sclerosis, or multiple sclerosis. Syringomyelia and Friedreich's ataxia may also present with bilateral ankle clonus. However, if there are cranial nerve signs, one must consider a brain stem tumor as well as other degenerative diseases of the brain and brain stem.

DIAGNOSTIC WORKUP

Ankle clonus is a significant clinical sign, especially when it is unilateral. Therefore, if a brain disorder is suspected, a CT scan or MRI of the brain should be done. If a spinal cord lesion is suspected, then a CT scan at the appropriate level of the spinal cord should be done. If there are no findings on the examination to indicate a level, then of course the entire spine would have to be covered. MRI is a more cost-effective method for the cervical and thoracic levels of the cord. The spinal tap with analysis of the fluid for myelin basic protein and gamma globulin levels should be done if multiple sclerosis is suspected. In addition, somatosensory evoked potentials (SSEPs) and visual evoked potentials (VEPs) should also be done if multiple sclerosis is suspected. Finally, the most cost-effective approach to a patient with ankle clonus is to refer the patient to a neurologic specialist.

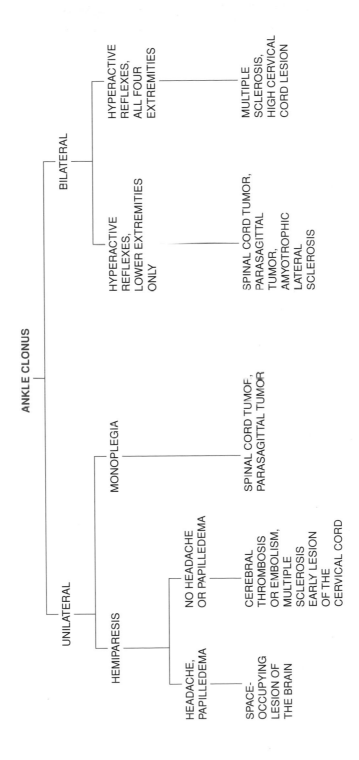

ANKLE CLONUS

UNILATERAL

HEMIPARESIS

HEADACHE, PAPILLEDEMA

SPACE-OCCUPYING LESION OF THE BRAIN

NO HEADACHE OR PAPILLEDEMA

CEREBRAL THROMBOSIS OR EMBOLISM, MULTIPLE SCLEROSIS EARLY LESION OF THE CERVICAL CORD

MONOPLEGIA

SPINAL CORD TUMOF, PARASAGITTAL TUMOR

BILATERAL

HYPERACTIVE REFLEXES, LOWER EXTREMITIES ONLY

SPINAL CORD TUMOR, PARASAGITTAL TUMOR, AMYOTROPHIC LATERAL SCLEROSIS

HYPERACTIVE REFLEXES, ALL FOUR EXTREMITIES

MULTIPLE SCLEROSIS, HIGH CERVICAL CORD LESION

CASE HISTORY

A 32-year-old white female presents to your office with the chief complaint of anorexia and weight loss over the past 3 months. Following the algorithm, you ask about a history of drug or alcohol use or abuse. There is no cough or night sweats to suggest tuberculosis, carcinoma, or other pulmonary conditions.

Your examination fails to reveal an abdominal mass or hepatomegaly. You suspect anorexia nervosa, hypopituitarism, and adrenal insufficiency.

ASK THE FOLLOWING QUESTIONS:

1. **Is it acute or chronic?** Acute anorexia would most likely be due to an acute febrile disease or acute psychiatric disturbance.
2. **Is there a history of drug or alcohol ingestion?** Alcoholics frequently have a loss of appetite. Patients on aspirin and digitalis and many other drugs may lose their appetite.
3. **Is there an abdominal mass?** The abdominal mass may be either an enlarged liver or other mass. The most likely abdominal mass to produce anorexia as the only symptom would be an early pancreatic neoplasm. When the neoplasm advances, jaundice should be present. Other neoplasms may be felt and/or metastasize to the liver and cause hepatomegaly.
4. **Is there a cough?** If there is a chronic cough, one should consider tuberculosis or carcinoma of the lung.
5. **Is there hepatomegaly?** Hepatomegaly without any other masses present in the abdomen would certainly bring to mind cirrhosis. This could be of cardiac origin, so congestive heart failure should be ruled out. Also, the hepatomegaly may be related to a collagen disease or metastatic carcinoma.

DIAGNOSTIC WORKUP

If the general physical examination is normal, it may be wise to obtain a psychiatric consult at the outset. All patients with anorexia as the major sign should have a CBC, sedimentation rate, chemistry panel, thyroid profile [free thyroxine index (FT_4I) and thyroid-stimulating hormone-sensitive assay (S-TSH)], and a chest x-ray. A referral to a gastroenterologist may be wise if these are negative. However, if the clinician wishes to proceed on his own, then a search for a neoplasm should be conducted and should include an upper GI series, barium enema, abdominal CT scan, and bone scan. If these are negative, a gastroscopy or colonoscopy may be required.

A complete endocrinologic workup by an endocrinologist may be indicated if all the above studies are negative. Patients with a normal physical examination and normal diagnostic studies should be referred to a psychiatrist.

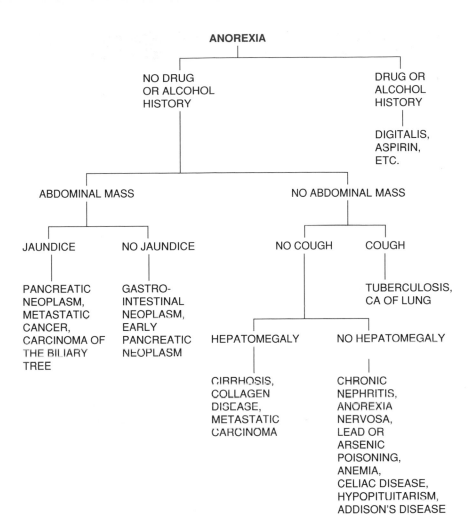

ASK THE FOLLOWING QUESTIONS:

1. **Is it acute or chronic?** Acute loss of smell would certainly suggest an acute upper respiratory infection (URI). It would also suggest recent exposure to toxic fumes or recent head injury. If the anosmia or unusual odor is intermittent, then one should consider psychomotor epilepsy.

2. **Is there a history of trauma?** A skull fracture, particularly if it involves the cribriform plate, may interrupt the olfactory nerves and cause anosmia.

3. **Is there a history of drug use or overuse of nasal sprays?** Captopril and penicillamine may cause anosmia. Overuse of alcohol or tobacco may also be the problem. Antirheumatic and antiproliferative drugs are also known to cause anosmia.

4. **Is the anosmia unilateral or bilateral?** If there is unilateral anosmia, one should consider an olfactory groove meningioma.

5. **Are there other neurologic signs?** Multifocal neurologic signs should suggest multiple sclerosis, and additional neurologic signs such as memory loss should suggest an olfactory groove meningioma or parietal lobe tumor.

6. **Are there signs of a systemic disease?** Many systemic diseases may cause anosmia, including hypothyroidism, diabetes, renal failure, hepatic failure, and pernicious anemia.

DIAGNOSTIC WORKUP

If the disorder is acute and associated with a URI, nothing needs to be done. However, if the condition has been of gradual onset, the nasopharyngeal examination is negative, and the history of drugs is negative, then a CT scan of the brain should be done. If this is negative, a workup for systemic disease should be done, and that should include a CBC and chemistry panel, thyroid profile, serum B_{12} and folic acid, glucose tolerance test, and liver profile. If the anosmia or unusual odors are intermittent, a wake-and-sleep EEG should be done.

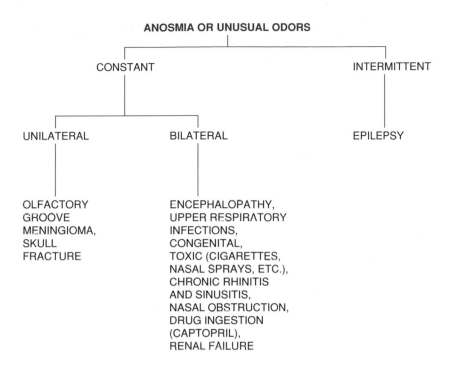

ANOSMIA OR UNUSUAL ODORS

CONSTANT   INTERMITTENT

UNILATERAL   BILATERAL   EPILEPSY

OLFACTORY GROOVE MENINGIOMA, SKULL FRACTURE

ENCEPHALOPATHY, UPPER RESPIRATORY INFECTIONS, CONGENITAL, TOXIC (CIGARETTES, NASAL SPRAYS, ETC.), CHRONIC RHINITIS AND SINUSITIS, NASAL OBSTRUCTION, DRUG INGESTION (CAPTOPRIL), RENAL FAILURE

ANURIA OR OLIGURIA

ASK THE FOLLOWING QUESTIONS:

1. **Has the patient been on any drugs?** Sulfonamides are notorious for causing renal failure, but one must also consider amphotericin B, gold compounds that might be administered in arthritis, and lead and other drugs or heavy metals.
2. **What is the blood pressure?** If there is hypertension and anuria, one should consider acute or chronic glomerulonephritis, polycystic kidneys, and acute tubular necrosis. If there is a low blood pressure, one should consider prerenal causes of anuria such as dehydration, blood loss, the acute abdomen, and other causes of shock.
3. **Is there cardiomegaly or chest pain?** If there is an enlarged heart, one should consider congestive heart failure. If there is chest pain, one should consider myocardial infarction or pulmonary infarction. If there is chest or abdominal pain with hypertension, then one should consider dissecting aneurysm.
4. **Is there enlargement of the kidneys?** Enlargement of both kidneys should suggest bilateral hydronephrosis or polycystic kidneys. Unilateral enlargement of the kidneys is not usually associated with anuria.
5. **Is there bladder enlargement?** Enlarged bladder would make one think of bladder neck obstructions due to prostatic hypertrophy or carcinoma or a urethral stricture. Occasionally, what is thought to be an enlarged bladder is actually a pelvic mass that is obstructing the ureters.
6. **Is there hematuria?** Hematuria would suggest glomerulonephritis, acute tubular necrosis, intravascular hemolysis, and nephrolithiasis.
7. **What has been the patient's recent intake of fluid?** Dehydration is a frequent cause of oliguria and anuria.

DIAGNOSTIC WORKUP

The first thing to determine is whether the patient really has anuria or oliguria. A Foley catheter should be passed and attached to drainage to determine the urine output. If there is obstructive uropathy due to bladder neck obstruction, obviously this will determine the diagnosis, as there will be a large volume of urine and it should be taken off gradually. Then studies of obstructive uropathy can be done, including cystoscopy and retrograde pyelography. If the obstructive uropathy is due to obstruction of the ureter, renal ultrasonography can be reliable in detecting the dilated calyces or dilated ureter.

If the patient presents with anuria and hypotension, the most important thing is to reestablish the blood pressure with a bolus of normal saline or dopamine drip. If the anuria does not cease at this point, high-dose furosemide or a mannitol infusion can be started. Meanwhile, a CBC, chemistry panel, urinalysis, spot urine sodium, serum protein electrophoresis, an ANA assay, an EKG, and chest x-ray should be done. A flat plate of the abdomen should give an idea of the kidney size but a CT scan of the abdomen is even better. The clinician should examine the urinary sediment himself, and this will identify cases of acute glomerulonephritis, lupus erythematosus, and acute tubular necrosis with considerable accuracy. The BUN and creatinine ratio are helpful in distinguishing pre-renal from renal azotemia.

If intravascular hemolysis is suspected, serum haptoglobins and serum hemoglobin tests should be done. Eosinophilia of the blood or urine will be found in drug-induced nephritis. Renal angiography and aortography should be done in cases of suspected dissecting aneurysm or bilateral renal artery stenosis. Abdominal ultrasound will also be helpful in diagnosing polycystic kidneys and pelvic masses that may be obstructing the ureter. A CT scan may be necessary as well.

In difficult cases, a renal biopsy may be necessary to diagnose the various collagen diseases and the various forms of glomerulonephritis. Referral to a nephrologist would be best at this point.

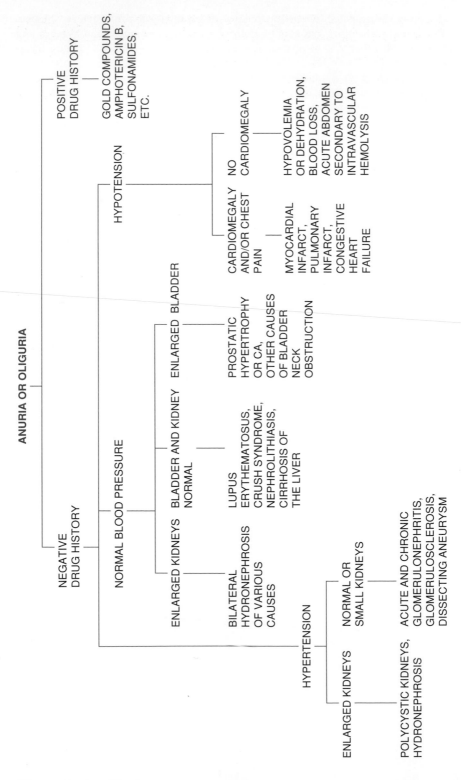

ANURIA OR OLIGURIA

- NEGATIVE DRUG HISTORY
  - NORMAL BLOOD PRESSURE
    - ENLARGED KIDNEYS
      - BILATERAL HYDRONEPHROSIS OF VARIOUS CAUSES
    - BLADDER AND KIDNEY NORMAL
      - LUPUS ERYTHEMATOSUS, CRUSH SYNDROME, NEPHROLITHIASIS, CIRRHOSIS OF THE LIVER
    - ENLARGED BLADDER
      - PROSTATIC HYPERTROPHY OR CA, OTHER CAUSES OF BLADDER NECK OBSTRUCTION
  - HYPERTENSION
    - NORMAL OR SMALL KIDNEYS
      - ACUTE AND CHRONIC GLOMERULONEPHRITIS, GLOMERULOSCLEROSIS, DISSECTING ANEURYSM
    - ENLARGED KIDNEYS
      - POLYCYSTIC KIDNEYS, HYDRONEPHROSIS
  - HYPOTENSION
    - CARDIOMEGALY AND/OR CHEST PAIN
      - MYOCARDIAL INFARCT, PULMONARY INFARCT, CONGESTIVE HEART FAILURE
    - NO CARDIOMEGALY
      - HYPOVOLEMIA OR DEHYDRATION, BLOOD LOSS, ACUTE ABDOMEN SECONDARY TO INTRAVASCULAR HEMOLYSIS
- POSITIVE DRUG HISTORY
  - GOLD COMPOUNDS, AMPHOTERICIN B, SULFONAMIDES, ETC.

ANXIETY

ASK THE FOLLOWING QUESTIONS:

1. **Is the anxiety intermittent or constant?** Intermittent anxiety suggests the possibility of psychomotor epilepsy, a pheochromocytoma, or insulinoma. It is also possible that the patient is suffering from an intermittent cardiac arrhythmia such as paroxysmal supraventricular tachycardia or atrial fibrillation.
2. **What is the patient's age?** Be alert for sexual abuse in children with anxiety. The young or middle-aged patient is more likely to be suffering from a psychiatric disorder, whereas the older patient may be suffering from cerebral arteriosclerosis or some other type of dementia.
3. **If there is tachycardia, is it sustained during sleep?** Tachycardia that is sustained during sleep would suggest hyperthyroidism, caffeine effects, or other drug effects.
4. **Is there associated weight loss?** Sustained tachycardia with weight loss makes hyperthyroidism a very likely possibility.
5. **What drugs or addictive substances is the patient on?** You wouldn't want to miss alcohol or cocaine abuse.

DIAGNOSTIC WORKUP

Patients with intermittent anxiety with long periods of calmness in between should have a wake-and-sleep EEG and possibly a CT scan to rule out a cerebral tumor. A 24-hr urine collection for catecholamines should also be done to rule out a pheochromocytoma. Twenty-four-hour Holter monitoring may be necessary to rule out a paroxysmal cardiac arrhythmia. In difficult cases, a 24-hr EEG or an EEG with nasopharyngeal electrodes inserted may be necessary.

Patients with constant anxiety should have a thyroid profile, a drug screen, and an EKG. If these are not revealing, perhaps 24-hr Holter monitoring may be of some value. With a negative workup, a referral to a psychiatrist is in order. It may be even wiser to consult a psychiatrist before undertaking an expensive workup.

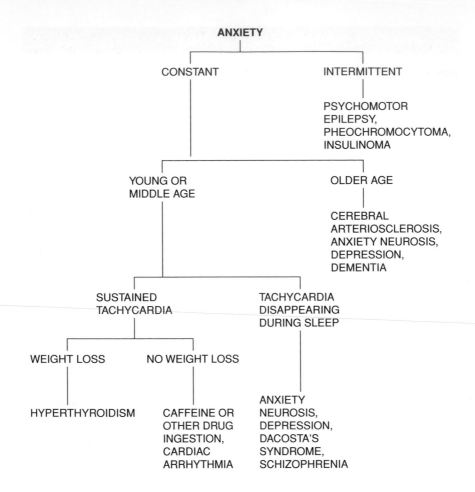

ANXIETY

CONSTANT   INTERMITTENT

INTERMITTENT → PSYCHOMOTOR EPILEPSY, PHEOCHROMOCYTOMA, INSULINOMA

CONSTANT →

YOUNG OR MIDDLE AGE   OLDER AGE

OLDER AGE → CEREBRAL ARTERIOSCLEROSIS, ANXIETY NEUROSIS, DEPRESSION, DEMENTIA

YOUNG OR MIDDLE AGE →

SUSTAINED TACHYCARDIA   TACHYCARDIA DISAPPEARING DURING SLEEP

SUSTAINED TACHYCARDIA →

WEIGHT LOSS   NO WEIGHT LOSS

WEIGHT LOSS → HYPERTHYROIDISM

NO WEIGHT LOSS → CAFFEINE OR OTHER DRUG INGESTION, CARDIAC ARRHYTHMIA

TACHYCARDIA DISAPPEARING DURING SLEEP → ANXIETY NEUROSIS, DEPRESSION, DACOSTA'S SYNDROME, SCHIZOPHRENIA

ASK THE FOLLOWING QUESTIONS:

1. **Is it intermittent?** Episodic aphasia, apraxia, or agnosia would suggest epilepsy, transient ischemic attacks, migraine, or hypertensive encephalopathy.
2. **Is it acute or gradual in onset?** Acute onset of aphasia, apraxia, or agnosia would suggest a cerebral vascular accident, or if there is fever, the onset of a cerebral abscess. It may also mark the onset of acute encephalitis. The gradual onset of aphasia, apraxia, and agnosia would suggest a tumor or other type of space-occupying lesion.
3. **Is there associated headache or papilledema?** Headaches with aphasia, apraxia, and agnosia might suggest migraine, but one should not forget a brain tumor. Obviously, papilledema is a sign of a space-occupying lesion.
4. **Is there significant dementia?** The development of dementia along with the aphasia, apraxia, and agnosia suggest Alzheimer's disease, Pick's disease, herpes encephalitis, multiple sclerosis, or Korsakoff's psychosis.

DIAGNOSTIC WORKUP

All patients should have a CBC, sedimentation rate, chemistry panel, a VDRL test, and a CT scan of the brain. The CT scan may demonstrate an infarct, a space-occupying lesion, a degenerative disease, or multiple sclerosis. If this is negative, a neurologist should be consulted before ordering MRI or a spinal tap.

If the patient presents with intermittent aphasia, apraxia, or agnosia, an EEG should be done to rule out epilepsy, and a carotid scan should be done to rule out carotid stenosis or carotid plaques with ulceration. Four vessel angiography may need to be considered, but a neurologist should be consulted before this is done.

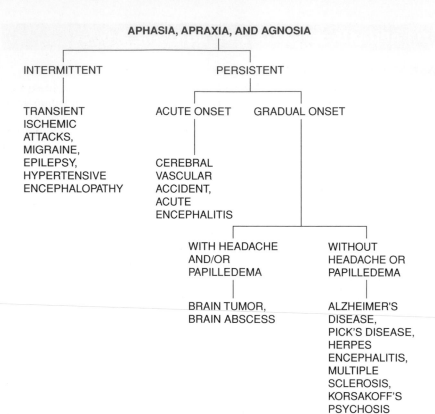

APHASIA, APRAXIA, AND AGNOSIA

INTERMITTENT

PERSISTENT

TRANSIENT
ISCHEMIC
ATTACKS,
MIGRAINE,
EPILEPSY,
HYPERTENSIVE
ENCEPHALOPATHY

ACUTE ONSET   GRADUAL ONSET

CEREBRAL
VASCULAR
ACCIDENT,
ACUTE
ENCEPHALITIS

WITH HEADACHE
AND/OR
PAPILLEDEMA

WITHOUT
HEADACHE OR
PAPILLEDEMA

BRAIN TUMOR,
BRAIN ABSCESS

ALZHEIMER'S
DISEASE,
PICK'S DISEASE,
HERPES
ENCEPHALITIS,
MULTIPLE
SCLEROSIS,
KORSAKOFF'S
PSYCHOSIS

⦿ ASCITES

ASK THE FOLLOWING QUESTIONS:

1. **Is there associated dyspnea?** If there is associated dyspnea, one should look for congestive heart failure, pulmonary emphysema, and other cardiopulmonary conditions.
2. **Is there hepatomegaly?** If there is associated hepatomegaly, certainly cirrhosis of the liver has to top the list of possibilities, but additional causes of ascites with hepatomegaly are constrictive pericarditis, the cardiomyopathies, Budd–Chiari syndrome, metastatic carcinoma, and hydatid cyst.
3. **Is there edema of the lower extremities or significant proteinuria?** Edema in the lower extremities along with significant proteinuria certainly suggests a nephrotic syndrome, whether it is due to glomerulonephritis, diabetes, or a collagen disease. It also suggests end-stage nephritis. If there is no significant proteinuria, then a primary peritoneal condition such as tuberculous peritonitis or peritoneal carcinomatosis must be considered. Remember, a large ovarian cyst can simulate ascites.
4. **Is there a history of a primary tumor elsewhere?** GI tumors may spread to the peritoneal surface and cause ascites, but a malignant melanoma may do the same thing.

DIAGNOSTIC WORKUP

Ultrasonography may help confirm the presence of ascites and differentiate it from other conditions such as pregnancy or ovarian cysts. A peritoneal tap with analysis of the fluid to determine whether it is a transudate or exudate and cell block studies as well as amylase, culture and sensitivity should be done; an elevated amylase indicates pancreatic disease. A CBC, chemistry panel, urinalysis, and sedimentation rate need to be done in all cases, and the urinary sediment should be examined under the microscope.

To rule out congestive heart failure, venous pressure and circulation time, EKG, pulmonary function studies, echocardiography, and chest x-ray should be done. To rule out pulmonary emphysema, pulmonary function studies and chest x-rays should be done. To rule out liver disease, a liver profile may be done along with a serum protein electrophoresis and a CT scan of the liver. A tuberculin test can be done to rule out tuberculous peritonitis, but the ascitic fluids should be studied with an AFB smear and culture. Guinea pig inoculation is sometimes necessary for a positive diagnosis. Laparoscopy is useful in differentiating peritoneal carcinomatosis from tuberculous peritonitis. A CT scan of the abdomen should be done to determine if there is peritoneal carcinomatosis or a primary malignancy of the GI tract and other structures in the abdomen. An upper GI series and barium enema may need to be done. Also, colonoscopy and gastroscopy may need to be done.

As the diagnostic tests become more expensive, the clinician should consider a referral to a gastroenterologist, nephrologist, or hepatologist before proceeding.

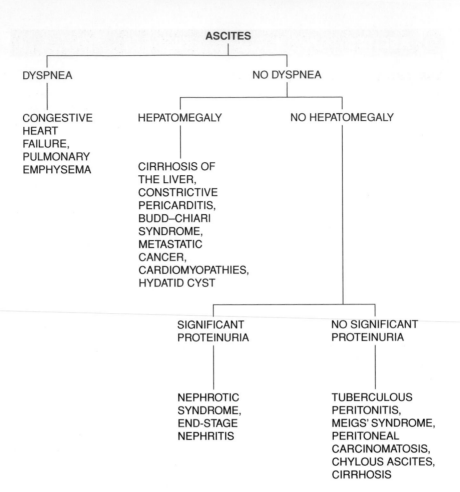

ASCITES

DYSPNEA

CONGESTIVE
HEART
FAILURE,
PULMONARY
EMPHYSEMA

NO DYSPNEA

HEPATOMEGALY

CIRRHOSIS OF
THE LIVER,
CONSTRICTIVE
PERICARDITIS,
BUDD–CHIARI
SYNDROME,
METASTATIC
CANCER,
CARDIOMYOPATHIES,
HYDATID CYST

NO HEPATOMEGALY

SIGNIFICANT
PROTEINURIA

NEPHROTIC
SYNDROME,
END-STAGE
NEPHRITIS

NO SIGNIFICANT
PROTEINURIA

TUBERCULOUS
PERITONITIS,
MEIGS' SYNDROME,
PERITONEAL
CARCINOMATOSIS,
CHYLOUS ASCITES,
CIRRHOSIS

ASPARTATE AMINOTRANSFERASE ELEVATION

ASK THE FOLLOWING QUESTIONS:

1. **Is the patient receiving heparin therapy?** As many as 27% of patients taking heparin have an elevated aspartate aminotransferase [AST, or serum glutamine-oxaloacetic transaminase (SGOT)], and 60% have an elevated alanine aminotransferase (ALT).

2. **Are the results of liver function tests abnormal?** This indicates that the elevated AST is due to liver disease.

3. **Is the creatine phosphokinase (CPK) or troponins elevated?** An elevated CPK would indicate that the elevated AST is related to muscle damage or disease or a myocardial infarction. Further differentiation of these two conditions is made by ordering CPK isoenzymes and an EKG.

4. **What is the arm-to-tongue circulation time?** This is increased in congestive heart failure.

5. **Is the serum amylase elevated?** This would point to pancreatitis as the cause of the AST elevation. If all of the above related tests are normal, the AST elevation is most likely due to liver disease or renal infarction.

6. **Is the patient participating in risky sexual behavior?** In this case, look for Hepatitis B or C.

7. **What drugs is the patient on?** Isoniazid (INH), statins, alcohol, and depakote cause elevated AST.

DIAGNOSTIC WORKUP

Additional tests to order that will help pin down the diagnosis include a CBC, serum amylase, chemistry panel, lactic acid dehydrogenase (LDH) isoenzymes, γ-glutamyltransferase, urinalysis, serial EKGs, echocardiography, pulmonary function tests, chest x-ray, flat plate of the abdomen, electromyography (EMG), liver biopsy, and muscle biopsy. Consultation with a cardiologist or hepatologist would be prudent before ordering expensive diagnostic tests.

ASPARTATE AMINOTRANSFERASE ELEVATION

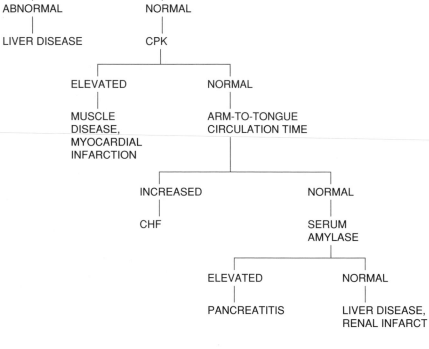

CASE HISTORY

A 67-year-old white male complains of increasing loss of balance for several months. He denies headaches, vertigo, tinnitus or deafness. Neurologic examination discloses no nystagmus or papilledema but there is definite loss of vibratory and position sense in the lower extremities and a smooth tongue. You suspect pernicious anemia and you would be correct.

ASK THE FOLLOWING QUESTIONS:

1. **Is there vertigo, tinnitus, or deafness?** Any one of these three signs and symptoms should suggest Ménière's disease or other labyrinthine disease as well as eighth nerve pathology.
2. **Are there headaches, nystagmus, or papilledema?** These signs should suggest a cerebellar tumor or acoustic neuroma.
3. **Are there other neurologic signs?** If there are long tract signs such as hyperactive reflexes and loss of vibratory or position sense, one should consider multiple sclerosis, pernicious anemia, or basilar artery insufficiency. If there are glove and stocking hypoesthesia and hypoactive reflexes, one should consider peripheral neuropathy or tabes dorsalis.
4. **Is the ataxia worse in the dark?** This is a sign that the dorsal column or peripheral nerve is affected, and one should look for peripheral neuropathy, pernicious anemia, multiple sclerosis, and Friedreich's ataxia. One should also look for tabes dorsalis.
5. **Is there a secondary gain?** Hysterical patients and patients who are malingering will often show a completely normal neurologic examination, but be unable to walk or stand without staggering. The author has been particularly impressed with patients applying for long-term disability who stagger a great deal without support, but as soon as support in the form of a cane is given, their ataxia completely clears up.

DIAGNOSTIC WORKUP

A wise clinician should consider a neurologic referral at the outset. If there is vertigo, tinnitus, or deafness, then an audiogram and caloric testing should be done. If these suggest eighth nerve damage, then a CT scan or MRI of the brain should be done. Headaches, sustained nystagmus, or papilledema are other indications for a CT scan or MRI. If multiple sclerosis is suspected, MRI of the brain is very useful, as well as spinal fluid for gamma globulin and myelin basic protein. Perhaps VEP, brain stem evoked potential (BSEP), or SSEP studies should be done. If vascular disease is suspected, magnetic resonance angiography will allow assessment of the vertebral-basilar arteries. If this is not available, four-vessel cerebral angiography may be utilized. Patients with hypoactive reflexes and glove and stocking hypesthesia and hypalgesia will need a neuropathy workup (see page 356). When there is ataxia in the presence of a normal neurologic examination, referral to a psychologist for psychometric testing should be done.

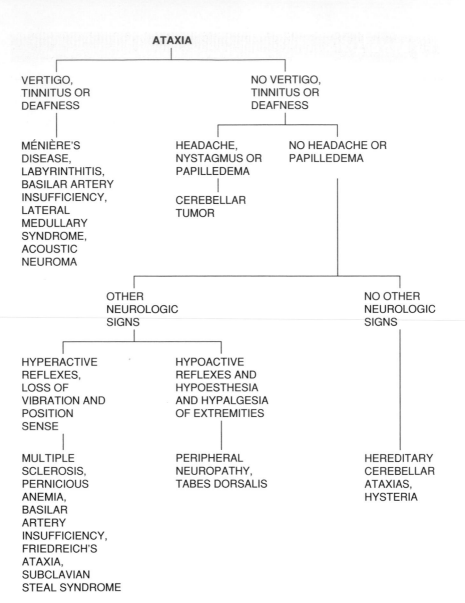

ATAXIA

VERTIGO, TINNITUS OR DEAFNESS

MÉNIÈRE'S DISEASE, LABYRINTHITIS, BASILAR ARTERY INSUFFICIENCY, LATERAL MEDULLARY SYNDROME, ACOUSTIC NEUROMA

NO VERTIGO, TINNITUS OR DEAFNESS

HEADACHE, NYSTAGMUS OR PAPILLEDEMA

CEREBELLAR TUMOR

NO HEADACHE OR PAPILLEDEMA

OTHER NEUROLOGIC SIGNS

HYPERACTIVE REFLEXES, LOSS OF VIBRATION AND POSITION SENSE

MULTIPLE SCLEROSIS, PERNICIOUS ANEMIA, BASILAR ARTERY INSUFFICIENCY, FRIEDREICH'S ATAXIA, SUBCLAVIAN STEAL SYNDROME

HYPOACTIVE REFLEXES AND HYPOESTHESIA AND HYPALGESIA OF EXTREMITIES

PERIPHERAL NEUROPATHY, TABES DORSALIS

NO OTHER NEUROLOGIC SIGNS

HEREDITARY CEREBELLAR ATAXIAS, HYSTERIA

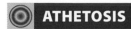
ATHETOSIS

Athetosis is an involuntary, smooth, sinuous, writhing movement of the upper limbs and, less commonly, the face and lower extremity. The pill-rolling of Parkinson's disease is an example. Athetosis is due to a lesion of the basal ganglia. It may be the result of cerebral palsy, encephalitis, Wilson's disease, Parkinson's disease, dystonia musculorum deformans, or a cerebral infarct.

DIAGNOSTIC WORKUP

Patients presenting with this complaint should have MRI, a serum copper and ceruloplasmin, a CBC, and liver function tests. A spinal tap should be performed if central nervous system lues is suspected.

ASK THE FOLLOWING QUESTIONS:

1. **Is it unilateral or bilateral?** Unilateral masses are usually enlarged lymph nodes due to some infectious process in the extremity served by the axillary nodes or the breast served by the axillary nodes. The unilateral mass may also be a tuberculous abscess, lipoma, a sebaceous cyst, metastatic carcinoma, or Hodgkin's disease. Rarely, it is due to an aneurysm. When the masses are bilateral, one should consider a systemic infection, leukemia, or advanced lymphoma. Rheumatoid arthritis and tuberculosis may be associated with bilateral axillary nodes.

2. **Is it painful or painless?** A painful axillary mass is usually an acute abscess or an acute inflammation of the lymph node due to infection on the extremity or breast supplied by the lymph node or hidradenitis suppurativa.

3. **Is there a discharge from the mass?** A discharge from an axillary mass usually means hidradenitis suppurativa.

4. **Is there fever?** Fever with a bilateral axillary mass would suggest an acute systemic infection or infectious mononucleosis. Fever with a unilateral axillary mass would suggest that there is mastitis, a breast abscess, or lymphangitis of the extremity supplied by the axillary lymph nodes.

5. **If the mass is unilateral, are there signs of an infection on the extremity or breast supplied by the axillary nodes?** In tularemia there will be a bubo on the extremity supplied by the axillary nodes, and in lymphadenitis there should be an infectious lesion on the extremity involved. If the lymphadenitis is due to mastitis, there should be a breast discharge or extreme tenderness and enlargement of the breast.

6. **Does the mass pulsate?** A pulsatile mass in the axilla is usually an aneurysm.

DIAGNOSTIC WORKUP

If the mass is fluctuant or exudes a discharge, then needle aspiration should be done and the material retrieved to have culture and sensitivity performed on it. The discharge may also be cultured for an organism. A surgeon may need to be consulted for diagnosis and treatment. All patients with bilateral axillary masses should have a CBC, sedimentation rate, chemistry panel, and urinalysis. Skin testing for tuberculosis, sarcoidosis, and various fungi should be done. A chest x-ray should be done to look for tuberculosis or malignancy. Mammography should be done in cases of unilateral axillary masses that suggest lymphadenopathy. In the final analysis, a biopsy of the mass may need to be done to make the diagnosis.

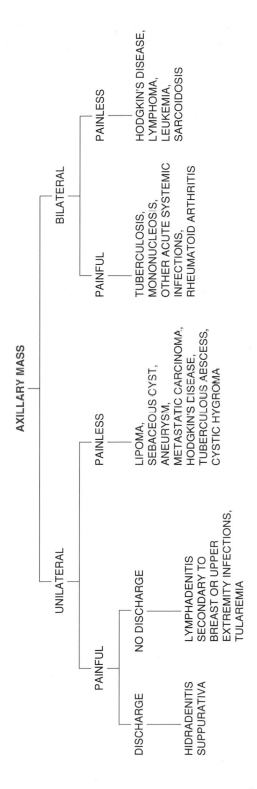

BABINSKI'S SIGN

ASK THE FOLLOWING QUESTIONS:

1. **Is the onset acute?** Babinski's sign of acute onset is due to trauma or vascular diseases in most cases. If there is a fever, one should consider an infectious process, most likely a cerebral abscess. Multiple sclerosis may also cause Babinski's sign of recent or acute onset.

2. **Is Babinski's sign unilateral or bilateral?** Unilateral Babinski's signs suggest a space-occupying lesion of the brain such as hematoma, abscess, or tumor. It also suggests a cerebral vascular accident. If Babinski's signs are bilateral, it may be due to a toxic or degenerative condition of the brain such as encephalitis. It may also be due to a spinal cord tumor or other space-occupying lesion of the spinal cord.

3. **Are there associated cranial nerve signs?** If there is associated central facial palsy on the ipsilateral side, one should consider an infarct or a space-occupying lesion of the opposite cerebral hemisphere. If there are cranial nerve signs aside from a facial palsy, one should consider a brain stem lesion, especially if they are contralateral.

4. **Are there hypoactive reflexes?** Babinski's sign with hypoactive reflexes, if it is of acute onset, would be considered a traumatic or vascular lesion of the brain if it is unilateral and an acute vascular or traumatic lesion of the spinal cord if it is bilateral. Hypoactive reflexes of relatively insidious onset should make one think of pernicious anemia or Friedreich's ataxia.

5. **Are there hyperactive reflexes?** Unilateral hyperactive reflexes of the upper and lower extremity with cranial nerve signs should bring to mind middle cerebral artery thrombosis or hemorrhage, carotid stenosis, and a space-occupying lesion of the brain. Hyperactive reflexes of the upper and lower extremities with no cranial nerve signs should suggest a high spinal cord tumor or a herniated cervical disk, especially if it is unilateral. Unilateral hyperactive reflexes of the lower extremity only would suggest an anterior cerebral artery thrombosis or parasagittal meningioma. Hyperactive reflexes of all extremities with cranial nerve signs should suggest a basilar artery thrombosis, brain stem tumor, or other lesion of the brain stem. Weakness and hyperactive reflexes of all four extremities without cranial nerve signs and without any sensory changes should suggest a primary lateral sclerosis, although multiple sclerosis may occasionally present in this manner.

6. **Are there sensory changes?** Hyperactive reflexes with sensory changes confined to the trunk and extremities would make one think of a spinal cord lesion such as multiple sclerosis, pernicious anemia, or Friedreich's ataxia, and, especially if it is unilateral, one would consider a space-occupying lesion of the spinal cord. Other considerations are transverse myelitis and anterior spinal artery occlusion.

7. **Is there involvement of the lower extremity only?** This is an important question to ask, as this would suggest a spinal cord tumor of the thoracic level or a parasagittal meningioma.

8. **Is there radicular pain?** The association of radicular pain in the cervical or thoracic area would make one think of a spinal cord tumor or other space-occupying lesion of the spinal cord.

9. **Is there associated fever?** The finding of fever along with a unilateral Babinski's sign should make one think of a cerebral abscess or an epidural abscess somewhere in the spinal column. The finding of fever with bilateral Babinski's signs should make one think of an encephalitis, particularly if there are disturbances of consciousness. However, fever may be associated with a cerebral vascular accident, so don't be misled.

DIAGNOSTIC WORKUP

It is wise to consult a neurologist at the outset. The diagnostic workup depends on other symptoms and signs that help the physician determine what level the neurologic lesion might be. If there is an acute unilateral Babinski's sign with hemiplegia and cranial nerve signs, a space-occupying lesion or vascular lesion of the brain must be considered. In that case, a CT scan or MRI of the brain should be done and this may be followed with a spinal tap and carotid scans if a vascular lesion is suspected. A spinal tap would not be done if there is any possibility of increased intracranial pressure.

If a cerebral vascular disease is suspected, then a source for an embolism should be looked for. Useful studies include echocardiography and possibly blood cultures and an EKG. If the patient's condition had an insidious onset and there are no cranial nerve signs, an MRI of the cervical or thoracic sign should be done to look for a tumor, multiple sclerosis, or degenerative diseases.

Babinski's sign associated with trauma and without cranial nerve signs should prompt one to do x-rays of the cervical, thoracic, and lumbar spine for fracture and other traumatic lesions. If there are associated disturbances of consciousness, one must look for a cerebral lesion, and MRI of the brain must be done in these traumatic conditions.

The fact that Babinski's sign is a definite sign of neurologic disease is reason enough to call a neurologic specialist in before undertaking any diagnostic studies. A neurologic consultation is much less expensive than a CT scan or MRI.

BABINSKI'S SIGN

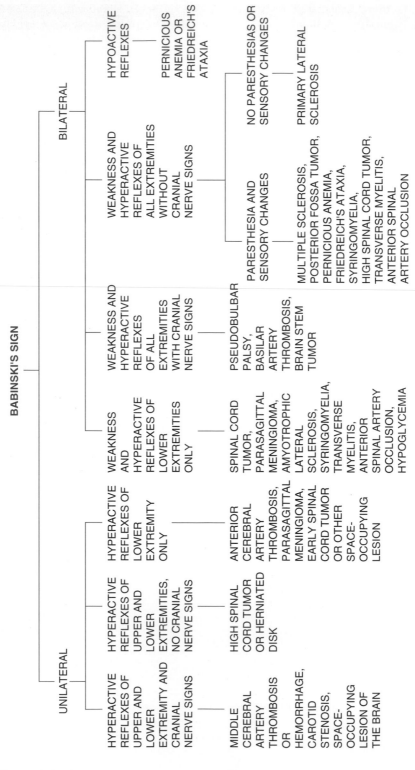

UNILATERAL

HYPERACTIVE REFLEXES OF UPPER AND LOWER EXTREMITY AND CRANIAL NERVE SIGNS

MIDDLE CEREBRAL ARTERY THROMBOSIS OR HEMORRHAGE, CAROTID STENOSIS, SPACE-OCCUPYING LESION OF THE BRAIN

HYPERACTIVE REFLEXES OF UPPER AND LOWER EXTREMITIES, NO CRANIAL NERVE SIGNS

HIGH SPINAL CORD TUMOR OR HERNIATED DISK

HYPERACTIVE REFLEXES OF LOWER EXTREMITY ONLY

ANTERIOR CEREBRAL ARTERY THROMBOSIS, PARASAGITTAL MENINGIOMA, EARLY SPINAL CORD TUMOR OR OTHER SPACE-OCCUPYING LESION

WEAKNESS AND HYPERACTIVE REFLEXES OF LOWER EXTREMITIES ONLY

SPINAL CORD TUMOR, PARASAGITTAL MENINGIOMA, AMYOTROPHIC LATERAL SCLEROSIS, SYRINGOMYELIA, TRANSVERSE MYELITIS, ANTERIOR SPINAL ARTERY OCCLUSION, HYPOGLYCEMIA

WEAKNESS AND HYPERACTIVE REFLEXES OF ALL EXTREMITIES WITH CRANIAL NERVE SIGNS

PSEUDOBULBAR PALSY, BASILAR ARTERY THROMBOSIS, BRAIN STEM TUMOR

BILATERAL

WEAKNESS AND HYPERACTIVE REFLEXES OF ALL EXTREMITIES WITHOUT CRANIAL NERVE SIGNS

NO PARESTHESIAS OR SENSORY CHANGES

PRIMARY LATERAL SCLEROSIS

PARESTHESIA AND SENSORY CHANGES

MULTIPLE SCLEROSIS, POSTERIOR FOSSA TUMOR, PERNICIOUS ANEMIA, FRIEDREICH'S ATAXIA, SYRINGOMYELIA, HIGH SPINAL CORD TUMOR, TRANSVERSE MYELITIS, ANTERIOR SPINAL ARTERY OCCLUSION

HYPOACTIVE REFLEXES

PERNICIOUS ANEMIA OR FRIEDREICH'S ATAXIA

BACK PAIN

CASE HISTORY

A 72-year-old black male presents to your office with a 3-month history of low back pain. Following the algorithm, you find there is no history of trauma, fever, or chills. The pain radiates down the back of both legs and he has had difficulty with urination for past month.

Your examination shows a suprapubic mass, a small nodule of the right lobe of the prostate, saddle hypesthesia, and hypalgesia, and absent Achilles reflexes bilaterally. The suprapubic mass disappears after you catheterize him and remove 625 cc of urine. You suspect a cauda equina tumor and you would be correct.

ASK THE FOLLOWING QUESTIONS:

1. **Is the pain of acute onset or gradual onset?** If it is acute onset, one must consider the possibility of epidural abscess, pyelonephritis, or other abdominal conditions as the cause of the back pain. If it is gradual onset, one should consider that it may be a tumor, particularly of the spinal cord or cauda equina, a pelvic tumor, or an aortic aneurysm that is compressing one of the nerve roots. In addition, chronic conditions such as lumbar spondylosis, rheumatoid spondylitis, and prostatitis must be considered.
2. **Is there a history of trauma?** If there is a history of trauma, one should consider a compression fracture of the spine, a sprain or herniated disk, as well as spondylolisthesis. Without a history of trauma, one should consider a tumor, herpes zoster, or dissecting aneurysm. Lumbar spondylosis might be silent for a while only to cause pain after a significant traumatic event.
3. **Is there radiation of the pain around the trunk or into the extremities?** Radiation of the pain would certainly be more likely to signify a space-occupying lesion of the spinal column such as a tumor, an epidural abscess, or a herniated disk. If there is no radiation, one would consider osteoarthritis or lumbar spondylosis and rheumatoid spondylitis.
4. **Finally, are there bladder symptoms associated with the pain?** If there are, then one must consider the possibility of a spinal cord tumor, cauda equina tumor, or kidney disease.

DIAGNOSTIC WORKUP

The first thing to do is rule out malingering. With the patient standing straight and one of your hands on his shoulder and the other on the opposite hip, rotate his body. If he complains of pain he is probably malingering. Next, measure the leg length. At least one-fourth of the patients with back pain have one leg shorter than the other. All patients with back pain need to have a CBC, urinalysis, and probably a urine culture, as well as a chemistry panel. A sedimentation rate and arthritis panel should be done if rheumatoid arthritis is suspected. All patients should also have plain x-rays of the thoracic and/or lumbar spine. It is very important to get anterior posterior views, as well as oblique and lateral views. A standing upright A-P will help diagnose a short leg syndrome as well. At this point, it is wise to observe the results of conservative therapy before ordering expensive diagnostic tests. If there is doubt about the diagnosis at this point, a neurologic or orthopedic specialist may be consulted. If there is radiation of the pain into the extremities or around the trunk and definite neurologic findings, one should proceed to a CT scan or MRI immediately. The CT scan costs about half as much as the MRI and usually will show any significant herniated disks, primary or metastatic tumor. Even without radiation of pain into the extremities or definite neurologic findings, a patient with persistent back pain should have a CT scan or MRI. Electromyography (EMG) will be useful in identifying radiculopathy.

When all these studies are negative, it might be wise to get a bone scan because this will show the increased uptake of the sacroiliac joints in rheumatoid spondylitis. Also, one should test for the HLA B27 antigen. In the event that all of the above studies are negative, the possibility of a non-neurologic condition or nonorthopedic condition causing the back pain should be considered. Perhaps abdominal ultrasound should be done to rule out an aortic aneurysm. Perhaps a pelvic tumor or prostatic tumor should be reconsidered. Perhaps there is a pancreatic tumor that is causing the back pain. Occasionally, combined myelography and CT scan is the only way to identify a lesion. Exploratory surgery is rarely necessary. Older patients should have a serum protein electrophoresis (for multiple myeloma) and acid phosphatase or PSA to rule out prostatic carcinoma.

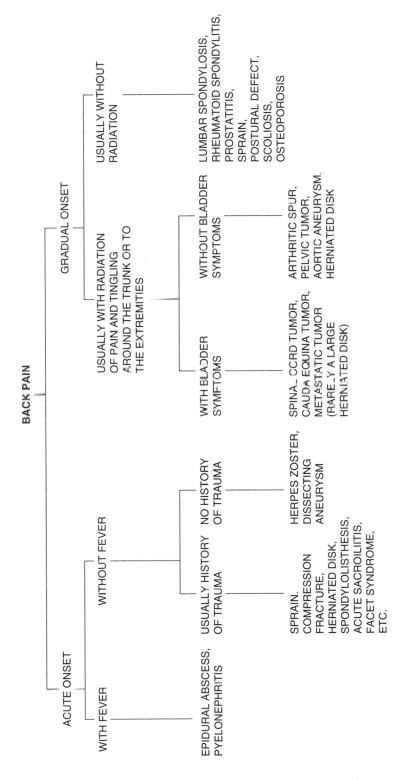

BACK PAIN

ACUTE ONSET

- WITH FEVER
  - EPIDURAL ABSCESS, PYELONEPHRITIS
- WITHOUT FEVER
  - USUALLY HISTORY OF TRAUMA
    - SPRAIN, COMPRESSION FRACTURE, HERNIATED DISK, SPONDYLOLISTHESIS, ACUTE SACROILIITIS, FACET SYNDROME, ETC.
  - NO HISTORY OF TRAUMA
    - HERPES ZOSTER, DISSECTING ANEURYSM

GRADUAL ONSET

- USUALLY WITH RADIATION OF PAIN AND TINGLING AROUND THE TRUNK OR TO THE EXTREMITIES
  - WITH BLADDER SYMPTOMS
    - SPINAL CORD TUMOR, CAUDA EQUINA TUMOR, METASTATIC TUMOR (RARELY A LARGE HERNIATED DISK)
  - WITHOUT BLADDER SYMPTOMS
    - ARTHRITIC SPUR, PELVIC TUMOR, AORTIC ANEURYSM, HERNIATED DISK
- USUALLY WITHOUT RADIATION
  - LUMBAR SPONDYLOSIS, RHEUMATOID SPONDYLITIS, PROSTATITIS, SPRAIN, POSTURAL DEFECT, SCOLIOSIS, OSTEOPOROSIS

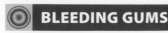

ASK THE FOLLOWING QUESTIONS:

1. **Are there abnormalities on examination of the teeth or gums?** The gums may be swollen, as in phenytoin use and early scurvy, and bleed on slight pressure, as in pyorrhea or other conditions. There may be ulceration of the tongue, gums, and buccal mucosa. There may be isolated dental caries that are causing bleeding. Excessive tartar may be noted on the teeth.

2. **Is there an enlarged spleen or a systemic rash?** The presence of an enlarged spleen should bring to mind Hodgkin's disease, leukemia, lupus erythematosus, thrombocytopenia purpura, and aplastic anemia. A systemic rash that is due to petechiae is common in any disorder that might cause thrombocytopenia.

3. **Is there a positive Rumpel–Leede test?** This would test for capillary fragility, and it may be positive in scurvy, thrombocytopenia purpura, leukemia, and other disorders that depress the platelet count. It will also be positive in disorders of platelet function such as von Willebrand's disease.

DIAGNOSTIC WORKUP

A CBC, sedimentation rate, chemistry panel, ANA titer, and coagulation profile are basic studies that need to be done. If these are negative, referral to a dentist or periodontist would be appropriate. X-rays of the teeth need to be done to look for dental caries, abscesses, and pyorrhea. X-rays of the teeth will also help identify scurvy. A plasma or platelet ascorbic acid level needs to be done if scurvy is suspected. If syphilis is suspected, a VDRL test needs to be done.

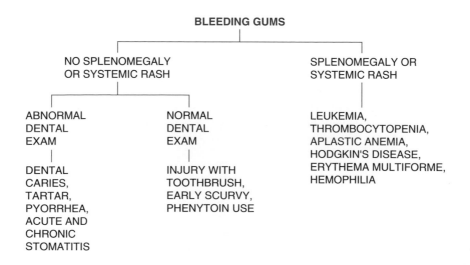

BLEEDING GUMS

NO SPLENOMEGALY OR SYSTEMIC RASH

ABNORMAL DENTAL EXAM

DENTAL CARIES, TARTAR, PYORRHEA, ACUTE AND CHRONIC STOMATITIS

NORMAL DENTAL EXAM

INJURY WITH TOOTHBRUSH, EARLY SCURVY, PHENYTOIN USE

SPLENOMEGALY OR SYSTEMIC RASH

LEUKEMIA, THROMBOCYTOPENIA, APLASTIC ANEMIA, HODGKIN'S DISEASE, ERYTHEMA MULTIFORME, HEMOPHILIA

BLINDNESS

CASE HISTORY

A 72-year-old Hispanic male is brought to the emergency room because of sudden onset of blindness in the left eye which has persisted for several hours. Your examination shows weakness and hypoactive reflexes in the right extremities but a normal ophthalmoscopic examination. There is a left carotid bruit, so you suspect a carotid artery thrombosis. A carotid duplex scan confirms your suspicions.

ASK THE FOLLOWING QUESTIONS:

1. **Is it transient?** Transient blindness may occur in transient ischemic attacks, epilepsy, migraine, and hypertension.
2. **Is it a sudden onset?** The sudden onset of blindness may occur in optic neuritis, retinal vein thrombosis, central retinal artery occlusion, vitreous hemorrhage, detached retina, carotid artery thrombosis, temporal arteritis, injuries to the optic nerve, retrobulbar neuritis, fracture of the skull, glaucoma, posterior cerebral artery occlusion, multiple sclerosis, and hysteria.
3. **Is it unilateral or bilateral?** Unilateral blindness may occur in glaucoma, vitreous hemorrhage, optic neuritis, retinal vein thrombosis, central retinal artery thrombosis, carotid artery thrombosis, temporal arteritis, injury to the optic nerve, fractured skull, brain tumors, retinoblastomas, and sphenoid ridge meningiomas. Bilateral blindness may occur in posterior cerebral artery occlusion, pituitary tumors, retinitis pigmentosa, hereditary optic atrophy, uveitis, toxic amblyopia, cataracts, glaucoma, multiple sclerosis, and iritis. Head trauma may cause transient cortical blindness in children.
4. **Is there papilledema?** The presence of papilledema should make one suspect optic neuritis, retinal vein thrombosis, and space-occupying lesions of the brain.
5. **Are there abnormalities on ophthalmoscopic examination?** Besides papilledema, there may be changes on the ophthalmoscopic examination in iritis, glaucoma, papillitis from optic neuritis, retinal vein thrombosis, central retinal artery occlusion, vitreous hemorrhage, detached retina, and retinoblastoma.

DIAGNOSTIC WORKUP

Referral to an ophthalmologist is usually the first step in a good workup. If one is not available, a careful eye examination including slit lamp examination, visual acuity evaluation, tonometry, and visual field studies should be done. If these are unrevealing, a referral to an ophthalmologist or neurologist should be made without further delay. Additional studies would include a CT scan or MRI of the brain and orbits, carotid scans, spinal tap, MRA, VEP studies, and four-vessel cerebral angiography. An EEG would be useful in diagnosing hysterical blindness and malingering.

BLINDNESS

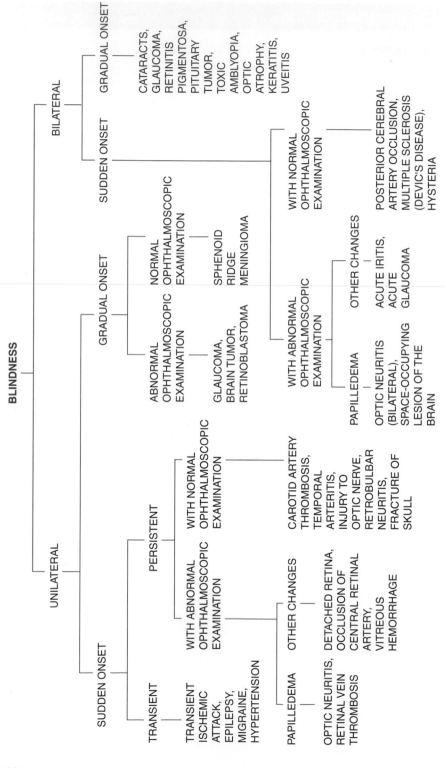

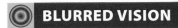

ASK THE FOLLOWING QUESTIONS:

1. **Is it unilateral or bilateral?** The presence of unilateral blurred vision should suggest such local ocular conditions as cataract, refractive error, iritis, glaucoma, keratitis, retinal detachment, foreign body, and optic neuritis. Transient blurred vision may occur in migraine and carotid artery insufficiency. Orbital fracture and vitreous hemorrhage may cause unilateral blurred vision also.

2. Bilateral blurred vision may result from cocaine use, methyl alcohol poisoning, tobacco, barbiturates, quinine, and other drugs. However, cataracts, glaucoma, chorioretinitis, retinitis pigmentosa, optic atrophy, papilledema, papillitis, optic neuritis, refractive error, pituitary tumors, posterior cerebral artery occlusion, concussion, migraine, and hysteria must also be considered.

3. **Is there a positive history for drug or alcohol ingestion?** If this history is positive, then cocaine, tobacco, barbiturates, methyl alcohol, quinine, and other drugs may be responsible.

4. **Is it sudden in onset?** Sudden onset of blurred vision should make one suspect migraine, optic neuritis, vitreous hemorrhage, iritis, keratitis, glaucoma, retinal detachment, foreign body, retrobulbar neuritis, orbital fracture, carotid artery insufficiency, and hysteria.

5. **Is the eye examination abnormal?** Local ocular diseases such as cataracts, refractive errors, iritis, keratitis, glaucoma, retinal detachment, foreign bodies, retinitis pigmentosa, chorioretinitis, and papilledema should be detected by the primary care physician.

DIAGNOSTIC WORKUP

A referral to an ophthalmologist is usually the first step in a workup. If an ophthalmologist is not available, a careful eye examination including slit lamp evaluation, tonometry, visual acuity evaluation, and visual fields should be done. A toxicology screen may be indicated by history. If these studies are unremarkable, referral to a neurologist may be made. Further studies would include a CT scan or MRI of the brain, carotid scans, spinal tap, VEP studies, and four-vessel cerebral angiography.

BLURRED VISION

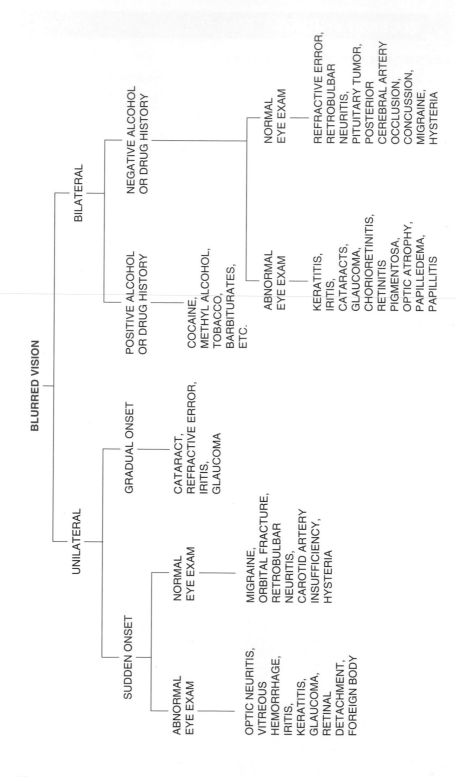

UNILATERAL

SUDDEN ONSET

ABNORMAL EYE EXAM

OPTIC NEURITIS, VITREOUS HEMORRHAGE, IRITIS, KERATITIS, GLAUCOMA, RETINAL DETACHMENT, FOREIGN BODY

NORMAL EYE EXAM

MIGRAINE, ORBITAL FRACTURE, RETROBULBAR NEURITIS, CAROTID ARTERY INSUFFICIENCY, HYSTERIA

GRADUAL ONSET

CATARACT, REFRACTIVE ERROR, IRITIS, GLAUCOMA

BILATERAL

POSITIVE ALCOHOL OR DRUG HISTORY

COCAINE, METHYL ALCOHOL, TOBACCO, BARBITURATES, ETC.

NEGATIVE ALCOHOL OR DRUG HISTORY

ABNORMAL EYE EXAM

KERATITIS, IRITIS, CATARACTS, GLAUCOMA, CHORIORETINITIS, RETINITIS PIGMENTOSA, OPTIC ATROPHY, PAPILLEDEMA, PAPILLITIS

NORMAL EYE EXAM

REFRACTIVE ERROR, RETROBULBAR NEURITIS, PITUITARY TUMOR, POSTERIOR CEREBRAL ARTERY OCCLUSION, CONCUSSION, MIGRAINE, HYSTERIA

ASK THE FOLLOWING QUESTIONS:

1. **Is there a history of trauma?** Trauma, of course, may cause fractures and subperiosteal hematomas.
2. **Is the patient a child or an adult?** Children are more likely to have Ewing's tumors, scurvy, rickets, syphilis, battered baby syndrome, osteosarcoma, osteomas, and osteochondromas. Adults are more likely to have a giant cell tumor, metastasis, osteomyelitis, osteogenic sarcoma, fibrosarcoma, multiple myeloma, generalized fibrocystic disease, Paget's disease, acromegaly, and chondromas.
3. **Are the lesions single or focal or are they multiple or diffuse?** Multiple and diffuse lesions in children are often due to scurvy, rickets, syphilis, and battered baby syndrome. Multiple lesions or diffuse lesions in adults are often due to metastasis, multiple myeloma, generalized fibrocystic disease, Paget's disease, acromegaly, and chondroma. Single lesions in children are more likely to be fracture, osteomyelitis, hematoma, Ewing's tumor, osteosarcoma, osteomas, and osteochondromas. Single lesions in adults are often due to a giant cell tumor, osteomyelitis, fracture, hematoma, osteogenic sarcoma, and fibrosarcoma, but may be due to a metastasis.
4. **Are the lesions usually painful?** Painful lesions in children are more likely to be due to fracture, osteomyelitis, hematoma, Ewing's tumors, scurvy, syphilis, battered baby syndrome, and rickets. Painful lesions in adults may be due to a giant cell tumor, metastasis, osteomyelitis, fracture, hematomas, osteogenic sarcoma, fibro-sarcomas, and multiple myeloma.

DIAGNOSTIC WORKUP

Routine diagnostic studies include a CBC, sedimentation rate, urinalysis, chemistry panel, arthritis panel, serum protein electrophoresis, and plain films of the involved bones. A skeletal survey may be necessary. If the diagnosis remains in doubt, consult an orthopedic surgeon at this point. Bone scans are often useful. A search for a primary tumor may require chest x-ray, upper GI series, barium enema, IVP, CT scan of the abdomen mammography, prostatic examination, PSA titer, thyroid scans, lymph node biopsy, and bone marrow examinations.

CT scans of the area may help differentiate the mass or swelling. Needle biopsy or exploratory surgery and bone biopsy may be necessary before deciding what surgical approach should be undertaken.

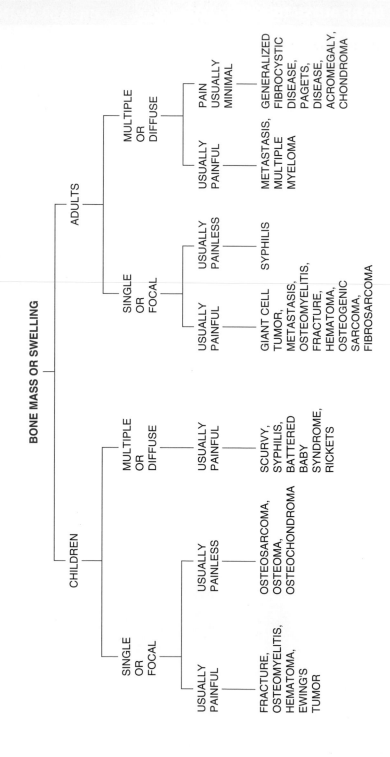

BONE MASS OR SWELLING

- CHILDREN
  - SINGLE OR FOCAL
    - USUALLY PAINFUL
      - FRACTURE, OSTEOMYELITIS, HEMATOMA, EWING'S TUMOR
    - USUALLY PAINLESS
      - OSTEOSARCOMA, OSTEOMA, OSTEOCHONDROMA
  - MULTIPLE OR DIFFUSE
    - USUALLY PAINFUL
      - SCURVY, SYPHILIS, BATTERED BABY SYNDROME, RICKETS
- ADULTS
  - SINGLE OR FOCAL
    - USUALLY PAINFUL
      - GIANT CELL TUMOR, METASTASIS, OSTEOMYELITIS, FRACTURE, HEMATOMA, OSTEOGENIC SARCOMA, FIBROSARCOMA
    - USUALLY PAINLESS
      - SYPHILIS
  - MULTIPLE OR DIFFUSE
    - USUALLY PAINFUL
      - METASTASIS, MULTIPLE MYELOMA
    - PAIN USUALLY MINIMAL
      - GENERALIZED FIBROCYSTIC DISEASE, PAGETS DISEASE, ACROMEGALY, CHONDROMA

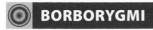

ASK THE FOLLOWING QUESTIONS:

1. **Is there abdominal distention?** If there is abdominal distention, an intestinal obstruction should be considered.
2. **Is there obvious diarrhea?** If there is diarrhea, one should look for malabsorption syndrome, lactase deficiency, and carcinoid syndrome. Other causes of chronic diarrhea are discussed on page 117.
3. **Is there flushing of the face?** If there is significant flushing of the face along with diarrhea, carcinoid syndrome is the most likely possibility.

DIAGNOSTIC WORKUP

If there is significant distention of the abdomen, a flat plate of the abdomen with lateral decubiti should be done to rule out intestinal obstruction. A stool for occult blood, culture, quantitative fat and ovum and parasites should be done. If there is flushing, a urine for 5-hydroxyindoleacetic acid (5-HIAA) should be done to rule out carcinoid syndrome. A lactose tolerance test may be indicated. After these tests are done, further workup can proceed. An upper GI series with an esophagogram, a small bowel series, and a barium enema would be next in line. If all these studies are negative, perhaps referral to a gastroenterologist or psychiatrist would be indicated. Endoscopy is rarely necessary.

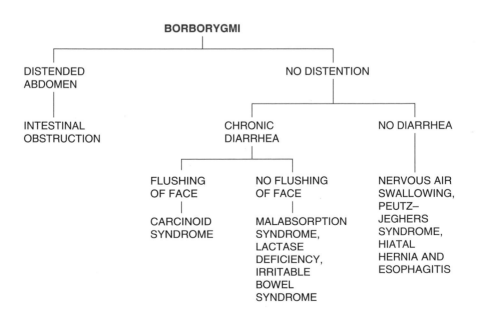

ASK THE FOLLOWING QUESTIONS:

1. **Is there fever?** If there is fever, one should look for yellow fever, diphtheria, cerebral abscess, or meningitis. Perhaps the fever and bradycardia are related to increased intracranial pressure from apoplexy.
2. **Are there episodes of syncope?** The addition of syncope should make one think of a sick sinus syndrome, complete heart block, vasovagal syncope, or carotid sinus syncope.
3. **Is there a heart murmur present?** Heart murmurs are found in complete heart block, but they are also a sign of aortic stenosis, which can cause bradycardia.
4. **Is there a history of drug ingestion?** Several drugs can induce bradycardia, the most notable being digitalis; propranolol, quinidine, calcium channel blockers, amitriptyline, and various cholinergic drugs also may induce bradycardia. Opium poisoning may cause bradycardia.
5. **Is there nonpitting edema?** Obviously, this is a sign of myxedema and should be looked for in any patient presenting with bradycardia.
6. **Is there chest pain?** An acute myocardial infarction may present with bradycardia, although it is more typical for tachycardia to be associated with this condition. Heart disease, most notably, Chagas disease, sarcoidosis, and Lyme disease, can cause a second- and third-degree block, which may result in bradycardia, but also various other types of arrhythmia that cause the slowing of the pulse.

DIAGNOSTIC WORKUP

If there is fever without any definite focal signs, a CBC, sedimentation rate, blood culture, chemistry panel, febrile agglutinins, and tests for other antibodies may be done. Digoxin levels are helpful for patients on this drug. If there is fever with nuchal rigidity, a spinal tap should be done, preferably after a CT scan. An EKG will need to be done on all patients, and if this shows simple sinus bradycardia and there is no history of drug ingestion, a thyroid profile should be done. If there is chest pain, serial EKGs and cardiac enzymes should be done. If there is a heart murmur, echocardiography would be an important ancillary study. If the EKG shows various types of arrhythmia, a cardiologist should be consulted for further evaluation. A trial of glucagon i.m or i.v. is helpful for beta-blocker overdose.

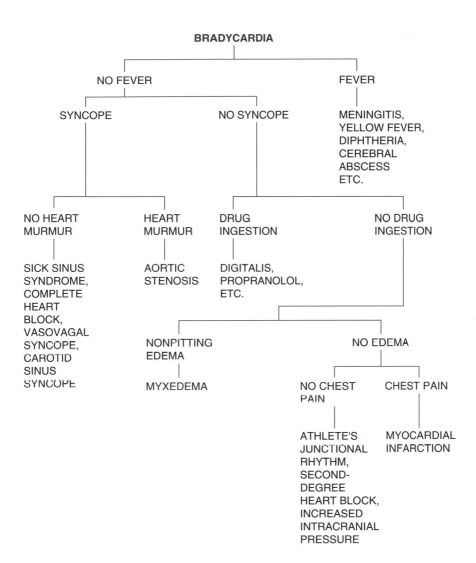

ASK THE FOLLOWING QUESTIONS:

1. **Is the discharge unilateral or bilateral?** If it is unilateral and watery or bloody, one should look for a neoplasm in the breast. If it is bilateral and milky, one should look for the various conditions that cause hyperprolactinemia or pregnancy.
2. **Is the discharge bloody?** A unilateral bloody discharge is most suggestive of carcinoma of the breast. Other types of lesions of the breast, such as Paget's disease, papillary cystadenoma, and epithelioma of the nipple, are causes of a bloody discharge also.
3. **Is there a focal mass in the breast?** A bloody discharge with a focal mass makes a neoplasm almost certain. If there is a focal mass, fever, and a non-bloody discharge, one should consider abscess.
4. **Is there fever?** Fever or chills along with a purulent discharge from the breast is most likely acute mastitis or an abscess.

DIAGNOSTIC WORKUP

If there is a bloody discharge, one should not hesitate to refer the patient to a general surgeon, who will probably order mammography and perform a biopsy. The type of biopsy may be either a fine-needle aspiration or fine-needle biopsy or excisional biopsy, but the general surgeon can decide which is appropriate for any given patient. A unilateral nonbloody discharge may be studied further by ordering tests for occult blood, cytology, and mammography before referral. If infection is suspected, order a CBC, culture of the discharge, and trial of antibiotic therapy. Remember that exploratory surgery may be the only way to get a diagnosis.

If the discharge is bilateral and milky, a serum prolactin should be ordered. If the prolactin is high, referral to an endocrinologist is probably the best step to take next. The endocrinologist will probably order a CT scan of the brain and pituitary and do further workup studies based on his examination.

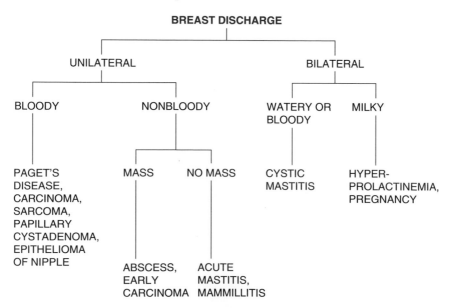

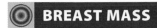
ASK THE FOLLOWING QUESTIONS:

1. **Is the mass tender?** A tender mass is most likely due to an infectious process such as mastitis or an abscess. However, chronic cystic mastitis may present with a tender mass. Also, advanced carcinoma of the breast usually produces a tender mass.
2. **Is there a discharge?** A bloody discharge from the breast means that the mass is most likely due to a malignant process. If there is a purulent discharge, abscess or mastitis must be considered. A watery discharge is often associated with chronic cystic mastitis, and this occasionally may become bloody.
3. **Does it transilluminate?** Cysts of the breasts and galactoceles customarily transilluminate. A mass that does not transilluminate is probably a benign or malignant tumor.
4. **Is there a deformity of the breast associated with the mass?** An orange peel appearance of the skin over a tumor certainly suggests that it is a carcinoma. Retraction of the skin or the nipple suggests carcinoma. Also, in carcinoma there may be necrosis and ulceration of the tissues overlying the tumor.
5. **Is there fever?** Fever would suggest an acute mastitis or abscess.

DIAGNOSTIC WORKUP

A breast mass is a clear indication for a referral to a general surgeon. The general surgeon will probably perform mammography and a biopsy before proceeding with surgery. If a cystic lesion is suspected, ultrasonography may be done, followed by fine-needle aspiration and biopsy. When there is a definite mass on physical examination, surgery is indicated even if mammography and other tests are negative.

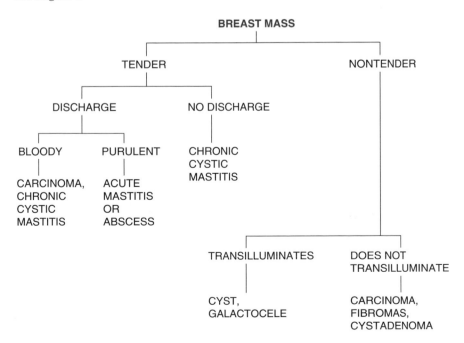

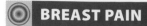

ASK THE FOLLOWING QUESTIONS:

1. **Is it unilateral or bilateral?** Unilateral breast pain should make one think of an infectious process or advanced carcinoma. Bilateral breast pain should make one think of pregnancy. This may be a normal pregnancy or an ectopic pregnancy.
2. **Is there an associated mass?** A tender breast mass is most likely a mastitis or abscess, but advanced carcinoma can also produce a tender breast mass. If there are tender masses in both breasts, chronic cystic mastitis should be considered.
3. **Is there a discharge?** A bloody discharge associated with a tender breast should make one think of a carcinoma. A non-bloody discharge suggests a breast abscess.
4. **Is there fever?** Fever associated with a tender breast or tender breast mass is most likely acute mastitis or abscess.

DIAGNOSTIC WORKUP

If there is a fever and discharge, a culture and sensitivity of the discharge should be done before beginning antibiotics. When there is a localized tender mass, referral to a general surgeon should be made. Patients with bilateral breast pain without any masses identified should have a pregnancy test. If this is negative and the pain is associated with the menstrual cycle, they should be treated as having premenstrual tension. A gynecologist may need to be consulted. If there is persistent bilateral breast pain in a young unmarried female, perhaps a psychiatrist should be consulted.

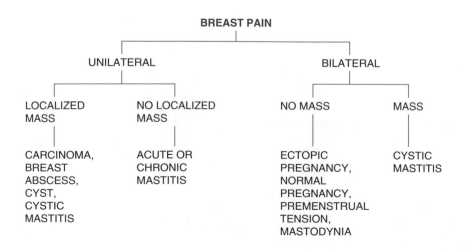

ASK THE FOLLOWING QUESTIONS:

1. **Is it acute or chronic?** An acute cardiac arrhythmia should make one consider a myocardial infarction first.
2. **Is the heart rate slow, normal, or fast?** A rapid cardiac arrhythmia may be associated with hyperthyroidism, congestive heart failure, or drug toxicity. A slow cardiac arrhythmia is more likely to be associated with heart block and syncope. A myocardial infarction may produce either the rapid or slow cardiac arrhythmia.
3. **Is the rhythm regular or irregular?** A tachycardia with a regular rhythm is more likely to be a supraventricular tachycardia or ventricular tachycardia. Carotid sinus massage can be used to distinguish sinus tachycardia from supraventricular arrhythmias. A tachycardia with an irregular rhythm is more likely to be atrial fibrillation, but atrial flutter can also cause a rapid irregular rhythm. Irregular premature contractions and ventricular premature contractions may be associated with rapid, slow, or normal cardiac rates. A slow, fairly regular heart rate is associated with complete heart block.
4. **Is there chest pain associated with the cardiac arrhythmia?** Chest pain should make one think of myocardial infarction, pericarditis, or coronary insufficiency.
5. **Is there fever?** If there is fever, one should consider rheumatic fever, subacute bacterial endocarditis, and thyroid storm.
6. **Is there a heart murmur associated with the arrhythmia?** A heart murmur associated with arrhythmia should make one think of rheumatic fever or subacute bacterial endocarditis, myocardiopathy, or acute congestive heart failure.
7. **Are there signs of congestive heart failure?** Hepatomegaly, jugular vein distention, crepitant rales and pitting edema of the extremities would make one think that congestive heart failure was the cause of the arrhythmia.
8. **Is there a thyroid enlargement?** An enlarged thyroid gland would certainly make one think of thyrotoxicosis.
9. **Is there hypertension?** Hypertension is another important cause of cardiac arrhythmias that should not be forgotten.

DIAGNOSTIC WORKUP

All patients should have an EKG, chest x-ray, and a CBC to rule out anemia. A thyroid profile should be done to look for both hyperthyroidism and hypothyroidism. In acute arrhythmias, serial EKGs and tests for cardiac enzymes need to be done to exclude an acute myocardial infarction. Venous pressure and circulation time or brain natriuretic peptide (BNP) should be determined to rule out congestive heart failure; pulmonary function tests may be helpful, as they may rule out both congestive heart failure and emphysema. Echocardiograms should be done to rule out valvular disease and cardiomyopathy. If there are paroxysmal arrhythmias, Holter monitoring needs to be done. An exercise tolerance test may allow the recording of an arrhythmia that is only induced on exercise. Signal-averaged EKG and electrophysiologic testing should also be considered. Patients on digitalis, quinidine, or other cardiac drugs should have blood levels of these drugs measured to determine if their levels are toxic. If there is a fever, blood cultures should be done to rule out bacterial endocarditis. Referral to a cardiologist can be made at any point in the diagnostic workup.

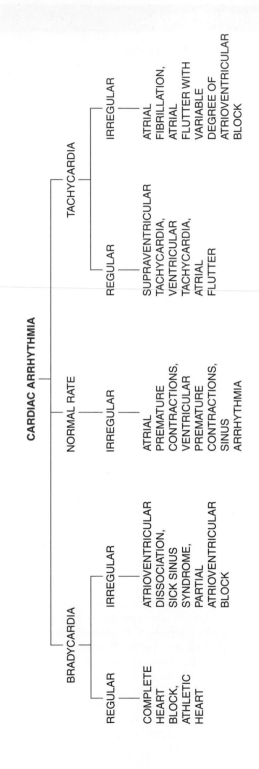

CARDIAC ARRHYTHMIA

BRADYCARDIA

REGULAR

COMPLETE
HEART
BLOCK,
ATHLETIC
HEART

IRREGULAR

ATRIOVENTRICULAR
DISSOCIATION,
SICK SINUS
SYNDROME,
PARTIAL
ATRIOVENTRICULAR
BLOCK

NORMAL RATE

IRREGULAR

ATRIAL
PREMATURE
CONTRACTIONS,
VENTRICULAR
PREMATURE
CONTRACTIONS,
SINUS
ARRHYTHMIA

TACHYCARDIA

REGULAR

SUPRAVENTRICULAR
TACHYCARDIA,
VENTRICULAR
TACHYCARDIA,
ATRIAL
FLUTTER

IRREGULAR

ATRIAL
FIBRILLATION,
ATRIAL
FLUTTER WITH
VARIABLE
DEGREE OF
ATRIOVENTRICULAR
BLOCK

ASK THE FOLLOWING QUESTIONS:

1. **Could the murmur be extracardiac in origin?** Extracardiac murmurs include the pericardial friction rub and cardiorespiratory murmurs.
2. **Is the murmur continuous?** A continuous murmur is most often due to a patent ductus arteriosus or combined valvular stenosis and insufficiency. However, arteriovenous aneurysms and ruptured aneurysm of the sinus of Valsalva must also be considered.
3. **Is the murmur systolic or diastolic?** Diastolic murmurs include aortic regurgitation and mitral stenosis and are always organic. Many systolic murmurs are functional in nature.
4. **Is there associated cardiomegaly?** An enlarged heart associated with the murmur makes it more likely that it is pathologic. One would consider mitral regurgitation, aortic regurgitation, and aortic stenosis and various forms of congenital heart disease.
5. **Is there hepatomegaly?** Hepatomegaly associated with the murmur would make one think of congestive heart failure or tricuspid regurgitation and tricuspid stenosis.
6. **Is there associated fever?** Cardiac murmurs occurring with fever suggest acute rheumatic fever and subacute bacterial endocarditis.
7. **Is there dyspnea?** Dyspnea associated with a cardiac murmur suggests congestive heart failure
8. **Is there chest pain?** If there is chest pain associated with a cardiac murmur, one must consider pericarditis and myocardial infarction.
9. **Is there an enlarged thyroid or intention tremor?** These findings suggest hyperthyroidism.
10. **Is there cyanosis or clubbing?** These findings suggest congenital heart disease.

DIAGNOSTIC WORKUP

If the murmur is believed to be organic, the most cost-effective approach would be to consult a cardiologist at the outset. If the astute clinician wishes to pursue the diagnostic workup on his own, it is suggested that a CBC, sedimentation rate, chemistry panel, VDRL test, and thyroid profile should be done for the initial blood work. In addition, a chest x-ray including obliques, to rule out congestive heart failure, phonocardiograms, and EKG should be performed. These findings may provide a diagnosis. If there is fever, a streptozyme test, antistreptolysin-O (ASO) titer, and serial blood culture should be performed. If congestive heart failure is suspected, venous pressure and circulation time and BNP should be determined. Pulmonary function studies are also helpful. Echocardiography will be extremely helpful in diagnosing the various forms of valvular disease and will also help in identifying a pericardial effusion, congestive heart failure, or the various cardiomyopathies. Cardiac catheterization and angiography and angiocardiography will identify the various congenital heart lesions and valvular disease. These studies, however, are most important when surgery is being considered.

CARDIAC MURMURS

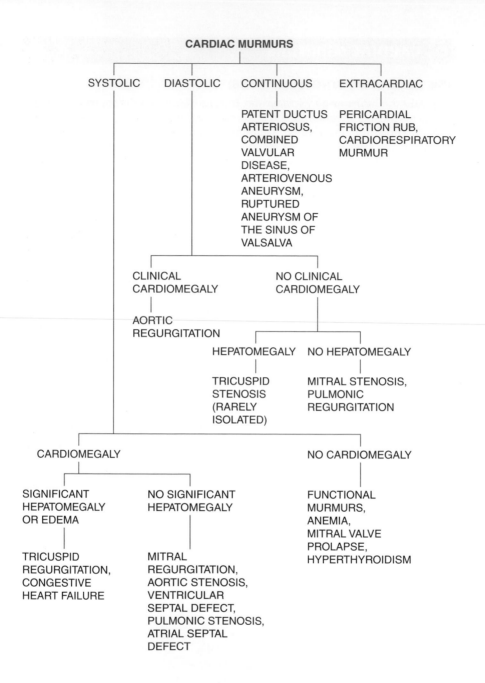

SYSTOLIC   DIASTOLIC   CONTINUOUS   EXTRACARDIAC

CONTINUOUS → PATENT DUCTUS ARTERIOSUS, COMBINED VALVULAR DISEASE, ARTERIOVENOUS ANEURYSM, RUPTURED ANEURYSM OF THE SINUS OF VALSALVA

EXTRACARDIAC → PERICARDIAL FRICTION RUB, CARDIORESPIRATORY MURMUR

DIASTOLIC → CLINICAL CARDIOMEGALY / NO CLINICAL CARDIOMEGALY

CLINICAL CARDIOMEGALY → AORTIC REGURGITATION

NO CLINICAL CARDIOMEGALY → HEPATOMEGALY / NO HEPATOMEGALY

HEPATOMEGALY → TRICUSPID STENOSIS (RARELY ISOLATED)

NO HEPATOMEGALY → MITRAL STENOSIS, PULMONIC REGURGITATION

SYSTOLIC → CARDIOMEGALY / NO CARDIOMEGALY

CARDIOMEGALY → SIGNIFICANT HEPATOMEGALY OR EDEMA / NO SIGNIFICANT HEPATOMEGALY

SIGNIFICANT HEPATOMEGALY OR EDEMA → TRICUSPID REGURGITATION, CONGESTIVE HEART FAILURE

NO SIGNIFICANT HEPATOMEGALY → MITRAL REGURGITATION, AORTIC STENOSIS, VENTRICULAR SEPTAL DEFECT, PULMONIC STENOSIS, ATRIAL SEPTAL DEFECT

NO CARDIOMEGALY → FUNCTIONAL MURMURS, ANEMIA, MITRAL VALVE PROLAPSE, HYPERTHYROIDISM

CARDIOMEGALY

ASK THE FOLLOWING QUESTIONS:

1. **Is there a murmur?** Cardiomegaly with cardiac murmurs suggests valvular disease, but it also suggests congestive heart failure and advanced cardiomyopathies. One should also be sure that the murmur is not a pericardial friction rub.
2. **Is there fever?** Fever with cardiomegaly should suggest rheumatic heart disease and bacterial endocarditis. However, it may also suggest an acute myocarditis or acute pericarditis.
3. **Is there chest pain?** Cardiomegaly with chest pain would certainly suggest a myocardial infarction, but it may also suggest an acute pericarditis.
4. **Is there hepatomegaly?** Cardiomegaly and hepatomegaly suggest congestive heart failure. Hepatomegaly may also suggest one of the systemic diseases that causes a myocardiopathy such as amyloidosis.
5. **Is there edema?** The presence of peripheral edema would suggest congestive heart failure, and if it is nonpitting, it would suggest myxedema.
6. **Is there hypertension?** Cardiomegaly with hypertension would suggest that the cardiomegaly is due to left ventricular enlargement from the chronic hypertension.
7. **Is there cyanosis?** Cardiomegaly with cyanosis, particularly if there is an associated murmur, suggests congenital heart disease of the cyanotic type.

DIAGNOSTIC WORKUP

A CBC, sedimentation rate, ANA, chemistry panel, VDRL test, thyroid profile, EKG, and chest x-ray should be done on all patients. An echocardiogram will be helpful in diagnosing valvular disease, myocardiopathies, congestive heart failure, and pericardial effusion. If congestive heart failure is suspected, BNP, venous pressure and circulation time can be measured, and one should do pulmonary function studies. If there is fever, then one would want to do a streptozyme test, ASO titer, and serial blood cultures. If there is hypertension, a hypertensive workup may be indicated (see page 248). Patients with cyanosis need a workup for congenital heart disease, which will probably include cardiac catheterization and angiocardiography.

Most prudent physicians will refer the patient with cardiomegaly to a cardiologist before pursuing this extensive diagnostic workup.

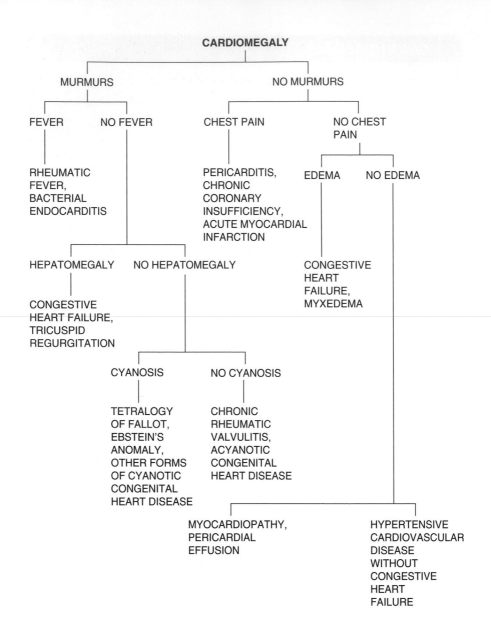

CHEST DEFORMITY

Many deformities of the chest may be observed on inspection of the patient and provide a clue to lung or systemic disease. Scoliosis may be a clue to syringomyelia, old poliomyelitis, muscular dystrophy, and Friedreich's ataxia. The "rachitic rosary" seen in rickets is due to swelling of the costochondral junctions. Expansion of one side of the chest may be seen in acute pneumothorax. A barrel chest is typical of emphysema. Empyema may produce a localized swelling of the chest. An aortic aneurysm may cause a pulsatile swelling of the upper anterior chest. Hodgkin's disease, carcinoma of the lung, tuberculosis, actinomycosis, and various benign tumors of the lung will cause localized swellings in the chest.

DIAGNOSTIC WORKUP

Plain films of the chest, thoracic spine, and ribs will usually be diagnostic of chest deformities. Sputum culture and sensitivity, pleural fluid analysis, culture, and CT scans will be helpful in confusing cases. Referral to a pulmonologist will also help clear up the confusion.

⊚ CHEST PAIN

ASK THE FOLLOWING QUESTIONS:

1. **Is the chest pain acute or chronic?** If it is acute, one must consider acute myocardial infarction, dissecting aneurysm, pulmonary embolism, pneumothorax, pericarditis, and fractures. If the chest pain is chronic, one must consider chronic coronary insufficiency, esophagitis, hiatal hernia, and various chest wall conditions. The endocardium is the source of chest pain in mitral valve prolapsed.

2. **Is the pain constant or intermittent?** Constant pain suggests acute myocardial infarction, pulmonary infarction, dissecting aneurysm, and pneumonia. Intermittent pain would suggest coronary insufficiency, Tietze's disease, and DaCosta's syndrome. Intermittent chest pain at rest may be due to Prinzmetal angina.

3. **Is there associated significant hypertension?** Significant hypertension would make one think of dissecting aneurysm, but it is also found occasionally in acute myocardial infarction.

4. **Is the pain relieved by antacids?** Relief by antacids should prompt one to consider reflux esophagitis and hiatal hernia.

5. **Is the pain precipitated or increased by breathing?** The pain of pleurisy, costochondritis, rib fractures, and pneumothorax is precipitated or increased by breathing. In costochondritis there is tenderness of the costochondral junctions.

6. **Is there associated hemoptysis?** Hemoptysis should make one consider a pulmonary embolism.

7. **Is there fever and purulent sputum?** Fever and purulent sputum should make one consider pneumonia.

8. **Is there dyspnea?** Dyspnea should make one consider pneumothorax, pulmonary embolism, and pneumonia, as well as congestive heart failure secondary to acute myocardial infarction.

9. **Is it aggravated by movement?** Aggravation of the chest pain by movement should suggest pericarditis. Remember, myocardial infarctions may also have extension into the pericardium and must be considered at times.

10. **Is it relieved by nitroglycerin?** Relief by nitroglycerin should suggest a coronary insufficiency, but esophagospasm may be relieved by nitroglycerin also. Relief with 5 to 10 cc of lidocaine viscus will help diagnose reflux esophagitis.

DIAGNOSTIC WORKUP

All patients should have a CBC, sedimentation rate, chemistry panel, VDRL test, chest x-ray, and EKG. If there is sputum, a smear and culture should be done as soon as possible.

If a myocardial infarction is suspected, then serial EKGs and tests for the isoenzyme of creatine kinase (CK-MB) should be done if the initial EKG and enzymes do not show any significant changes. Serum cardiac troponin levels may also be diagnostic of a myocardial infarct. Thallium-201 scintigraphy is useful in diagnosing both myocardial infarction and coronary insufficiency. Exercise tolerance tests may help diagnose coronary insufficiency. Immediate coronary angiography should be undertaken if the condition deteriorates and in the cases of ST segment elevation myocardial infarction (STEMI). This can be followed by immediate balloon angioplasty, reperfusion therapy, or bypass surgery.

If a pulmonary embolism is suspected, arterial blood gases and a ventilation-perfusion scan should be done or a spiral CT of the chest and may also pick up a dissecting aneurysm. D-dimer testing of whole blood is a sensitive test of pulmonary embolus. Pulmonary angiography may need to be done if these are negative and pulmonary embolism is still strongly suspected. Ultrasonography of the lower extremities will be helpful in picking up an embolic source as will an MRI of the pelvis.

If esophageal disease is suspected, an upper GI series with esophagogram should be done; this can be followed by esophagoscopy and gastroscopy if needed. A Bernstein test (acid perfusion of the esophagus) may reproduce the exact pain and distinguish esophageal reflux from a cardiac source of the pain. Ambulatory pH monitoring may also diagnose reflux esophagitis.

If pericarditis is suspected, echocardiography and possibly a CT scan of the chest and pericardium may be necessary. Coronary angiography may be necessary to diagnose coronary insufficiency. Echocardiography is also helpful in diagnosing mitral valve prolapse and the various myocardiopathies. Twenty-four-hr Holter monitoring is useful in diagnosing many causes of intermittent chest pain.

Referral to a cardiologist or pulmonologist may be appropriate at any point in this workup. Dissecting aneurysm may be confirmed by a CT scan, transesophageal echocardiography, or MRI of the chest.

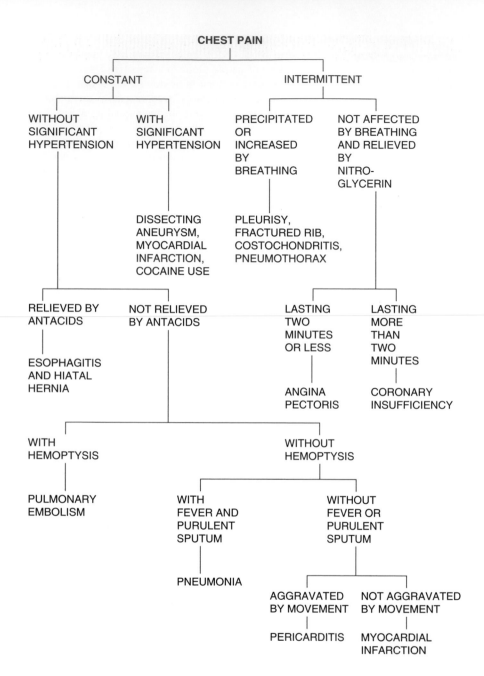

CHEST PAIN

CONSTANT | INTERMITTENT

CONSTANT:

WITHOUT SIGNIFICANT HYPERTENSION | WITH SIGNIFICANT HYPERTENSION

WITH SIGNIFICANT HYPERTENSION →
DISSECTING ANEURYSM, MYOCARDIAL INFARCTION, COCAINE USE

WITHOUT SIGNIFICANT HYPERTENSION:

RELIEVED BY ANTACIDS | NOT RELIEVED BY ANTACIDS

RELIEVED BY ANTACIDS →
ESOPHAGITIS AND HIATAL HERNIA

NOT RELIEVED BY ANTACIDS:

WITH HEMOPTYSIS | WITHOUT HEMOPTYSIS

WITH HEMOPTYSIS →
PULMONARY EMBOLISM

WITHOUT HEMOPTYSIS:

WITH FEVER AND PURULENT SPUTUM | WITHOUT FEVER OR PURULENT SPUTUM

WITH FEVER AND PURULENT SPUTUM →
PNEUMONIA

WITHOUT FEVER OR PURULENT SPUTUM:

AGGRAVATED BY MOVEMENT | NOT AGGRAVATED BY MOVEMENT

AGGRAVATED BY MOVEMENT →
PERICARDITIS

NOT AGGRAVATED BY MOVEMENT →
MYOCARDIAL INFARCTION

INTERMITTENT:

PRECIPITATED OR INCREASED BY BREATHING | NOT AFFECTED BY BREATHING AND RELIEVED BY NITRO-GLYCERIN

PRECIPITATED OR INCREASED BY BREATHING →
PLEURISY, FRACTURED RIB, COSTOCHONDRITIS, PNEUMOTHORAX

NOT AFFECTED BY BREATHING AND RELIEVED BY NITROGLYCERIN:

LASTING TWO MINUTES OR LESS | LASTING MORE THAN TWO MINUTES

LASTING TWO MINUTES OR LESS →
ANGINA PECTORIS

LASTING MORE THAN TWO MINUTES →
CORONARY INSUFFICIENCY

CHEST TENDERNESS

ASK THE FOLLOWING QUESTIONS:

1. **Is there a history of trauma?** Fractured or bruised ribs head the list of traumatic conditions that can cause chest tenderness. Intercostal myositis and burns may cause tenderness.
2. **Are there significant signs of systemic diseases?** Signs of petechiae or ecchymoses elsewhere may suggest blood dyscrasia. Splenomegaly and hepatomegaly may also suggest a systemic disease. Evidence of arthritic changes of the joints may suggest ankylosing spondylitis.
3. **Is there a rash in the area of the tenderness?** A rash in the area of tenderness suggests herpes zoster. At times only a few vesicles or bullae may be present, and it is easy to miss this diagnosis in the early stages.
4. **Are there abnormalities on auscultation and percussion of the lung?** The pleura and pericardium may elicit a friction rub that will indicate pericarditis or pleurisy. Flatness or dullness to percussion may indicate pleural effusion, lobar pneumonia, or empyema. There may be a murmur beneath the area of tenderness suggesting an aortic aneurysm.

DIAGNOSTIC WORKUP

In any case of unexplained tenderness of the chest, x-rays of the chest and the ribs will be extremely useful in the diagnosis. If a systemic disease is suspected, a CBC and sedimentation rate, chemistry panel, and arthritis profile should be done. If cardiac disease is suspected, serial EKGs and serial cardiac enzymes may be necessary. A bone scan may diagnose subtle fractures or metastatic neoplasm of the ribs. A CT scan may be helpful in mediastinal tumors. Trigger point injections may help diagnose costochondritis. In confusing cases, a cardiologist should be consulted.

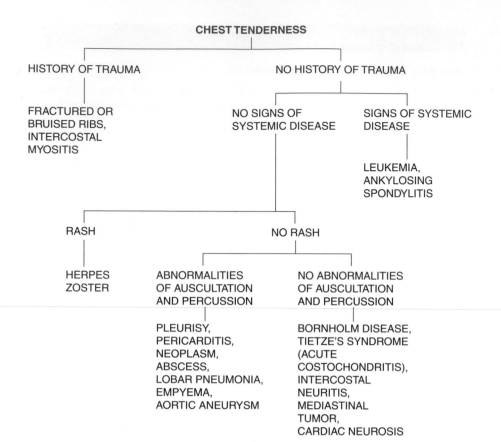

CHEST TENDERNESS

HISTORY OF TRAUMA

FRACTURED OR
BRUISED RIBS,
INTERCOSTAL
MYOSITIS

NO HISTORY OF TRAUMA

NO SIGNS OF
SYSTEMIC DISEASE

SIGNS OF SYSTEMIC
DISEASE

LEUKEMIA,
ANKYLOSING
SPONDYLITIS

RASH

HERPES
ZOSTER

NO RASH

ABNORMALITIES
OF AUSCULTATION
AND PERCUSSION

PLEURISY,
PERICARDITIS,
NEOPLASM,
ABSCESS,
LOBAR PNEUMONIA,
EMPYEMA,
AORTIC ANEURYSM

NO ABNORMALITIES
OF AUSCULTATION
AND PERCUSSION

BORNHOLM DISEASE,
TIETZE'S SYNDROME
(ACUTE
COSTOCHONDRITIS),
INTERCOSTAL
NEURITIS,
MEDIASTINAL
TUMOR,
CARDIAC NEUROSIS

ASK THE FOLLOWING QUESTIONS:

1. **Is there a heart murmur?** The presence of a heart murmur would suggest bacterial endocarditis.
2. **Is there jaundice?** The presence of jaundice should suggest ascending cholangitis and cholecystitis. Viral hepatitis is not usually associated with chills.
3. **Is there frequency or burning of urination?** The presence of frequency or burning of urination should suggest pyelonephritis, perinephric abscess, and prostatic abscess.
4. **Is there hepatomegaly?** The presence of an enlarged liver usually without jaundice is indicative of amebic abscess. The liver may be palpable, but not significantly enlarged in subdiaphragmatic abscess.
5. **Are there neurologic signs?** Neurologic findings would indicate a brain abscess, sinus thrombosis, various forms of encephalitis, and epidural abscess. Don't forget that an epidural abscess of the spine may have its onset with chills. This type of abscess should be looked for in diabetics.
6. **Is there cough or rales?** The presence of cough or rales should prompt a search for a lung abscess, lobar pneumonia, bronchiectasis, and tuberculosis.
7. **Is there bone pain or a bone mass?** These findings are typical of osteomyelitis.
8. **Are there no focal signs of infection?** Without focal signs of infection, one should suspect septicemia, malaria, acute hemolytic anemias, relapsing fever, subdiaphragmatic abscess, and dental abscesses. However, chills may occur at the onset of any acute infection.

DIAGNOSTIC WORKUP

This is identical to the diagnostic workup for acute fever on page 177.

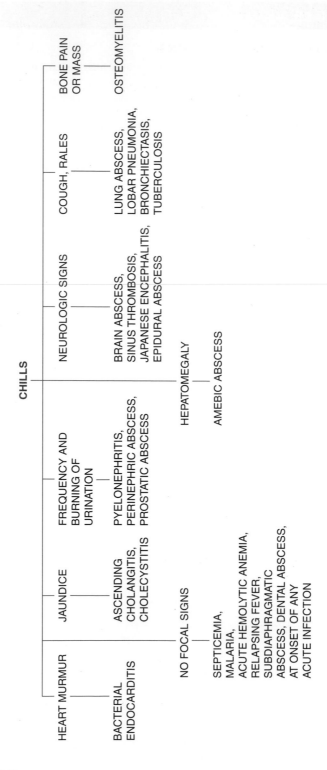

CHILLS

HEART MURMUR — BACTERIAL ENDOCARDITIS

JAUNDICE — ASCENDING CHOLANGITIS, CHOLECYSTITIS

FREQUENCY AND BURNING OF URINATION — PYELONEPHRITIS, PERINEPHRIC ABSCESS, PROSTATIC ABSCESS

HEPATOMEGALY — AMEBIC ABSCESS

NEUROLOGIC SIGNS — BRAIN ABSCESS, SINUS THROMBOSIS, JAPANESE ENCEPHALITIS, EPIDURAL ABSCESS

COUGH, RALES — LUNG ABSCESS, LOBAR PNEUMONIA, BRONCHIECTASIS, TUBERCULOSIS

BONE PAIN OR MASS — OSTEOMYELITIS

NO FOCAL SIGNS — SEPTICEMIA, MALARIA, ACUTE HEMOLYTIC ANEMIA, RELAPSING FEVER, SUBDIAPHRAGMATIC ABSCESS, DENTAL ABSCESS, AT ONSET OF ANY ACUTE INFECTION

ASK THE FOLLOWING QUESTIONS:

1. **What is the patient's age?** Children are likely to develop Sydenham's chorea, Tourette's syndrome, or Wilson's disease. Huntington's chorea and senile chorea usually occur in adults.
2. **Is there associated fever or joint pains?** The presence of fever or joint pains would make one think of Sydenham's chorea, encephalitis lethargica, or systemic lupus erythematosus.
3. **Is there a family history?** A family history will be found in patients with Huntington's chorea, Tourette's syndrome, and Wilson's disease.
4. **Is there a history of drug ingestion?** Several drugs can lead to choreiform movements, including the phenothiazines, levodopa, anticonvulsants, and birth control pills.

DIAGNOSTIC WORKUP

A toxicology screen is usually the first thing to be done. A sedimentation rate, ASO titer, streptozyme test, and EKG will help diagnose Sydenham's chorea. Serum copper and ceruloplasmin will help diagnose Wilson's disease. An ANA assay may be done in patients suspected of having lupus erythematosus. Young adults with high-risk sexual behavior require human immunodeficiency virus (HIV) testing. If these tests are unrewarding, a neurologist should be consulted.

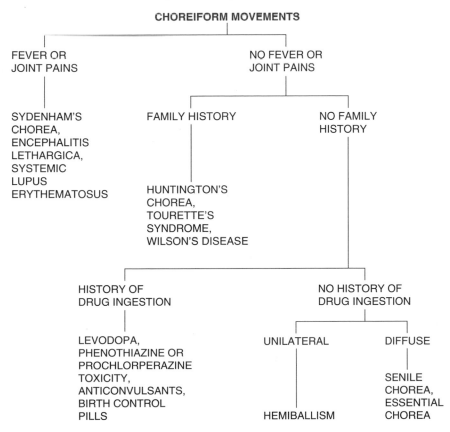

CHOREIFORM MOVEMENTS

CASE HISTORY

A 42-year-old executive is found to have clubbing on a routine physical. Following the algorithm, you look for cyanosis, heart murmurs, and cardiomegaly and find none of these. There is a history of chronic productive cough but no fever, chills, or night sweats. A CT Scan of the chest reveals bronchiectasis.

ASK THE FOLLOWING QUESTIONS:

1. **Is there cyanosis?** Cyanosis should make one think of cyanotic congenital heart disease and pulmonary arteriovenous aneurysms.
2. **Is there a cough or dyspnea?** A cough or shortness of breath should make one think of a pulmonary condition such as bronchiectasis, chronic interstitial fibrosis, asbestosis, emphysema, or carcinoma of the lung. Lung abscesses and tuberculosis must also be considered, although they are less frequent.
3. **Is there a fever?** A fever along with the clubbing should make one think of empyema, lung abscess, tuberculosis, or subacute bacterial endocarditis.

DIAGNOSTIC WORKUP

An EKG and chest x-ray will identify the most common causes of clubbing. A CBC, sedimentation rate, and chemistry panel should also be done routinely. If there is fever, a sputum smear, culture and sensitivity, and blood culture should be done. An upper GI series, an esophagogram, and a barium enema will identify most GI disorders. Cyanotic congenital heart disease will require further workup, including a cardiology consultation, cardiac catheterization, and angiocardiography. A thoracentesis may be necessary to diagnose empyema. Sputum cytology is the first step if a neoplasm is suspected. Bronchoscopy may be necessary to diagnose carcinoma of the lung. A CT scan of the chest can be used to diagnose bronchiectasis.

If a more extensive workup is necessary, referral to a pulmonologist or cardiologist should be considered.

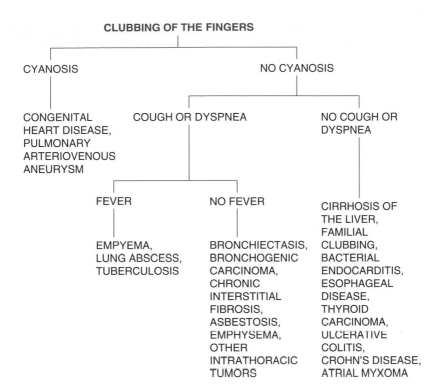

CLUBBING OF THE FINGERS

CYANOSIS

NO CYANOSIS

CONGENITAL HEART DISEASE, PULMONARY ARTERIOVENOUS ANEURYSM

COUGH OR DYSPNEA

NO COUGH OR DYSPNEA

FEVER

NO FEVER

CIRRHOSIS OF THE LIVER, FAMILIAL CLUBBING, BACTERIAL ENDOCARDITIS, ESOPHAGEAL DISEASE, THYROID CARCINOMA, ULCERATIVE COLITIS, CROHN'S DISEASE, ATRIAL MYXOMA

EMPYEMA, LUNG ABSCESS, TUBERCULOSIS

BRONCHIECTASIS, BRONCHOGENIC CARCINOMA, CHRONIC INTERSTITIAL FIBROSIS, ASBESTOSIS, EMPHYSEMA, OTHER INTRATHORACIC TUMORS

ASK THE FOLLOWING QUESTIONS:

1. **Is there a history of drug or alcohol ingestion?** This is a very important question to ask, as many cases of coma are due to acute alcohol intoxication, delirium tremens, opium poisoning, barbiturate poisoning, and other toxic cerebral depressants.

2. **Is there a history of trauma?** Most of the time it will be obvious that the patient has suffered a blow to the head. However, there are many times when one must contact the family or other people who witnessed the onset of the coma to determine if there was trauma.

3. **Are there focal neurologic signs?** Focal neurologic signs would make one think of a stroke, brain abscess, brain tumor, or epidural or subdural hematoma.

4. **Is there papilledema?** Papilledema certainly would indicate a possible space-occupying lesion such as a brain tumor, brain abscess, or subdural hematoma.

5. **Is there a sweet odor to the breath?** A sweet odor to the breath should make one think of a diabetic coma or alcoholism.

6. **Is there fever?** If there is fever, one should be thinking of meningitis, subarachnoid hemorrhage, or acute encephalitis. However, aspiration pneumonia, urinary tract infection (UTI), or septicemia may explain the fever.

7. **Is there nuchal rigidity?** The presence of nuchal rigidity suggests a meningitis or subarachnoid hemorrhage.

8. **Are there sibilant or crepitant rales on examination of the lung?** Sibilant rales would suggest the possibility that pulmonary emphysema is responsible for the coma, whereas crepitant rales would suggest that there is congestive heart failure or possibly pneumonia.

DIAGNOSTIC WORKUP

When one encounters a patient with coma, the first thing to do is to establish an airway. Next, the blood pressure is taken. If there are any signs of shock, an intravenous access is established, and the shock is treated appropriately. A cardiology and surgical consult are obtained. Blood should then be drawn for a CBC, type and cross-match, sedimentation rate, chemistry panel, electrolytes, serum osmolality to rule out hyperosmolar nonketotic diabetic coma, blood ammonia level, and blood alcohol levels. Before removing the syringe, 50 cc of 50% dextrose is given unless the patient is suspected of having hyperosmolar nonketotic diabetic coma. Urinalysis and urine drug screen must be done also. Administer naloxone IV if opiod intoxication is suspected. Arterial blood gas analysis should be done. If the situation is urgent or emergent, a CT scan of the brain is done before the results of the laboratory tests are available. If the laboratory tests are inconclusive, a CT scan must be done anyway.

If all of the above studies are negative, a spinal tap is done for cell count, protein, glucose, VDRL test, smear, and culture and sensitivity. This is especially true when there is fever or nuchal rigidity.

If the diagnosis is still in doubt, blood tests for other toxic materials, such as the lead level, and blood cultures and EEG are done. A neurologist or neurosurgeon is usually consulted as soon as one is available.

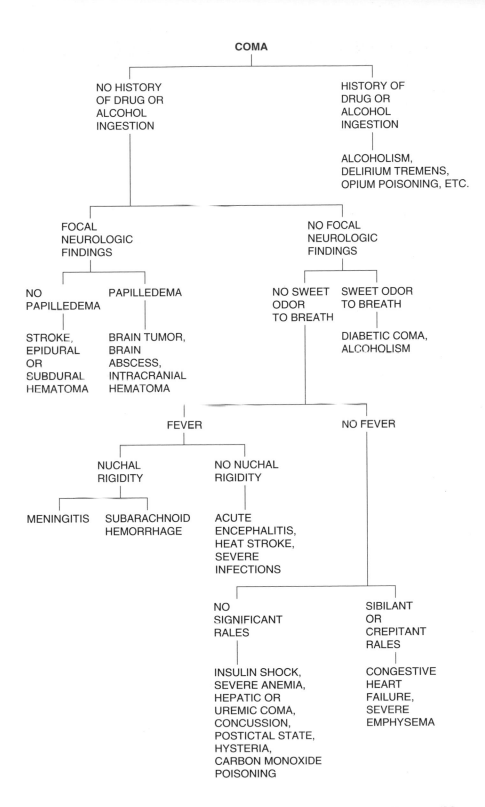

ASK THE FOLLOWING QUESTIONS:

1. **Is the constipation acute or chronic?** If the constipation is acute and there is abdominal pain or vomiting, one must consider the possibility of intestinal obstruction. An examination may disclose an empty rectum, in which case it is more likely complete intestinal obstruction; or there may be some feces in the rectum, in which case there may be incomplete intestinal obstruction. If the constipation is a chronic problem, one should investigate the patient's diet and emotional status and toilet habits over the life span.

2. **What kind of a diet is the patient on?** Many patients today eat on the run, and they eat mostly fast foods, which are devoid of fiber. Frequently, they don't take the time to go to the bathroom. Some patients are on special diets to lose weight or have a fear of gaining weight; therefore, they don't eat well at all. If what the patient labels as constipation is simply infrequent bowel movements, but the bowel movements are normal in consistency, this is not really true constipation.

3. **Does the patient take drugs of any kind?** Patients should be questioned first about chronic use of laxatives. Americans have the misconception that they must have a bowel movement everyday and, therefore, they get in the habit of using something to stimulate the bowels, which can lead them to believe they have chronic constipation. Chronic narcotic use can lead to constipation, as can the use of antispasmodics for ulcer or urinary incontinence.

4. **Associated symptoms?** We have already mentioned that abdominal pain and vomiting may be a sign of acute intestinal obstruction, and occasionally this is a sign of a chronic intestinal obstruction. If there is alternating diarrhea and constipation, one must consider the possibility of irritable bowel syndrome or a colon carcinoma. Blood in the stool along with painful defecation may indicate hemorrhoids and anal fissure. A person who is suffering from these conditions may delay moving his bowels for fear of the pain that accompanies this situation, and the hard stool that caused the hemorrhoids and anal fissure in the first place perpetuates the condition because it contributes to the constipation. If blood is found in the stool, well mixed with the stool, and defecation is basically painless, then colon carcinoma and diverticulitis must be considered. Blood and mucus in the stool would indicate an irritable bowel syndrome.

5. **What are the findings on physical examination?** The finding of an empty rectum indicates an intestinal obstruction. The finding of an abdominal mass or a rectal mass would certainly indicate carcinoma of the colon. Rectal examination may disclose hemorrhoids or anal fissure as causing the chronic constipation and allows one to test the stool for occult blood.

DIAGNOSTIC WORKUP

If the constipation is acute, a flat plate of the abdomen and a CBC would be in order to determine if the patient has intestinal obstruction. The workup of chronic constipation should include stool for occult blood, sigmoidoscopy, barium enema, or a colonoscopy. A chemistry panel and other diagnostic studies may be necessary to rule out systemic causes of constipation such as diabetes, hypothyroidism, and various conditions associated with hypercalcemia. If diagnostic tests yield no positive findings, referral to a psychiatrist or a gynecologist may be in order. A trial of a fiber diet may be helpful. At the same time, one should eliminate chronic laxative usage. Anorectal manometry will help diagnose rectal and anal sphincter dysfunction. Defecography will help diagnose anorectal dysfunction also. A neurologist should be consulted if urinary retention is also a problem.

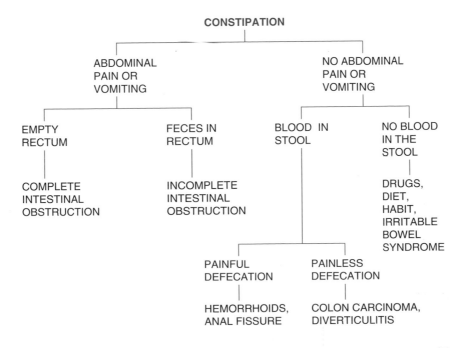

ASK THE FOLLOWING QUESTIONS:

1. **Are the episodes of loss of consciousness really seizures?** Real seizures, especially grand mal, present with incontinence and/or tongue biting and post-ictal somnolence. Hysterical seizures with actual tonic or clonic movements may occur, but there is no tongue biting or incontinence or post-ictal somnolence. Syncope usually is not accompanied by convulsive movements, but it occasionally can be after the drop in blood pressure or anoxia to the brain that has continued for a period of time. If there are no convulsive movements to the blackouts, then the possibility of syncope must be considered (page 468). In addition, cerebrovascular accidents, narcolepsy, and breath-holding attacks must be considered when there are no definite convulsive movements.

2. **Is there a history of drug or alcohol abuse?** Alcohol withdrawal seizures and seizures due to cocaine abuse are becoming more common. Patients frequently lie about their use of illicit drugs or alcohol. In young adults and teenagers, a urine drug screen should be done.

3. **Is there fever?** Fever should make one think of meningitis or encephalitis, or if it has been extended over a longer period of time, a cerebral abscess. In children, one should consider the possibility of febrile convulsions.

4. **What type of seizure disorder is it?** If there are convulsions, are they focal or jacksonian type? That would certainly suggest a space-occupying lesion as opposed to a generalized convulsion. Loss of awareness with no actual collapse for 1 minute or less is suggestive of a petit mal type seizure. In these seizures, the patient just simply stares. Longer attacks of loss of awareness are more likely to be due to complex partial seizures and occasionally an observer will note unusual behavior during these episodes. The patient may note unusual odors.

5. **Are there focal neurologic signs and papilledema?** These findings are more typical of a space-occupying lesion such as a cerebral tumor, cerebral abscess, or a subdural hematoma.

DIAGNOSTIC WORKUP

All patients should receive a CBC, urinalysis, sedimentation rate, ANA, VDRL test, and chemistry panel. Do a serum prolactin to rule out hysterical seizures. (It's only elevated in real seizures). Patients with high-risk behavior should have HIV testing. In older patients, a chest x-ray should be done to look for the possibility of a primary lung tumor. A urine drug screen is useful especially in young adults. All patients also need a wake-and-sleep EEG. Ambulatory EEG monitoring can now be done in the hospital or an outpatient setting with a digitrace device. In the elderly, a carotid duplex scan or magnetic resonance angiography may be needed to distinguish transient ischemic attacks from epilepsy. There is some argument over whether a CT scan or MRI should be done on all patients with definite convulsions. The author believes that a CT scan should be done on all patients, even those without focal neurologic signs or papilledema. Isotope brain scans, arteriography, and pneumoencephalography are no longer indicated unless something is found on the CT scan that needs further clarification. A spinal tap should also be done when there is fever or when central nervous system lues or multiple sclerosis are suspected. Visual evoked potential (VEP) and brain stem evoked potential

(BSEP) tests may also help diagnose multiple sclerosis. It should be noted that seizures occur in 7% of cases with multiple sclerosis. In patients with frequent attacks, a trial of anticonvulsant drugs may be diagnostic.

A consultation with a neurologic specialist can be done at any point in this workup. Certainly, it would be very important to have it done early if there are focal neurologic signs or papilledema.

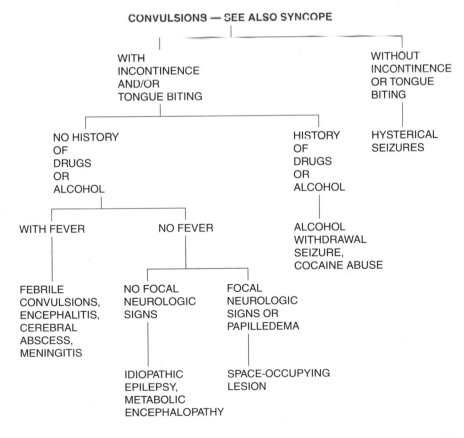

CONVULSIONS — SEE ALSO SYNCOPE

WITH INCONTINENCE AND/OR TONGUE BITING

WITHOUT INCONTINENCE OR TONGUE BITING

NO HISTORY OF DRUGS OR ALCOHOL

HISTORY OF DRUGS OR ALCOHOL

HYSTERICAL SEIZURES

WITH FEVER

NO FEVER

ALCOHOL WITHDRAWAL SEIZURE, COCAINE ABUSE

FEBRILE CONVULSIONS, ENCEPHALITIS, CEREBRAL ABSCESS, MENINGITIS

NO FOCAL NEUROLOGIC SIGNS

FOCAL NEUROLOGIC SIGNS OR PAPILLEDEMA

IDIOPATHIC EPILEPSY, METABOLIC ENCEPHALOPATHY

SPACE-OCCUPYING LESION

ASK THE FOLLOWING QUESTIONS:

1. **Is it acute or chronic?** Acute onset of a cough would suggest an acute URI, viral pneumonia, or bronchopneumonia. A chronic cough is more suggestive of pneumoconiosis, chronic bronchitis, emphysema, bronchiectasis, tuberculosis, carcinoma of the lung, or bronchial asthma.

2. **Is there exposure to toxic fumes?** The most common toxic fume is cigarette smoke. However, if one asks the patient's occupation, one might find that he is a miner and therefore pneumoconiosis comes to mind. One might find that he is an aircraft maker or shipbuilder, in which case berylliosis and asbestosis would come to mind; or that he is a farmer and therefore farmer's lung would come to mind.

3. **Is there significant sputum production?** If so, what is the nature of the sputum? Purulent sputum would suggest a pneumonia, abscess, tuberculosis, or bronchiectasis; bloody sputum would suggest carcinoma of the lung, tuberculosis, and bronchiectasis; mucoid sputum would suggest asthma. Advanced AIDS may manifest as a productive cough due to pneumocystis jiroveci. If the sputum is foamy, one would consider congestive heart failure, mitral stenosis, and inhalation of poison gas.

4. **Is there fever?** If there is fever associated with the cough, obviously one would suspect an infectious process to be present. This could be viral or bacterial. Most likely the patient has bronchopneumonia, but the possibility of an abscess or pulmonary infarct would still have to be entertained.

5. **What other symptoms and signs are associated with the cough?** The first thing to be considered would be dyspnea. In acute cases dyspnea would be a sign of congestive heart failure, pulmonary embolism, and, of course, advancing pneumonia. In chronic cases, dyspnea would be a sign of emphysema, chronic pulmonary fibrosis, and chronic congestive heart failure. Wheezing would be a sign of asthma or congestive heart failure, but of course it is also found in pulmonary emphysema. Cardiomegaly would suggest congestive heart failure and if there is an associated murmur, that makes congestive heart failure even more likely. If there is hepatosplenomegaly, one would suspect a systemic disease involving the lungs such as periarteritis nodosa or other collagen diseases.

6. **Is the patient taking drugs?** Angiotensin-converting enzyme (ACE) inhibitors such as captopril are well known to cause cough.

DIAGNOSTIC WORKUP

If there is nasal stuffiness and a postnasal drip, a trial of antihistamines or decongestants is indicated before starting an expensive workup. All patients require a CBC and differential count, a sedimentation rate, and a chemistry panel. For chronic cough a 24-hr sputum volume should be ordered. A sputum for routine smear and culture should be done, and in chronic cases a sputum for acid-fast bacilli (AFB) culture and smear must be done. In children, collect a specimen of gastric aspirate for AFB culture. One should keep a high index of suspicion for *Mycoplasma pneumoniae* and Legionnaire's disease. A therapeutic trial of a macrolide is useful in suspected cases of mycoplasma or Legionnaire's. Also, sputum for fungi culture should be done in chronic cases. For diagnosing TB, a skin test may be done but recently a quantiferon blood test has received attention.

Asthma can be further elucidated and confirmed by doing a sputum for eosinophils. Carcinoma of the lung can be confirmed with a sputum for Pap smear. If there is fever, blood cultures may be useful and febrile agglutinins should also be done. An x-ray of the chest with anteroposterior, lateral, and apical lordotic views should be done, and when a tumor is suspected, tomography should be done or a CT scan. In the cases of chronic cough, skin testing for coccidioidomycosis, cystoplasmosis, tuberculosis, and blastomycosis should be done. A Kveim test to rule out sarcoidosis may be necessary. When these tests fail to make a diagnosis, bronchoscopy and possibly bronchograms to look for a bronchiectasis should be done. Lung biopsy may also be necessary. Pulmonary function tests should be done in suspected cases of emphysema and asthma. Allergy skin testing is extremely valuable in cases of asthma. Look for alpha-1-antitrypsin deficiency in difficult cases. If congestive heart failure is suspected, echocardiography would be valuable. A trial of diuretics may also assist in the diagnosis. If reflux esophagitis is suspected, prolonged monitoring of esophageal pH may be diagnostic. A trial of therapy with an H_2 antagonist or proton pump inhibitor may also be diagnostic.

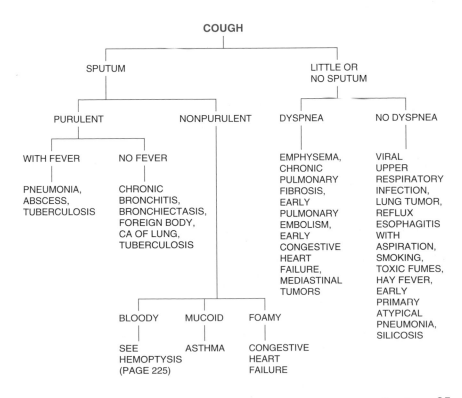

There are usually physiologic cramps occurring during menstruation and not associated with pathology of the female reproductive organs. If there is associated menorrhagia, the differential diagnosis of this symptom should be consulted (page 311).

Menstrual cramps occur more frequently in the virginal uterus, but may establish themselves after the first pregnancy. All women have experienced menstrual cramps at some time in their life. These cramps may be the first sign of endometriosis, pelvic inflammatory disease, or ectopic pregnancy.

CASE HISTORY

A 67-year-old black male complains of severe muscular cramps for the past year, especially at night. Following the algorithm, you ask about drug or alcohol use and find there is none.

On examination, he has normal peripheral and femoral pulses and a blood pressure of 110/70. The cramps are not isolated to one extremity and he has a positive Trousseau's sign. You correctly suspect hypoparathyroidism and other causes of hypocalcemia.

ASK THE FOLLOWING QUESTIONS:

1. **Is there a history of drug ingestion?** Many drugs produce muscular cramps. The most notable are the diuretics.
2. **Are there absent or diminished peripheral pulses?** Absent or diminished peripheral pulses suggest the cramps are due to ischemia from peripheral arteriosclerosis or arterial embolism.
3. **Are the femoral pulses diminished?** Diminished femoral pulses suggest a Leriche syndrome or saddle embolism of the terminal aorta.
4. **Is there hypertension?** Hypertension suggests aldosteronism and chronic glomerulonephritis.
5. **Are the cramps limited to one extremity?** Limitation of the cramps to one extremity suggests an occupational neurosis (professional cramps).
6. **Is there a positive Chvostek's and/or Trousseau's sign?** These are signs of tetany, as might be associated with hypoparathyroidism, uremia, alkalosis, and other causes of hypocalcemia.
7. **Is there fever?** Fever is associated with dehydration, heat stroke, and many infectious diseases that cause cramps.

DIAGNOSTIC WORKUP

All patients should have a CBC, sedimentation rate, chemistry panel, electrolytes, and urinalysis. If there is associated diminished or absent peripheral pulses, then Doppler studies and arteriography should be done. If the cramps are acute in onset, time should not be wasted in performing these studies. Magnetic resonance angiography is an excellent alternative to invasive angiography, but it is expensive. If there is associated hypertension, then 24-hr urine aldosterone and plasma renin studies should be done. If there are positive Trousseau's and/or Chvostek's signs, a thorough investigation for hypoparathyroidism should be done. A single serum calcium and phosphorus and alkaline phosphatase are not enough, but repeated studies should be done. In addition, 24-hr urine collection for calcium and serum parathyroid hormones should be done. An endocrinologist should probably be consulted if there is any doubt about the existence of hypoparathyroidism or any of the other causes of hypocalcemia.

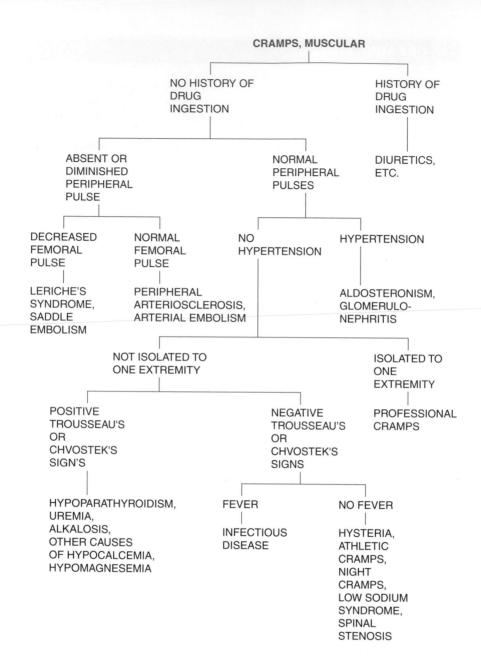

CRAMPS, MUSCULAR

NO HISTORY OF DRUG INGESTION

HISTORY OF DRUG INGESTION

ABSENT OR DIMINISHED PERIPHERAL PULSE

NORMAL PERIPHERAL PULSES

DIURETICS, ETC.

DECREASED FEMORAL PULSE

NORMAL FEMORAL PULSE

NO HYPERTENSION

HYPERTENSION

LERICHE'S SYNDROME, SADDLE EMBOLISM

PERIPHERAL ARTERIOSCLEROSIS, ARTERIAL EMBOLISM

ALDOSTERONISM, GLOMERULO-NEPHRITIS

NOT ISOLATED TO ONE EXTREMITY

ISOLATED TO ONE EXTREMITY

POSITIVE TROUSSEAU'S OR CHVOSTEK'S SIGN'S

NEGATIVE TROUSSEAU'S OR CHVOSTEK'S SIGNS

PROFESSIONAL CRAMPS

HYPOPARATHYROIDISM, UREMIA, ALKALOSIS, OTHER CAUSES OF HYPOCALCEMIA, HYPOMAGNESEMIA

FEVER

NO FEVER

INFECTIOUS DISEASE

HYSTERIA, ATHLETIC CRAMPS, NIGHT CRAMPS, LOW SODIUM SYNDROME, SPINAL STENOSIS

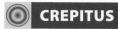

The most classic example of crepitus is subcutaneous emphysema following a chest injury, especially a fractured rib. This may also occur around a tracheotomy site. Crepitus is felt over arthritic joints, especially when there is synovitis. In tenosynovitis of the wrist, there is often a marked crepitus over the flexor tendons. A grating sound or crepitus may be felt over fractured bones if an effort is made to move the two portions of fractured bones. Palpation of a malignant bone tumor will elicit crepitus if the bone cortex has been penetrated. In patients with gas gangrene, crepitus may be felt over the infected area due to subcutaneous gas.

DIAGNOSTIC WORKUP

This will depend on the type of crepitus felt. Plain films will verify the presence of gas, fractures, and tumors. Undoubtedly, other symptoms and signs will be present to key the rest of the diagnostic workup using the pages in this book.

CYANOSIS

ASK THE FOLLOWING QUESTIONS:

1. **Is there a history of drug ingestion?** Potassium chlorate, sulfanilamide, and coal tar products are only a few of the drugs that may cause methemoglobinemia and sulfhemoglobinemia.
2. **Is the cyanosis limited to one extremity?** If the cyanosis is limited to one extremity, one should suspect an arterial embolism or phlebothrombosis.
3. **Is the cyanosis limited to the extremities or is it generalized?** Cyanosis that is limited to the extremities only suggests Raynaud's disease, Raynaud's phenomena, shock, and acrocyanosis.
4. **Is there associated dyspnea?** If there is significant dyspnea, one should consider a pulmonary or cardiac origin for the cyanosis such as cyanotic congenital heart disease, pulmonary emphysema, pulmonary fibrosis, or pulmonary embolism.
5. **Is the patient a child or an adult?** Certain causes of cyanosis are limited to children, such as laryngismus stridulus, laryngotracheitis, and acute subglottic laryngitis.
6. **Is there a heart murmur or cardiomegaly?** A heart murmur or cardiomegaly suggests rheumatic carditis, congenital heart disease, or congestive heart failure.

DIAGNOSTIC WORKUP

It is wise to order a cardiology consult at the outset. Arterial blood gases, EKG, chest x-ray, and pulmonary function studies will diagnose most cases that are due to pulmonary or cardiac causes. If there is a history of drug ingestion, the blood should be drawn for methemoglobin and sulfhemoglobin testing. If a pulmonary embolism is suspected, a ventilation-perfusion scan or spiral CT scan and pulmonary arteriography may need to be done. If a peripheral embolism is suspected, angiography of the vessel involved will be diagnostic. Sputum or nose and throat cultures will be useful in diagnosing the infectious diseases associated with cyanosis.

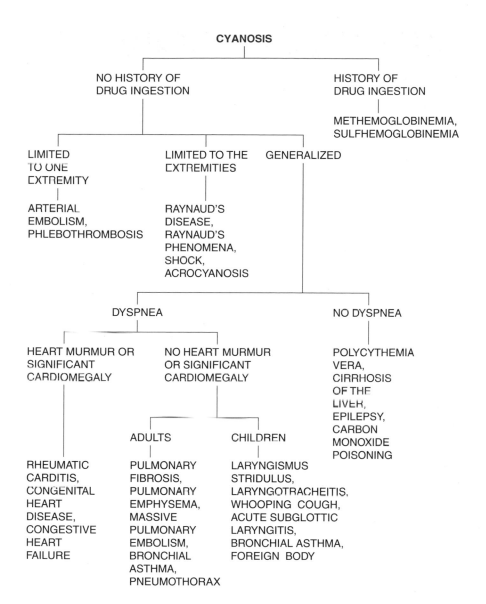

CASE HISTORY

A 48-year-old white female complains of progressive loss of hearing and tinnitus in her left ear over the past 2 years.

Following the algorithm, you find she has had occasional attacks of vertigo during that time. There is a family history of neurofibromatosis. Your examination reveals no other neurologic signs but she has coffee-colored areas of discoloration on her abdomen and thorax. What is your diagnosis?

ASK THE FOLLOWING QUESTIONS:

1. **Is it unilateral or bilateral?** Unilateral deafness may be due to local conditions such as wax, a foreign body, otitis media, or ruptured drum, or it may be due to neurologic conditions such as Ménière's disease, acoustic neuroma, or multiple sclerosis. Bilateral deafness is more likely due to otosclerosis, acoustic trauma, presbycusis, or drug toxicity.
2. **Are there abnormalities on otoscopic examination of the ear?** It is very important to do a thorough examination of the ear, as one may find wax, foreign body, otitis media, cholesteatoma, or ruptured drum.
3. **Is there associated vertigo?** The presence of vertigo should make one think of Ménière's disease or some neurologic condition such as acoustic neuroma, multiple sclerosis, or basilar artery insufficiency.
4. **What are the results of the Rinne test?** Normally, the Rinne test should show a 2 to 1 ratio of air to bone hearing. In otosclerosis, the ratio approaches 1 to 1, but in sensory neural deafness the ratio is preserved at 2 to 1. In unilateral deafness, the Weber test is helpful. This will lateralize to the affected ear if the problem is a conductive deafness, and it will lateralize to the good ear if the problem is a sensory neural deafness.

DIAGNOSTIC WORKUP

Audiometry and caloric testing or electronystagmography should be done in almost all cases in which the ear examination is normal. It is probably wise to consult an otolaryngologist at this point. Tympanography will be helpful in diagnosing subtle cases of serous otitis media. X-rays of the mastoids, petrous bones, and internal auditory canal should be done for chronic otitis media, cholesteatoma, and acoustic neuroma. If an acoustic neuroma is suspected, however, an MRI of the brain and auditory canals must be done. If basilar artery insufficiency is suspected, four-vessel cerebral angiography should be done. Magnetic resonance angiography is an excellent noninvasive alternative for diagnosing vertebral-basilar artery disease. If multiple sclerosis is suspected, MRI of the brain, BSEP and VEP studies, and a spinal tap for spinal fluid analysis may be done.

Rather than performing these tests, the most cost-effective approach would be to refer the patient to a neurologist if other focal neurologic findings are evident.

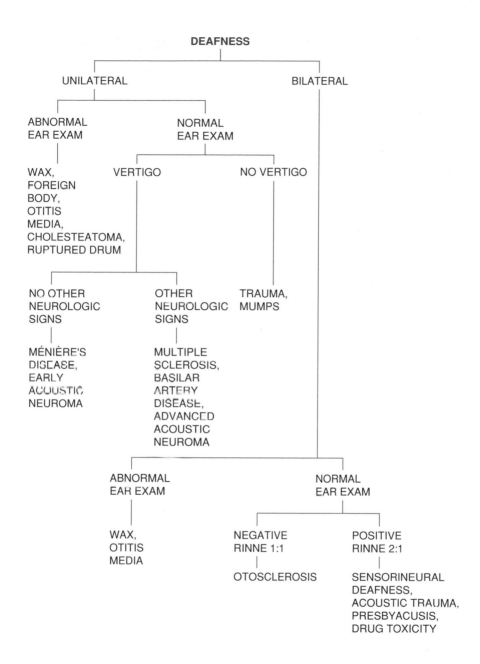

DELAYED PUBERTY

ASK THE FOLLOWING QUESTIONS:

1. **Is there a positive drug history?** Boys and girls may take anabolic steroids or androgens and thyroid hormones. These hormones may cause a delay in puberty.
2. **Is there a significant weight loss?** Significant weight loss would suggest anorexia nervosa, hyperthyroidism, celiac disease, cystic fibrosis, and uncontrolled diabetes among other conditions.
3. **Is there a short stature?** The presence of a short stature would suggest pituitary tumors, hypothalamic syndromes, gonadal dysgenesis, adrenal tumors, hyperplasia, hypothyroidism, and ovarian tumors.
4. **Is there a hemianopic field defect?** The presence of a hemianopic field defect would suggest a pituitary tumor. The presence of a normal or tall stature would suggest constitutional delayed puberty among other more rare conditions.

DIAGNOSTIC WORKUP

Before proceeding with an expensive diagnostic workup, it is perhaps best to consult an endocrinologist. If one is not available, routine tests would be a CBC, chemistry panel, and thyroid profile. Blood tests for a serum FSH, LH, and testosterone or estradiol may be done, although urine gonadotropins may be a cheaper screening test.

Pelvic ultrasound and CT scans of the abdomen and pelvis will help identify ovarian and adrenal tumors and abnormal configuration of the uterus. CT scans of the brain will help identify pituitary tumors. If all these studies are negative, a psychiatrist may need to be consulted. Remember, the family may be in more need of the psychiatrist than the child.

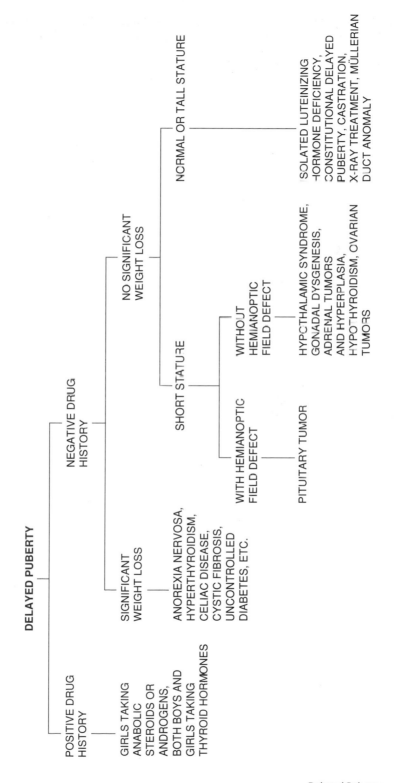

DELAYED PUBERTY

POSITIVE DRUG HISTORY

GIRLS TAKING ANABOLIC STEROIDS OR ANDROGENS, BOTH BOYS AND GIRLS TAKING THYROID HORMONES

NEGATIVE DRUG HISTORY

SIGNIFICANT WEIGHT LOSS

ANOREXIA NERVOSA, HYPERTHYROIDISM, CELIAC DISEASE, CYSTIC FIBROSIS, UNCONTROLLED DIABETES, ETC.

NO SIGNIFICANT WEIGHT LOSS

SHORT STATURE

WITH HEMIANOPTIC FIELD DEFECT

PITUITARY TUMOR

WITHOUT HEMIANOPTIC FIELD DEFECT

HYPOTHALAMIC SYNDROME, GONADAL DYSGENESIS, ADRENAL TUMORS AND HYPERPLASIA, HYPOTHYROIDISM, OVARIAN TUMORS

NORMAL OR TALL STATURE

ISOLATED LUTEINIZING HORMONE DEFICIENCY, CONSTITUTIONAL DELAYED PUBERTY, CASTRATION, X-RAY TREATMENT, MÜLLERIAN DUCT ANOMALY

ASK THE FOLLOWING QUESTIONS:

1. **Is there associated fever?** Delirium with fever may simply indicate a self-limited infectious process, but it should bring to mind encephalitis and meningitis as well as cerebral abscess and cerebral hemorrhage.

2. **Is there a history of trauma?** A history of head trauma would make one suspect a subdural or epidural hematoma and concussion.

3. **Is there a history of drug or alcohol ingestion?** This is probably the most important single question to ask in the average case coming into the emergency room these days without a good history. Very often, the problem is alcoholism or various popular drugs such as cocaine, lysergic acid diethylamide (LSD), and phencyclidine (PCP).

4. **Are there focal neurologic signs?** Focal neurologic signs along with the delirium would make one think of subdural or epidural hematoma, cerebral abscess, or cerebral hemorrhage. Remember, a cerebral thrombosis or embolism may present with delirium also.

5. **Is there nuchal rigidity?** If there is nuchal rigidity, the patient may have meningitis or subarachnoid hemorrhage.

6. **Is there a sweet odor to the breath?** A sweet odor to the breath should make one think of diabetic coma or alcoholism.

7. **What is the response to intravenous thiamine?** If the patient responds to intravenous thiamine, the diagnosis is usually Wernicke's encephalopathy or Korsakoff's syndrome.

8. Intermittent delirium should suggest psychomotor epilepsy and transient global amnesia.

DIAGNOSTIC WORKUP

Routine laboratory tests include a CBC, sedimentation rate, ANA, chemistry panel including electrolytes and BUN and VDRL tests, a blood alcohol level, urinalysis, and urine drug screen. A CT scan of the brain and EEG is also usually indicated. Acute delirium may be an indication to administer intravenous glucose and thiamine. If there is fever, blood cultures and a spinal tap for analysis and culture need to be done. Arterial blood gases and carboxyhemoglobin should be determined. Generally, a neurologist or neurosurgeon should be consulted early.

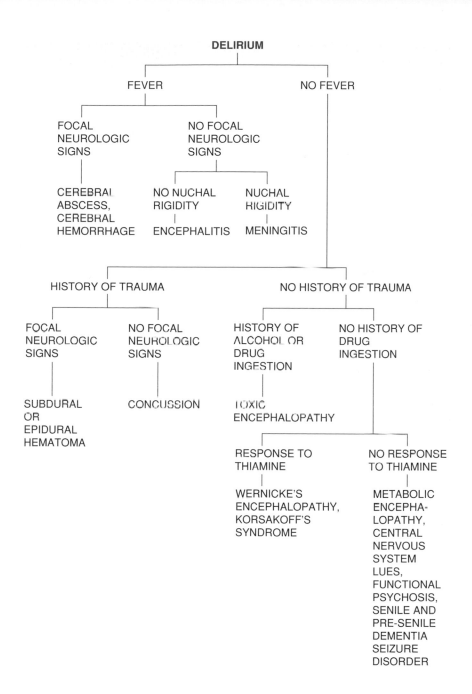

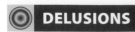

ASK THE FOLLOWING QUESTIONS:

1. **Is there a history of drug or alcohol ingestion?** Many drugs may be associated with delusions, especially cocaine, PCP, and LSD. The confabulations of Korsakoff's psychosis may be confused with delusions.
2. **Is there impairment of memory?** If there is impairment of memory, an organic psychosis should be suspected, such as senile and pre-senile dementia or general paresis. When there is no impairment of memory, the problem is probably a psychiatric disorder such as schizophrenia or manic-depressive psychosis.

DIAGNOSTIC WORKUP

If there is a history of alcohol or drug ingestion, a blood alcohol level and urine for drug screen should be done. A CT scan, EEG, and spinal fluid analysis will often need to be done before referring a patient to a psychiatrist for further evaluation.

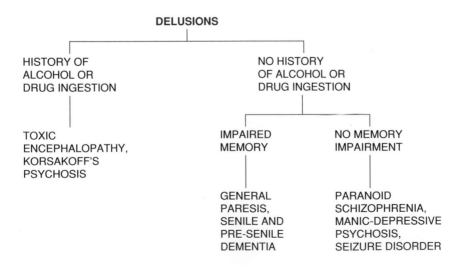

CASE HISTORY

A 68-year-old Hispanic is brought to your office for evaluation because his family says, he has become very forgetful lately. Following the algorithm, you ask about alcohol abuse, and inquire about the medication he is taking. He has an occasional glass of wine and is on no medication other than an occasional aspirin for headache.

Your examination reveals no papilledema or focal neurologic signs. Serum B_{12} and folic acid are normal. A trial of vitamin B complex fails to initiate improvement. The patient continues to insist he is okay. What is your diagnosis?

ASK THE FOLLOWING QUESTIONS:

1. **Is there a history of drug or alcohol ingestion?** Chronic barbiturate intoxication, ergotism, and other psychotropic or antidepressant drugs may cause dementia. Alcoholism may cause dementia in the form of Korsakoff's psychosis or Wernicke's encephalopathy.
2. **Is there headache, papilledema, or focal neurologic signs?** The most important condition to rule out in this category would be a space-occupying lesion, but normal pressure hydrocephalus, cerebral arteriosclerosis, acute cerebrovascular accident, and general paresis may present with focal neurologic signs.
3. **Is there a response to niacin, thiamine, vitamin B_{12}, or thyroid?** Response to these drugs would indicate that the patient has pellagra, Korsakoff's psychosis, pernicious anemia, or myxedema. However, laboratory tests should be done before administering the medications. Laboratory tests include serum B_{12} and folic acid, and a thyroid profile. Unfortunately, most laboratories do not have a test for niacin or thiamine.
4. **Is there insight?** In patients with cerebral arteriosclerosis, the patient notices that his memory is slipping. This is also true of acquired immunodeficiency syndrome (AIDS).
5. **Are there extrapyramidal tract signs?** Extrapyramidal tract signs should suggest Huntington's chorea or Parkinson's disease.
6. **Are there pyramidal tract signs or myoclonus?** Pyramidal tract signs are seen in general paresis and Jakob–Creutzfeldt syndrome, but also myoclonus is seen in Jakob–Creutzfeldt syndrome.

DIAGNOSTIC WORKUP

Routine laboratory tests include a CBC, sedimentation rate, chemistry panel, VDRL test, HIV antibody titer, ANA, blood alcohol level, urine drug screens, thyroid profile, serum B_{12}, and folic acid. A CT scan should probably be done in all cases. An EEG may be helpful in demonstrating drug intoxication. A spinal tap may need to be done to diagnose central nervous system lues. The best test for that is the fluorescent treponema antibody absorption test (FTA-ABS). MRI may be useful in distinguishing Alzheimer's disease from cerebral arteriosclerosis, as in cerebral arteriosclerosis small infarcts may be demonstrated. A radioiodinated serum albumin (RISA) cisternography study is useful to diagnose normal pressure hydrocephalus. Arterial blood gases should be drawn. Psychiatric testing will help differentiate organic brain syndrome from other psychiatric disorders and malingering. A neurologist or psychiatrist should be consulted before ordering expensive diagnostic tests. In mild cognitive disturbances, consider a trial of antidepressants or hormone therapy especially in postmenopausal women.

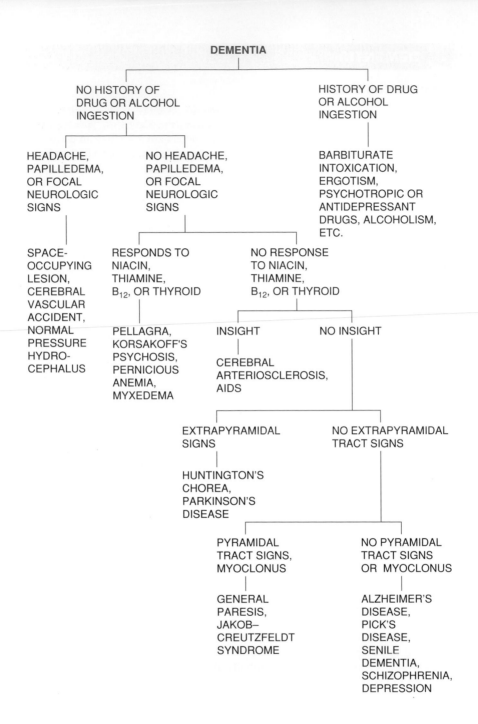

DEMENTIA

NO HISTORY OF DRUG OR ALCOHOL INGESTION

HISTORY OF DRUG OR ALCOHOL INGESTION

HEADACHE, PAPILLEDEMA, OR FOCAL NEUROLOGIC SIGNS

NO HEADACHE, PAPILLEDEMA, OR FOCAL NEUROLOGIC SIGNS

BARBITURATE INTOXICATION, ERGOTISM, PSYCHOTROPIC OR ANTIDEPRESSANT DRUGS, ALCOHOLISM, ETC.

SPACE-OCCUPYING LESION, CEREBRAL VASCULAR ACCIDENT, NORMAL PRESSURE HYDRO-CEPHALUS

RESPONDS TO NIACIN, THIAMINE, B_{12}, OR THYROID

NO RESPONSE TO NIACIN, THIAMINE, B_{12}, OR THYROID

PELLAGRA, KORSAKOFF'S PSYCHOSIS, PERNICIOUS ANEMIA, MYXEDEMA

INSIGHT

NO INSIGHT

CEREBRAL ARTERIOSCLEROSIS, AIDS

EXTRAPYRAMIDAL SIGNS

NO EXTRAPYRAMIDAL TRACT SIGNS

HUNTINGTON'S CHOREA, PARKINSON'S DISEASE

PYRAMIDAL TRACT SIGNS, MYOCLONUS

NO PYRAMIDAL TRACT SIGNS OR MYOCLONUS

GENERAL PARESIS, JAKOB–CREUTZFELDT SYNDROME

ALZHEIMER'S DISEASE, PICK'S DISEASE, SENILE DEMENTIA, SCHIZOPHRENIA, DEPRESSION

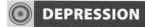

DEPRESSION

ASK THE FOLLOWING QUESTIONS:

1. **Is there associated headache, papilledema, dementia, or focal neurologic signs?** These findings would suggest a space-occupying lesion. This is something the clinician does not want to miss.
2. **Are there endocrine changes?** A number of endocrinologic diseases may present with depression, including Cushing's disease, myxedema, hyperthyroidism, and menopause.
3. **Is there marked loss of appetite, weight, and libido?** Endogenous depression, unipolar depression, and the depressive phase of manic-depressive psychosis may present with these findings. On the other hand, neurotic-depressive reaction usually is not associated with significant loss of appetite, weight, or libido.
4. **What drugs or addictive substances is the patient on?** Remember, patients are reluctant to admit the latter.

DIAGNOSTIC WORKUP

If the patient is suicidal, one should not hesitate to make a psychiatric referral or plan hospitalization immediately. To rule out organic causes, routine laboratory studies include a CBC, sedimentation rate, chemistry panel, urine drug screen, VDRL test, and thyroid profile. If Cushing's syndrome is suspected, a 24-hr urine-free cortisol and cortisol suppression test should be done. If menopause is suspected, order a serum FSH and estradiol level. A trial of estrogen therapy may be warranted in women or a trial of testosterone in men. A CT scan of the brain should probably be done in all cases to exclude a brain tumor, especially if there is no response to treatment! Office tests to evaluate nonorganic depression include the Beck Depression Inventory and the Hamilton Depression Scale. A referral to a psychiatrist should also be considered early if the depression is severe or if there is suicidal ideation.

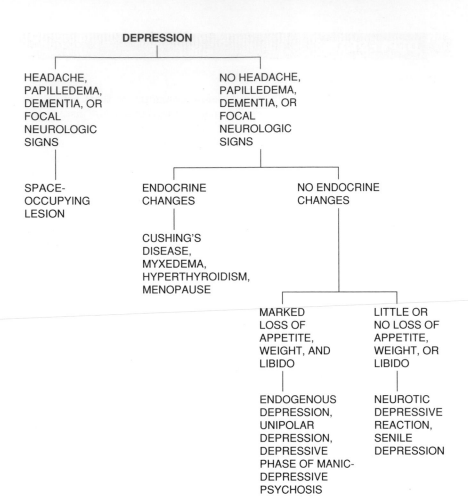

DEPRESSION

- HEADACHE, PAPILLEDEMA, DEMENTIA, OR FOCAL NEUROLOGIC SIGNS
  - SPACE-OCCUPYING LESION
- NO HEADACHE, PAPILLEDEMA, DEMENTIA, OR FOCAL NEUROLOGIC SIGNS
  - ENDOCRINE CHANGES
    - CUSHING'S DISEASE, MYXEDEMA, HYPERTHYROIDISM, MENOPAUSE
  - NO ENDOCRINE CHANGES
    - MARKED LOSS OF APPETITE, WEIGHT, AND LIBIDO
      - ENDOGENOUS DEPRESSION, UNIPOLAR DEPRESSION, DEPRESSIVE PHASE OF MANIC-DEPRESSIVE PSYCHOSIS
    - LITTLE OR NO LOSS OF APPETITE, WEIGHT, OR LIBIDO
      - NEUROTIC DEPRESSIVE REACTION, SENILE DEPRESSION

◎ DIAPHORESIS

ASK THE FOLLOWING QUESTIONS:

1. **Is there a history of drug or alcohol ingestion?** Many drugs can cause diaphoresis, but caffeine and nicotine head the list. Alcohol can be associated with significant diaphoresis also. Organophosphate intoxication is associated with profuse diaphoresis.
2. **Is there associated fever?** Obviously, infectious disease is a very important cause of diaphoresis, particularly when the fever breaks. Look for tuberculosis, malaria, acute rheumatic fever, and bacterial endocarditis. Thyroid storm can be associated with fever also.
3. **Is there associated chest pain or hypotension?** Chest pain with diaphoresis would make one think of an acute myocardial infarction, but this combination is also found in coronary insufficiency. Shock, whatever the cause, produces significant diaphoresis.
4. **Is there associated weight loss, hypertension, or both?** Weight loss and hypertension should make one think of hyperthyroidism and pheochromocytoma. Peripheral neuropathy is also associated with sweating because of involvement of the autonomic nervous system.
5. **Is there associated weight gain?** The triad of obesity, diaphoresis, and increased appetite is typical of an insulinoma. Diabetics taking excessive insulin will also sweat.
6. **Is there a rash?** Several skin diseases may cause hyperhidrosis.

DIAGNOSTIC WORKUP

Routine diagnostic studies include a CBC, sedimentation rate, chemistry panel, electrolytes, thyroid profile, blood alcohol level, EKG, and chest x-ray. Serial EKGs and cardiac enzymes should be done if a myocardial infarction is suspected. A 24-hr urine collection for catecholamines can be done if a pheochromocytoma is suspected. A glucose tolerance test, a 36- to 72-hr fast, and insulin tolerance test may be done for an insulinoma. If infectious disease is strongly suspected, a workup for fever of unknown origin can be done (see page 177).

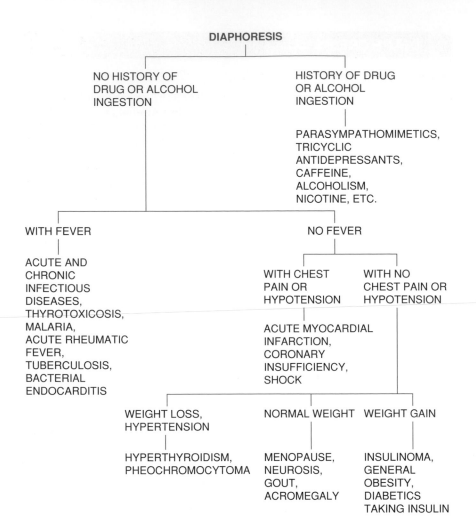

DIARRHEA, ACUTE

ASK THE FOLLOWING QUESTIONS:

1. **Is there blood in the stool?** From the algorithm, blood in the stool should indicate that there is *Salmonella, Shigella, Campylobacter jejuni,* ulcerative colitis, Crohn's disease, and amebic dysentery. Without blood in the stool, it is more likely that the acute diarrhea is due to a staphylococcal toxin, giardiasis, traveler's diarrhea, a virus, or contaminated food.

2. **Is there a fever?** Fever, especially with an elevated white count and blood in the stool, would suggest *Salmonella, Shigella, C. jejuni,* or ulcerative colitis in its acute stage. The absence of fever would suggest amebic dysentery or giardiasis, although there may be fever in amebic dysentery in the severe cases. Even traveler's diarrhea and toxic staphylococcal gastroenteritis do not usually give more than a low-grade temperature at best. Pseudomembranous colitis may result in a significant elevation of the temperature once the patient becomes severely dehydrated.

3. **Is there severe vomiting?** Severe vomiting is seen in toxic staphylococcal gastroenteritis! This follows 2 to 4 hrs after eating food poisoned with the toxin. Traveler's diarrhea and viral gastroenteritis may also cause severe vomiting, as may food that is contaminated. On the other hand, there is little or no vomiting in giardiasis and pseudomembranous colitis.

4. **Did several members of the family experience acute diarrhea also?** This is a key question because it indicates whether there is a possibility of toxic staphylococcal gastroenteritis, botulism or the possibility of a contagious condition such as infection with *Salmonella, Shigella,* or *Campylobacter.* If only one member of the family was suffering from diarrhea and everyone is eating the same food, then it is less likely to be a contagious condition, and one must consider ulcerative colitis, pseudomembranous colitis, and conditions listed under chronic diarrhea.

5. **Was there recent foreign travel?** Recent foreign travel would suggest the possibility of traveler's diarrhea, cholera, shigellosis, salmonellosis, and giardiasis.

6. **Is there neurologic symptomatology?** This should point one in the direction of botulism, and generally a little epidemiologic research will disclose that other people in the community have been suffering from the same condition.

DIAGNOSTIC WORKUP

The first thing to do is a stool for occult blood. This will help distinguish those patients who are having obvious infectious disease of the large intestine or maybe even the small intestine. It will also make one suspicious of ulcerative colitis. All patients need a stool culture and stool for ova and parasites. A stool for *Giardia* antigen can also be done. Serologic studies will not be of much help in the acute condition, but they may help later on in cases of salmonellosis and amebiasis. The clinician himself should do a methylene blue smear for leukocytes and examine a wet saline preparation of the stool. If there is a history of antibiotic use, a stool should be tested for *Clostridium difficile* toxin B. Leukocytes on a smear suggest bacterial cause and a culture should be done. The laboratory should be alerted if *Campylobacter* or *Yersinia* is suspected because special culture media are needed. If the diarrhea persists or if there is blood, sigmoidoscopy or colonoscopy should be performed. It is always important to examine the rectum for hemorrhoids and anal fissures that may be causing the positive stool for occult blood. When the diarrhea persists and becomes chronic, the diagnostic workup should include the studies that are listed under chronic diarrhea (page 117).

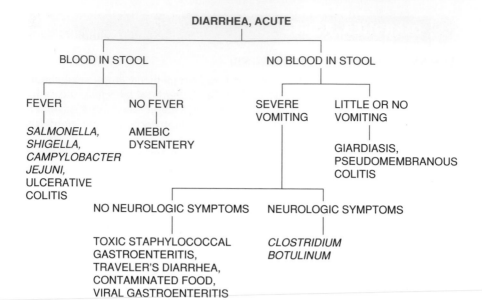

DIARRHEA, ACUTE

BLOOD IN STOOL

FEVER

SALMONELLA,
SHIGELLA,
CAMPYLOBACTER
JEJUNI,
ULCERATIVE
COLITIS

NO FEVER

AMEBIC
DYSENTERY

NO BLOOD IN STOOL

SEVERE
VOMITING

LITTLE OR NO
VOMITING

GIARDIASIS,
PSEUDOMEMBRANOUS
COLITIS

NO NEUROLOGIC SYMPTOMS

TOXIC STAPHYLOCOCCAL
GASTROENTERITIS,
TRAVELER'S DIARRHEA,
CONTAMINATED FOOD,
VIRAL GASTROENTERITIS

NEUROLOGIC SYMPTOMS

CLOSTRIDIUM
BOTULINUM

ASK THE FOLLOWING QUESTIONS:

1. **Is there a positive drug or alcohol history?** It is well known that alcohol can cause diarrhea, as do drugs in common use, such as digitalis, diuretics, beta-blockers, aspirin, colchicine, and other nonsteroidal anti-inflammatory drugs. Perhaps there is overuse of laxatives. Remember, patients may lie about the use of laxatives.
2. **Is there blood in the stool?** Blood in the stool certainly is significant for ulcerative colitis, Crohn's disease, carcinoma, and diverticulitis, but it is also found in amebiasis and the Zollinger–Ellison syndrome.
3. **Is there a lot of mucus in the stool?** Mucus is often found in ulcerative colitis, Crohn's disease, and irritable bowel syndrome.
4. **Is there evidence of steatorrhea?** Large volumes of stools that are partially formed or formed and float in the commode suggest steatorrhea. Stool analysis can be done, as is discussed later.
5. **Is there an abdominal mass?** A mass in the right lower quadrant would suggest carcinoma or diverticulitis. Tenderness in the left lower quadrant with or without a significant mass would be suggestive of ulcerative colitis, diverticulitis, and irritable bowel syndrome. A mass in the area of the ascending or descending colon or the transverse colon should be looked for also, as these would suggest carcinoma.
6. **Are there signs of systemic disease?** Many systemic diseases may cause diarrhea. Among them are thyrotoxicosis, in which case one would be looking for a thyroid tumor and a tremor and tachycardia; carcinoid syndrome, which would cause considerable flushing; Addison's disease, which would cause hyperpigmentation of the skin; and pellagra, which may cause dermatitis and dementia.
7. **Does significant diarrhea persist on fasting?** Diarrhea that persists after fasting suggests a secretory diarrhea from a polypeptide-secreting tumor, such as villous adenoma, a gastrinoma, or a carcinoid tumor.

DIAGNOSTIC WORKUP

Most patients will be diagnosed by a stool culture, stool for occult blood, and stool for ovum and parasites, along with a sigmoidoscopy and barium enema. Giardiasis may be best diagnosed by the finding of *Giardia* antigen in the stool. Perform a Hydrogen breath test if lactose intolerance is suspected. In patients who have been on antibiotics, the stool should be tested for *C. difficile* toxin B. If a systemic disease is suspected, CBC, sedimentation rate, chemistry panel, and thyroid profile should be done. An HIV antibody test may be indicated depending on the history. A urine test for 5-HIAA will uncover a carcinoid syndrome. A serum gastrin will usually reveal a gastrinoma. If these tests do not provide a diagnosis, the most cost-effective approach at this point is to refer the patient to a gastroenterologist who will undoubtedly perform a colonoscopy as part of the workup. Small bowel aspiration and biopsy will be useful in diagnosing *Giardia* infection or celiac sprue; angiography will confirm mesenteric ischemia or infarcts. A swallowed string test may pick up Giardia, but when all else fails, a trial of metronidazole will be diagnostic.

If a gastroenterologist is not available, the clinician may proceed with a quantitative 24-hr stool analysis for fat. If there is 10 g or more of fat in the stool in a day, then steatorrhea can be diagnosed and one can proceed with the workup of steatorrhea (page 457). If there is less than 7 g of fat per day in the stool, the stool volume after fasting should be done. If it is large and we have ruled out surreptitious laxative abuse, a polypeptide-secreting tumor should be considered. Here again, it would be best to refer the patient to a gastroenterologist. If the volume after a fast is small, the problem is most likely lactose or other food intolerance or an irritable bowel syndrome. Occasionally, the problem is dysfunction of the anal sphincter. Once again, a GI specialist is probably best consulted for workup of a dysfunctional anal sphincter.

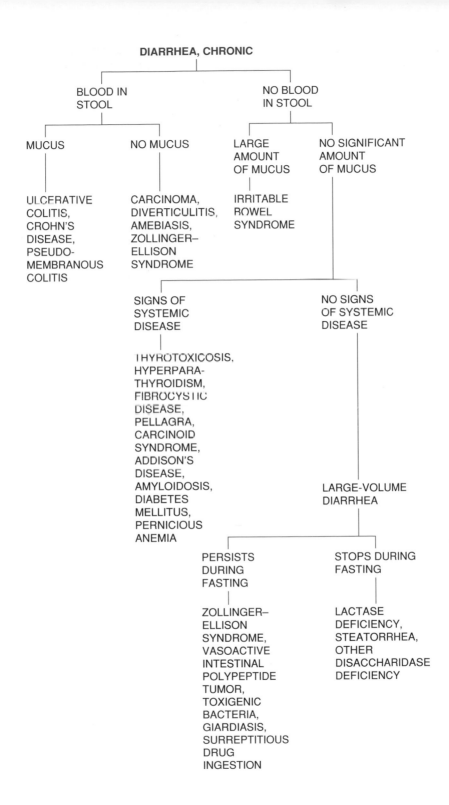

DIFFICULTY URINATING

ASK THE FOLLOWING QUESTIONS:

1. **Is there pain on urination?** The presence of pain on urination should suggest cystitis, urethritis, urethral caruncle, vesicular calculus, urethral stricture, and acute prostatitis.
2. **Are there focal neurologic signs?** The presence of focal neurologic signs should suggest multiple sclerosis, poliomyelitis, cauda equina tumor, acute spinal cord injury, tabes dorsalis, and diabetic neuropathy.
3. **Is the prostate enlarged?** The presence of an enlarged prostate would suggest benign prostatic hypertrophy or an advanced malignancy. A small nodular prostate may suggest an early carcinoma of the prostate. Chronic prostatitis would present with a normal-sized or small prostate that is firm.

DIAGNOSTIC WORKUP

It should go without saying that a complete physical, rectal, and neurologic examination should be done at the outset. A pelvic examination is essential in females. Routine laboratory tests include a CBC, sedimentation rate, urinalysis, VDRL test, urine culture, colony count, and sensitivity. If there is a urethral discharge, a Gram stain and culture for gonococcus should be done. If this is negative, a culture for chlamydia should be done. The patient should be catheterized for residual urine. Alternatively, ultrasonography may be done to demonstrate residual urine. If there is a significant amount of residual urine, referral to a urologist for cystoscopy and cystometric testing is done. A CT scan of the pelvis may be indicated but not before consulting a urologist.

If there are focal neurologic signs, a neurologist is consulted. An enlarged prostate or a prostate that is nodular should be an indication for a consultation with a urologist and ordering a PSA titer.

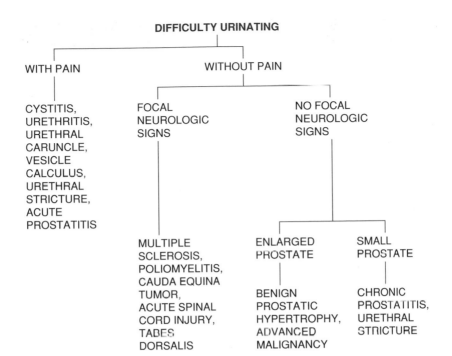

DIFFICULTY URINATING

WITH PAIN

CYSTITIS,
URETHRITIS,
URETHRAL
CARUNCLE,
VESICLE
CALCULUS,
URETHRAL
STRICTURE,
ACUTE
PROSTATITIS

WITHOUT PAIN

FOCAL
NEUROLOGIC
SIGNS

MULTIPLE
SCLEROSIS,
POLIOMYELITIS,
CAUDA EQUINA
TUMOR,
ACUTE SPINAL
CORD INJURY,
TABES
DORSALIS

NO FOCAL
NEUROLOGIC
SIGNS

ENLARGED
PROSTATE

BENIGN
PROSTATIC
HYPERTROPHY,
ADVANCED
MALIGNANCY

SMALL
PROSTATE

CHRONIC
PROSTATITIS,
URETHRAL
STRICTURE

ASK THE FOLLOWING QUESTIONS:

1. **Is it unilateral?** Diplopia that is unilateral is rare, but it can be encountered in ectopia lentis as associated with Marfan's disease as well as in congenital double pupil, cataracts, and corneal opacities.

2. **Is it intermittent?** Intermittent diplopia would make one think of myasthenia gravis, but remember, Eaton–Lambert syndrome can do the same thing.

3. **Is there associated proptosis?** If there is associated proptosis, one should consider hyperthyroidism or pituitary exophthalmos, especially if it is bilateral. However, when it is associated with chemosis and ecchymosis, one should consider an infectious process.

4. **Is there chemosis, ecchymosis, or periorbital edema?** These findings should make one think immediately of cavernous sinus thrombosis, but an arteriovenous aneurysm can produce unilateral chemosis, ecchymosis, and exophthalmos.

5. **Are there associated long tract neurologic signs?** The findings of associated pyramidal tract or other long tract signs would make one think of a brain stem infarct or a brain stem tumor. Advanced intercranial pressure will put pressure on the sixth nerve and cause diplopia. Multiple sclerosis and basilar artery thrombosis on insufficiency may cause long tract signs along with extraocular muscle palsies.

6. **Is there fever or chills?** Findings of fever and chills and diplopia should make one think of an orbital abscess, a brain abscess, or a cavernous sinus thrombosis. There is also the possibility of diphtheria.

DIAGNOSTIC WORKUP

An expensive diagnostic workup may be avoided by referring the patient to an ophthalmologist or a neurologist at the outset. If there is associated exophthalmos, a free T_4 and TSH is ordered. If the diplopia is intermittent, a Tensilon test would be indicated. If there are fever and chills, one should do a CBC, sedimentation rate, possibly blood cultures, skull x-ray, and x-rays of the sinuses. However, under these circumstances, it will usually be necessary to perform a CT scan of the brain, sinuses, and orbits. If there is chemosis or ecchymosis, a cavernous sinus thrombosis is likely, and immediate admission to the hospital and administration of antibiotics after blood culture has been drawn are indicated. MRI of the brain may be necessary to diagnose multiple sclerosis and some of the brain stem infarcts.

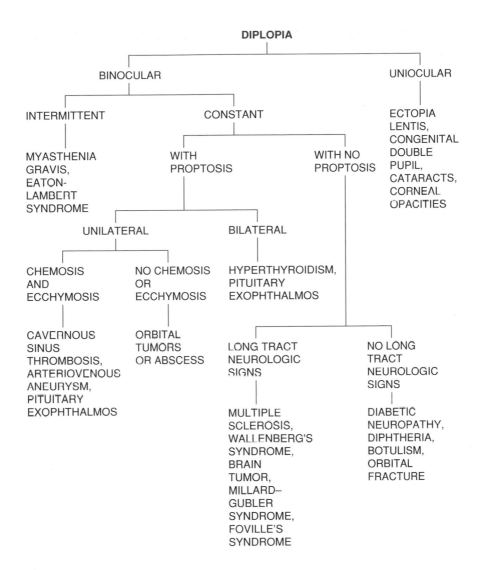

ASK THE FOLLOWING QUESTIONS:

1. **Is it true vertigo?** True vertigo is characterized by the fact that the subject feels he or his environment is turning. One other form of true vertigo is lateral pulsion, in which the subject feels as if he is moving to the left or right or may be moving forward or backward. True vertigo is a sign of neurologic or otologic disease, whereas dizziness that is not true vertigo is more likely a sign of cardiovascular disease, drug toxicity, or hypoglycemia.

2. **Is there associated tinnitus or deafness?** The presence of tinnitus or deafness, especially if the ear examination is negative, is a sign of a more serious otologic or neurologic condition. Disorders such as cholesteatoma, acoustic neuroma, and Ménière's disease must be considered. On the other hand, vertigo without tinnitus or deafness should prompt consideration of benign positional vertigo and vestibular neuronitis.

3. **Are there other neurologic findings?** The finding of abnormalities of other cranial nerves or the long tracts, such as the pyramidal tracts, would suggest multiple sclerosis, an advanced brain stem tumor, acoustic neuroma, or basilar artery insufficiency.

4. **Are there findings on otoscopic examination?** A normal neurologic examination with an abnormal ear examination would suggest otitis media, cholesteatoma, or petrositis.

5. **Is there tachypnea during the attack?** If there is hyperventilation during the attack, then hyperventilation syndrome should be considered.

6. **Is there a history of trauma?** A history of trauma would suggest a postconcussion syndrome.

7. **Are there abnormalities of the blood pressure?** If the dizziness is really lightheadedness, hypertension may be present, but hypertension may also cause true vertigo. Hypotension is more likely to cause lightheadedness, which is not true vertigo. Be sure to take the blood pressures while the patient is lying down and again after rapidly arising to the standing position.

8. **Are there abnormal cardiac findings?** A thorough cardiovascular examination should be done. Irregularities of the heartbeat, heart murmurs, or cardiac enlargement will suggest cardiac arrhythmia, aortic stenosis and insufficiency, mitral stenosis, prolapse of the mitral valve, and congestive heart failure. A slow pulse may indicate heart block or a sick sinus syndrome.

9. **Is there pallor?** Moderate to severe anemia will cause lightheadedness and dizziness, but usually not true vertigo.

DIAGNOSTIC WORKUP

If there is true vertigo, an audiogram and a caloric test or electronystagmography should be done. Hallpike's maneuver should also be done to exclude benign positional vertigo. If these are abnormal, an x-ray of the mastoids, petrous bones, and internal auditory canals should be done. At this point a neurologist should be consulted. If an acoustic neuroma is strongly suspected, an MRI of the brain stem and auditory canals should be done. If the MRI of the brain is negative, a spinal fluid examination can be done to exclude such disorders as central nervous system lues and multiple sclerosis. An MRI of the brain needs to be done to distinguish multiple sclerosis. BSEPs, VEPs, and SSEPs will also be helpful in making the diagnosis of multiple sclerosis, along with the spinal fluid analysis mentioned above. A wake-and-sleep EEG needs to be done to exclude temporal lobe epilepsy. If migraine or migraine equivalents are suspected, perhaps a trial of beta-blockers would help make this diagnosis. If vertebral-basilar artery ischemia is suspected, magnetic resonance angiography may be indicated.

If the dizziness is not true vertigo, a CBC and chemistry panel, thyroid profile, and 5-hr glucose tolerance test should be done at the outset. Additional studies in the form of 24-hr blood pressure monitoring, Holter monitoring, and echocardiography all have a valuable place in the diagnostic workup of dizziness without true vertigo. Perhaps a tilt table test should be ordered to rule out orthostatic hypotension. However, a referral to a cardiologist is wise before undertaking these expensive studies. If all studies are negative, perhaps a psychiatrist should be consulted.

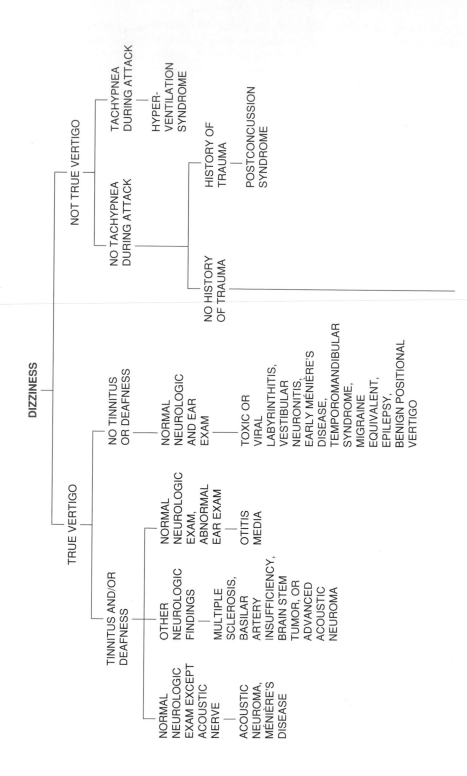

DIZZINESS

TRUE VERTIGO

TINNITUS AND/OR DEAFNESS

NORMAL NEUROLOGIC EXAM EXCEPT ACOUSTIC NERVE

ACOUSTIC NEUROMA, MÉNIÈRE'S DISEASE

OTHER NEUROLOGIC FINDINGS

MULTIPLE SCLEROSIS, BASILAR ARTERY INSUFFICIENCY, BRAIN STEM TUMOR, OR ADVANCED ACOUSTIC NEUROMA

NO TINNITUS OR DEAFNESS

NORMAL NEUROLOGIC EXAM, ABNORMAL EAR EXAM

OTITIS MEDIA

NORMAL NEUROLOGIC AND EAR EXAM

TOXIC OR VIRAL LABYRINTHITIS, VESTIBULAR NEURONITIS, EARLY MÉNIÈRE'S DISEASE, TEMPOROMANDIBULAR SYNDROME, MIGRAINE EQUIVALENT, EPILEPSY, BENIGN POSITIONAL VERTIGO

NOT TRUE VERTIGO

NO TACHYPNEA DURING ATTACK

NO HISTORY OF TRAUMA

HISTORY OF TRAUMA

POSTCONCUSSION SYNDROME

TACHYPNEA DURING ATTACK

HYPER-VENTILATION SYNDROME

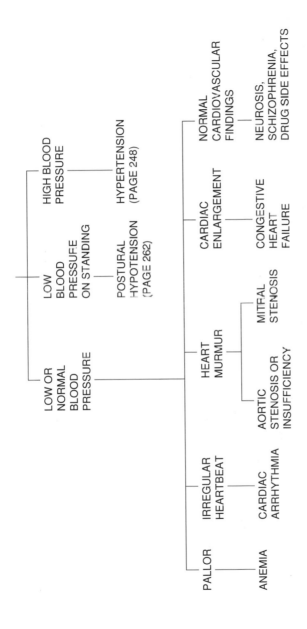

PALLOR

IRREGULAR
HEARTBEAT

LOW OR
NORMAL
BLOOD
PRESSURE

HIGH BLOOD
PRESSURE

ANEMIA

CARDIAC
ARRHYTHMIA

AORTIC
STENOSIS OR
INSUFFICIENCY

HEART
MURMUR

MITRAL
STENOSIS

LOW
BLOOD
PRESSUFE
ON STANDING

POSTURAL
HYPOTENSION
(PAGE 262)

HYPERTENSION
(PAGE 248)

CARDIAC
ENLARGEMENT

CONGESTIVE
HEART
FAILURE

NORMAL
CARDIOVASCULAR
FINDINGS

NEUROSIS,
SCHIZOPHRENIA,
DRUG SIDE EFFECTS

ASK THE FOLLOWING QUESTIONS:

1. **Is there loss of consciousness?** If there is loss of consciousness, the differential diagnosis for syncope should be considered (page 468).
2. **Are there other neurologic signs and symptoms?** Focal neurologic signs and symptoms should make one think of basilar artery insufficiency, cerebral arteriosclerosis, Ménière's disease, and cerebellar atrophy. A brain tumor should also be considered if there are focal signs.
3. **Is there hypotension, cardiomegaly, or a heart murmur?** These findings should make one think of orthostatic hypotension, aortic stenosis and insufficiency, and cardiac arrhythmia.

DIAGNOSTIC WORKUP

Basic studies for the workup of drop attacks are CBC, sedimentation rate, chemistry panel, VDRL test, chest x-ray, tilt table test, and EKG. These will help identify anemia, hypoglycemia, and cardiovascular diseases. An EEG should also be done to rule out epilepsy. If there are focal neurologic signs, a CT scan or MRI should be done. Remember, the MRI is double the cost of a CT scan and the diagnostic yield is only slightly higher. A neurologist should be consulted to help decide which study is appropriate. A 5-hr glucose tolerance test can be done to help diagnose hypoglycemia. Four-vessel angiography or MRA is necessary to diagnose vertebral-basilar disease. Holter monitoring will be useful to diagnose complete heart block and other cardiac arrhythmias. If the chest x-ray or EKG has revealed possible cardiac findings, a referral to a cardiologist would be wise.

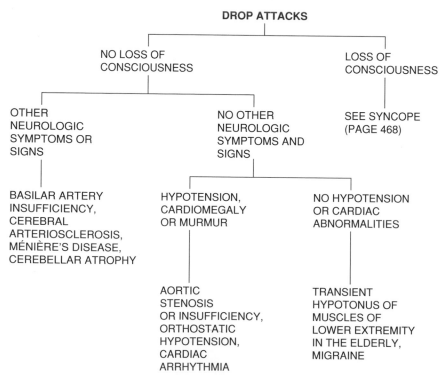

DWARFISM

ASK THE FOLLOWING QUESTIONS:

1. **Is there disproportion of the trunk and extremities?** These findings would suggest achondrodysplasia.
2. **Is there obesity?** The finding of obesity would suggest Fröhlich's syndrome, Laurence–Moon–Bardet–Biedl syndrome, and Brissaud's infantilism.
3. **Is there appearance of wasting and/or malnutrition?** The presence of wasting or other signs of malnutrition suggests chronic nephritis, congenital heart disease, progeria, malnutrition, and rickets.
4. **Is there an unusual appearance to the skull or face?** These findings suggest mongolism, cretinism, microcephaly, hydrocephalus, and cleidocranial dysostosis, among other conditions.
5. **Are there abnormal secondary sex characteristics?** The development of secondary sex characteristics is impaired in Turner's syndrome and pituitary dwarfism.

DIAGNOSTIC WORKUP

Routine studies should include a CBC, sedimentation rate, urinalysis, chemistry panel, thyroid profile, VDRL test, quantitative stool fat, a sweat test, and x-rays of the skull and long bones.

If Turner's syndrome is suspected, a buccal smear for sex chromogen may be done. If pituitary dwarfism is suspected, a CT scan of the skull may be helpful. Hypothyroidism can be distinguished by a delayed bone age. Additional endocrine tests include a serum growth hormone level before and after exercise, a resting somatomedin-C level, and an overnight dexamethasone suppression test. In patients suspected of having rickets and hypoparathyroidism, 24-hr urine calcium test may be done. However, it is best to consult a pediatrician, endocrinologist, or orthopedic surgeon before proceeding with expensive diagnostic tests.

DWARFISM

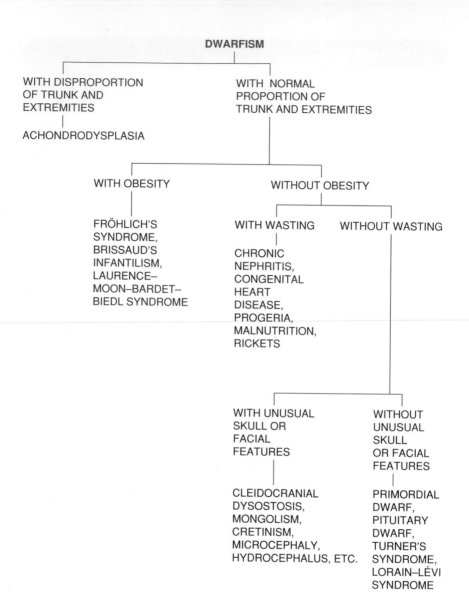

WITH DISPROPORTION OF TRUNK AND EXTREMITIES

ACHONDRODYSPLASIA

WITH NORMAL PROPORTION OF TRUNK AND EXTREMITIES

WITH OBESITY

FRÖHLICH'S SYNDROME, BRISSAUD'S INFANTILISM, LAURENCE–MOON–BARDET–BIEDL SYNDROME

WITHOUT OBESITY

WITH WASTING

CHRONIC NEPHRITIS, CONGENITAL HEART DISEASE, PROGERIA, MALNUTRITION, RICKETS

WITHOUT WASTING

WITH UNUSUAL SKULL OR FACIAL FEATURES

CLEIDOCRANIAL DYSOSTOSIS, MONGOLISM, CRETINISM, MICROCEPHALY, HYDROCEPHALUS, ETC.

WITHOUT UNUSUAL SKULL OR FACIAL FEATURES

PRIMORDIAL DWARF, PITUITARY DWARF, TURNER'S SYNDROME, LORAIN–LÉVI SYNDROME

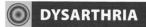

ASK THE FOLLOWING QUESTIONS:

1. **Is it intermittent?** Intermittent dysarthria should make one think of myasthenia gravis, epilepsy, and transient ischemic attacks.
2. **Is there associated ataxia or nystagmus?** The findings of nystagmus or ataxia should make one think of a cerebellar disorder such as multiple sclerosis, drug intoxication, or cerebellar ataxia.
3. **Is there a history of drug or alcohol ingestion?** Alcohol and phenytoin (Dilantin®) are just two of the toxic substances that may affect speech.
4. **Is there tremor or rigidity?** If there is tremor or rigidity, one should suspect Parkinson's disease, hepatolenticular degeneration, and phenothiazine toxicity.

DIAGNOSTIC WORKUP

The yield for diagnoses of dysarthria is high for a blood alcohol level and urine drug screen. If the dysarthria is intermittent, an EEG and Tensilon test or acetylcholine receptor antibody titer should be done. If transient ischemic attacks are suspected, a carotid scan should be done, but the only way to completely exclude this possibility is by doing four-vessel cerebral angiography. A CT scan or MRI should be done in all cases of persistent dysarthria. A neurologist can help decide which study would be most appropriate. If Wilson's disease is suspected, a test for serum copper and ceruloplasmin should be done. A spinal tap may help diagnose multiple sclerosis and intracranial hemorrhage.

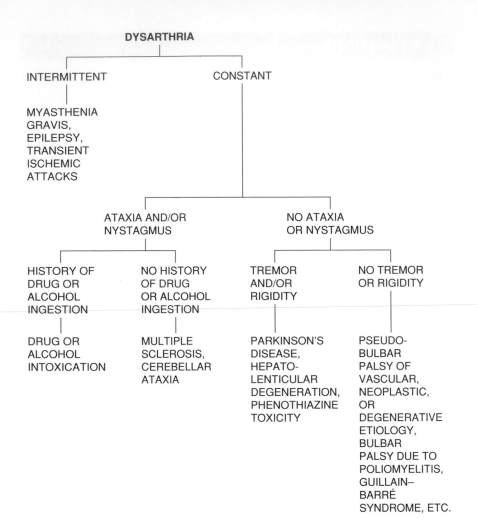

DYSARTHRIA

INTERMITTENT

CONSTANT

MYASTHENIA
GRAVIS,
EPILEPSY,
TRANSIENT
ISCHEMIC
ATTACKS

ATAXIA AND/OR
NYSTAGMUS

NO ATAXIA
OR NYSTAGMUS

HISTORY OF
DRUG OR
ALCOHOL
INGESTION

NO HISTORY
OF DRUG
OR ALCOHOL
INGESTION

TREMOR
AND/OR
RIGIDITY

NO TREMOR
OR RIGIDITY

DRUG OR
ALCOHOL
INTOXICATION

MULTIPLE
SCLEROSIS,
CEREBELLAR
ATAXIA

PARKINSON'S
DISEASE,
HEPATO-
LENTICULAR
DEGENERATION,
PHENOTHIAZINE
TOXICITY

PSEUDO-
BULBAR
PALSY OF
VASCULAR,
NEOPLASTIC,
OR
DEGENERATIVE
ETIOLOGY,
BULBAR
PALSY DUE TO
POLIOMYELITIS,
GUILLAIN–
BARRÉ
SYNDROME, ETC.

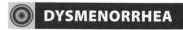 **DYSMENORRHEA**

ASK THE FOLLOWING QUESTIONS:

1. **Are there abnormalities on pelvic examination?** A tubo-ovarian mass on pelvic examination should suggest salpingo-oophoritis, endometriosis with a chocolate cyst, or ectopic pregnancy. Perhaps the uterus is abnormal, in which case one should suspect fibroids, endometrial carcinoma, uterine pregnancy, retroverted uterus, endometrial cast, or cervical polyp. A normal examination should suggest ovarian dysfunction, endocrine imbalance, and psychogenic causes.
2. **What is the age of the patient?** If the patient is young, she probably has a virginal uterus and may be considered to have primary dysmenorrhea. These cases are usually due to uterine hypoplasia, congenital malformations, ovarian dysfunction, or psychogenic causes.
3. **Does the patient have an IUD?** This may be the cause.

DIAGNOSTIC WORKUP

Routine studies should include a CBC, sedimentation rate, chemistry panel, and thyroid profile. If there is vaginal discharge, a smear and culture should be done for gonorrhea and chlamydia. A cervical and rectal culture for these organisms may also be necessary. If there is a tubo-ovarian mass or enlarged uterus, abdominal ultrasound or a CT scan of the abdomen may help in differentiating the cause. A pregnancy test should be done. The pregnancy test of choice is radioimmunoassay for the beta subunit of human chorionic gonadotropin (HCG), which will be positive within a week of fertilization. If a ruptured ectopic pregnancy is expected, a peritoneal tap or culdocentesis may help if abdominal ultrasound is not conclusive. Laparoscopy may also be helpful in the diagnosis. A fern test and basal body temperature may help diagnose endometriosis. An exploratory laparotomy may be the only way to make a diagnosis in cases of a pelvic mass. If the pelvic examination is perfectly normal, sometimes a course of progesterone hormones is useful in alleviating the problem. A dilation and curettage may also be done to address the problem. Referral to a gynecologist is usually made before doing expensive diagnostic tests.

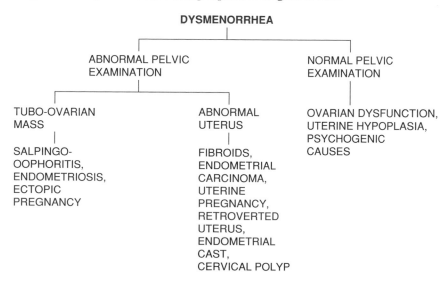

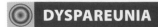

ASK THE FOLLOWING QUESTIONS:

1. **Does the history indicate that the difficulty is on penetration?** Difficulties on penetration usually point to a vulval or vaginal origin for the problem. In that case, bartholinitis, vulvitis, vulval dystrophy, cystitis, urethritis, and urethral caruncle should be suspected.
2. **Is the urinalysis abnormal?** An abnormal urinalysis may indicate cystitis or a bladder calculus.
3. **Are there abnormalities on rectal examination?** Hemorrhoids, anal fissures, and impacted feces may cause dyspareunia.
4. **Is the pelvic examination totally normal?** If this is true, one would consider functional dyspareunia, or it may be that the patient does not have dyspareunia at all and simply has no sexual desire or dislikes the sexual act.

DIAGNOSTIC WORKUP

It is extremely important to look for evidence of sexual abuse both on history and physical examination before undertaking an expensive workup. Routine studies include a CBC, sedimentation rate, urinalysis, urine culture and sensitivity, and vaginal smear and culture. A Pap smear should also be done. If pregnancy is suspected, a pregnancy test should be done. If there is a pelvic mass, pelvic ultrasound may be helpful. A referral to a gynecologist is usually made before ordering this study, however. If vulval dystrophy is suspected, a vaginal biopsy may be useful. If the vaginal examination is normal, perhaps a psychiatrist should be consulted.

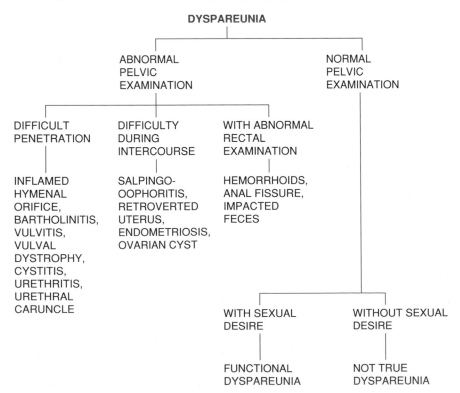

ASK THE FOLLOWING QUESTIONS:

1. **Are there abnormalities on oropharyngeal examination?** If so, then of course the cause may be local. This is particularly true if there are painful ulcerations of the mouth, glossitis, or tonsillitis. There may be neoplasms in the oropharynx or larynx that may be either obstructing swallowing or causing pain on swallowing.
2. **Is the dysphagia constant or intermittent?** Intermittent dysphagia would make one think of myasthenia gravis, and if there are other neurologic findings to suggest that, it would be the most likely working diagnosis. Without neurologic findings, a Schatzki ring may be present.
3. **Does the patient have difficulty swallowing both liquids and solids or only solids?** If the patient has difficulty with both liquids and solids, a diagnosis of achalasia, scleroderma, or diffuse esophageal spasm should be entertained. Patients who have difficulty swallowing solids only usually should be considered to have esophageal carcinoma until proven otherwise.
4. **Is heartburn present?** If there is heartburn as well as dysphagia, a diagnosis of reflux esophagitis with or without hiatal hernia should be entertained. Many conditions, including achalasia, diffuse esophageal spasm, and even advanced esophageal carcinoma, may be associated with pain on swallowing or chest pain.
5. **Is the patient male or female?** Dysphagia in a male is suggestive of esophageal carcinoma; this would be especially true with a history of significant smoking and drinking. Dysphagia in a female would suggest esophageal web, as in Plummer–Vinson syndrome.
6. **Is there significant weight loss?** Significant weight loss is very often associated with esophageal carcinoma, but not until it is advanced to a significant degree. One often forgets that weight loss is also associated with achalasia.
7. **Is there a history of syphilis?** Obviously, this would suggest an aortic aneurysm, and in considering aortic aneurysm, one should also consider other mediastinal masses that might be associated with this condition.
8. **Are there dermatologic signs and symptoms?** This would bring up the possibility of scleroderma.

DIAGNOSTIC WORKUP

In a patient with definite dysphagia, it is wise to consult a gastroenterologist at the outset! The most useful diagnostic test (and most inexpensive) is the barium swallow, and an upper GI series might be done as well. The barium swallow will often display fairly definitive features of carcinoma of the esophagus, esophageal diverticulum, achalasia, hiatal hernia, and esophagitis. The barium swallow, however, must be frequently followed by esophagoscopy to obtain a more definitive diagnosis and a tissue biopsy, particularly in the case of carcinoma of the esophagus. If both of these tests are negative, the possibility of myasthenia gravis should be considered, and a Tensilon test should be done. Esophageal manometry may detect achalasia or diffuse esophageal spasm. When a mediastinal mass is suspected, a CT scan of the mediastinum should be done. When all testing is negative, hysteria should be considered. Ultrasonography can be used to diagnose abnormal movements of the tongue and larynx. Videofluoroscopy is also useful in diagnosing oropharyngeal causes. Reflux esophagitis can be diagnosed with ambulatory pH monitoring. A therapeutic trial of a proton-pump inhibitor may be useful.

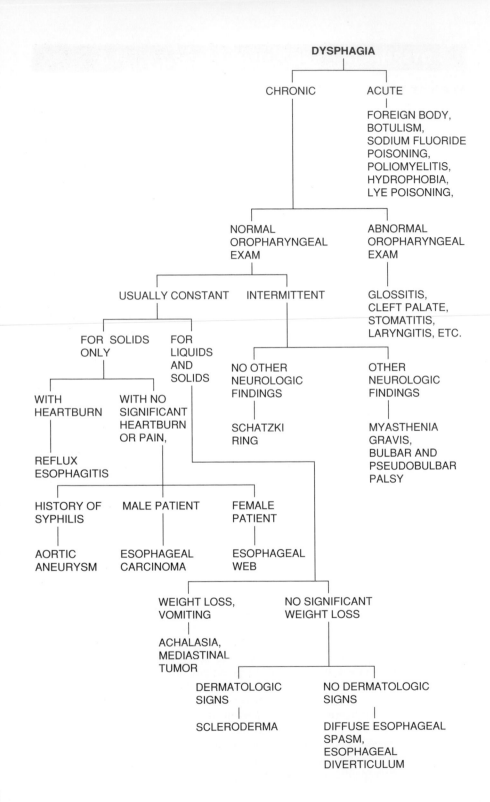

ASK THE FOLLOWING QUESTIONS:

1. **Is the dyspnea acute?** If the dyspnea is acute onset, one should ask if there is a drug history, particularly a history of mainlining narcotics. If so, adult respiratory distress syndrome should be considered. Furthermore, is there an embolic source for a possible pulmonary embolism? If the onset is gradual, one should move on to consider chronic diseases such as congestive heart failure and pulmonary emphysema and fibrosis. Exposure to heavy metals such as cadmium or mercury can cause severe lung damage, while bleach and phosphoric acid can cause ARDS.

2. **Is there fever or purulent sputum?** Obviously, fever and purulent sputum should make one think of pneumonia.

3. **What kind of rales are there?** If there are crepitant rales, one should consider congestive heart failure or pneumonia. If there are sibilant and sonorous rales or wheezing, one should consider bronchial asthma or pulmonary emphysema.

4. **Is there hepatomegaly?** Hepatomegaly would be a sign of congestive heart failure. However, in the acute stages it may not manifest immediately. Hepatomegaly may also be an indication of other systemic diseases that are associated with either lung disease or heart disease. The collagen diseases, in particular, come to mind.

5. **Is there an abnormal neurologic examination?** Look for myasthenia gravis and muscular dystrophy.

DIAGNOSTIC WORKUP

The basic workup of acute onset dyspnea should include a CBC to exclude anemia; a chest x-ray and arterial blood gases to exclude pneumothorax, pneumonia, and other pulmonic diseases; and an EKG and serial cardiac enzymes to exclude myocardial infarction and some of the causes of congestive heart failure. A sputum smear and culture should always be done when there is adequate sputum. Eosinophils should be sought. It is important to make sure that you have an adequate specimen and, therefore, leukocytes should be reported on the smear.

If there is chest pain accompanied by hemoptysis, a D-dimer, arterial blood gases and a ventilation–perfusion scan or spiral CT of the chest should be done to rule out pulmonary embolism. Even without chest pain and hemoptysis, a pulmonary embolism may need to be excluded. If the ventilation–perfusion scan is inconclusive, a pulmonary angiography may still need to be done in difficult cases. Look for an embolic source in the extremities or pelvis. If routine smears and cultures are negative, cultures for AFB and fungi may need to be done, especially when there is continuing purulent sputum. The clinician should also consider doing skin testing for these diseases.

If congestive heart failure is suspected, an arm-to-tongue circulation time, BNP and pulmonary function testing should also be done. Echocardiography may also be diagnostic. A therapeutic trial of a diuretic may be valuable. When there is significant wheezing, a trial of epinephrine 0.3 cc subcutaneously may clear up the confusion. If ARDS is suspected, look for sepsis from an abdominal source or IV drug abuse.

In chronic dyspnea, the chest x-ray and EKG should be complemented by pulmonary function testing, exercise testing, and arterial blood gases. Pulmonary function testing will be very useful in diagnosing asthma and distinguishing pulmonary emphysema from pulmonary fibrosis. A diagnosis of pulmonary fibrosis is substantiated by a reduction in a single-breath carbon monoxide–diffusing capacity. The advice of a pulmonologist should be sought when extensive pulmonary function testing, such as compliance and diffusing capacity, needs to be determined. Bronchoscopy may need to be done to exclude a foreign body, neoplasm, or bronchiectasis. Cardiac catheterization and pulmonary angiography may be needed to identify chronic recurrent pulmonary embolism, intracardiac shunts, and pulmonary hypertension. Dyspnea without objective findings on physical examination should prompt a referral to a psychiatrist.

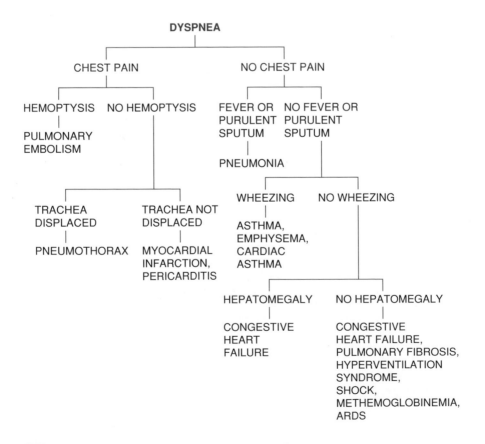

DYSURIA

ASK THE FOLLOWING QUESTIONS:

1. **Is there fever?** A significant fever would suggest either pyelonephritis, particularly in females, or acute prostatitis in males.

2. **Is the urine grossly bloody or are there a significant number of red cells on microscopic examination?** Grossly bloody urine in a young female should suggest acute cystitis, particularly if she has just returned from a honeymoon. In older patients it may indicate bladder carcinoma, but generally these patients have blood in their urine before they develop dysuria. Really significant blood in the urine may also indicate schistosomiasis or tuberculous cystitis. Dysuria and hematuria can occur in renal or vesicular calculi as well.

3. **Is there a urethral or vaginal discharge?** If either of these signs is present, one must consider that the patient may have gonorrhea until proven otherwise. Repeated negative smears and cultures for gonococcus should suggest that the patient may have female urethral syndrome or nonspecific urethritis due to chlamydia.

4. **Are there systemic symptoms?** If there are systemic symptoms, one must consider the possibility of Reiter's syndrome or collagen disease. One should not forget that systemic symptoms of arthritis and rash may also be present in gonorrhea.

5. **Is the pain very severe?** Severe pain, particularly a need to stay close to the restroom so one can empty one's bladder, may indicate tabes dorsalis, although this condition is rarely seen today.

DIAGNOSTIC WORKUP

Obviously, a urinalysis and Gram stain of the unspun urine should be done in all cases. If this is positive, treatment can be initiated. Urine cultures are only necessary for resistant or repeated episodes. I also recommend a urethral smear and a vaginal smear and culture if sufficient material can be obtained. This may mean massaging the prostate for an adequate specimen. Even four white cells per high-powered field on a urethral smear probably indicate urethritis. Cultures for both gonorrhea and chlamydia should be done. DNA probe testing has become a useful tool in detecting Chlamydia and Gonorrhea. In persistent cases of dysuria, a helical CT scan, ultrasonography, and a cystoscopy must be done. In children a voiding cystogram is essential. A urologist needs to be consulted before ordering these tests. Blood cultures should be done in cases of acute pyelonephritis. Cultures for anaerobic bacilli and tuberculosis may be necessary in persistent pyuria. It should go without saying that a rectal and vaginal examination should be done in all cases. However, this is frequently neglected. A therapeutic trial of antibiotics is useful. In particular, a course of ciprofloxacin is useful in diagnosing prostatitis.

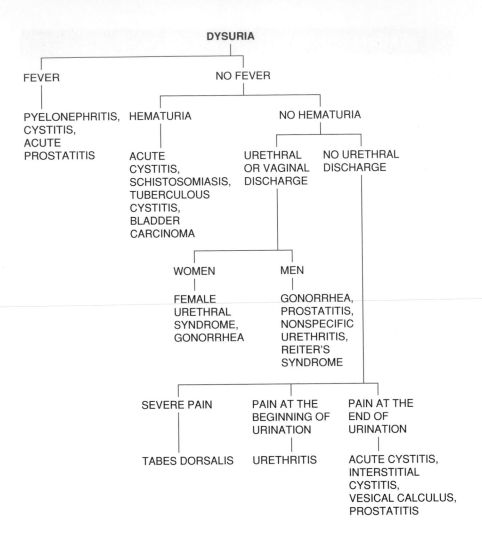

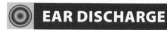

ASK THE FOLLOWING QUESTIONS:

1. **Is it acute?** Acute ear discharge suggests acute otitis media with rupture or an otitis externa, especially if it is painful. If the patient is diabetic, look for malignant otitis externa from a pseudomonas infection. A chronic discharge would suggest cholesteatoma, chronic otitis media, and possibly cerebrospinal fluid.

2. **Is it painful?** A painful ear with a discharge is most likely acute otitis media with rupture. It may, however, be due to otitis externa, a foreign body, or serous otitis media.

3. **Is there associated fever?** An ear discharge with fever suggests otitis media, mastoiditis, and petrositis.

4. **What is the character of the discharge?** A mucopurulent discharge suggests chronic otitis media and mastoiditis, whereas a fetid discharge with whitish debris suggests a cholesteatoma. If the discharge is clear, a cerebrospinal fluid otorrhea should be suspected.

DIAGNOSTIC WORKUP

The most important test to do is a smear, culture, and sensitivity of the discharge. If there is fever, a CBC, sedimentation rate, and chemistry panel should be done. The ears should be examined after thorough irrigation. X-rays of the mastoids and petrous bones should be done if a deep source for the discharge is suspected. Audiograms are helpful if there is hearing loss. If the discharge is thought to be cerebrospinal fluid, a RISA study and CT scan of the brain may need to be done. An ear, nose, and throat specialist should be consulted before ordering expensive diagnostic tests.

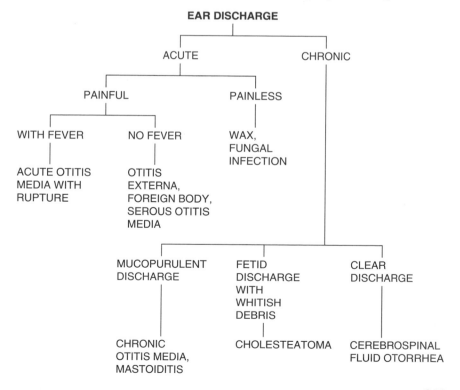

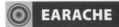

ASK THE FOLLOWING QUESTIONS:

1. **Are there abnormalities on the ear examination?** The ear examination may reveal severe otitis externa, an epithelioma of the pinna, a foreign body, or impacted wax. It may also show inflammation and bulging of the eardrum. Be sure to do pneumatic otoscopy for drum mobility. A vesicular rash of the drum and external auditory canal may indicate herpes zoster.

2. **Is there pain on moving the pinna?** Pain on moving the ear suggests otitis externa, foreign body, impacted wax, or keratosis obturans.

3. **Is there hearing loss?** Hearing loss with an abnormal drum would suggest serous or bacterial otitis media. It may also suggest a cholesteatoma. Hearing loss with a normal ear examination suggests aero-otitis.

4. **Could the pain be a referred pain?** Dental caries, dental abscesses, impacted teeth, tonsillitis, and temporomandibular joint syndrome may refer pain to the ear.

DIAGNOSTIC WORKUP

It should go without saying that diagnosis begins with an adequate otoscopic examination. If the drum is obscured by wax, gentle lavage after using Debrox® will usually clear the canal. If there is an exudate, a culture and sensitivity should be ordered. Perhaps a throat culture should be done also. X-rays of the mastoids and petrous bones should be done if the exudate is believed to be from a deeper source. Perhaps a CT scan is also needed. If there is hearing loss, an audiogram needs to be done and a tympanogram will be useful in diagnosing serous otitis media. A trial of carbamazepine (Tegretol®) or phenytoin (Dilantin®) may be useful in diagnosing glossopharyngeal neuralgia or tic douloureux. In children, a trial of antibiotics may be worthwhile especially if the drum is not visualized. If the discharge is thought to be cerebrospinal fluid, a CT scan and RISA study should be done.

Referral to an ear, nose, and throat specialist or neurologist should be considered before ordering expensive diagnostic tests.

EARACHE

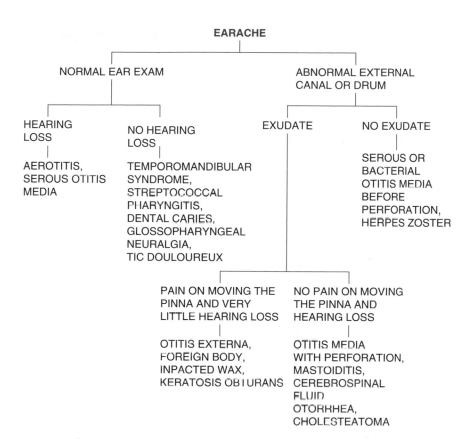

NORMAL EAR EXAM

- **HEARING LOSS**

  AEROTITIS, SEROUS OTITIS MEDIA

- **NO HEARING LOSS**

  TEMPOROMANDIBULAR SYNDROME, STREPTOCOCCAL PHARYNGITIS, DENTAL CARIES, GLOSSOPHARYNGEAL NEURALGIA, TIC DOULOUREUX

ABNORMAL EXTERNAL CANAL OR DRUM

- **EXUDATE**

  - **PAIN ON MOVING THE PINNA AND VERY LITTLE HEARING LOSS**

    OTITIS EXTERNA, FOREIGN BODY, INPACTED WAX, KERATOSIS OBTURANS

  - **NO PAIN ON MOVING THE PINNA AND HEARING LOSS**

    OTITIS MEDIA WITH PERFORATION, MASTOIDITIS, CEREBROSPINAL FLUID OTORRHEA, CHOLESTEATOMA

- **NO EXUDATE**

  SEROUS OR BACTERIAL OTITIS MEDIA BEFORE PERFORATION, HERPES ZOSTER

ASK THE FOLLOWING QUESTIONS:

1. **Does the edema pit on pressure?** Edema that pits on pressure is more likely to be due to heart, liver, or kidney disease. Edema that does not pit on pressure is more likely due to myxedema or lymphedema.
2. **Is there hepatomegaly?** If there is hepatomegaly, one should consider liver disease such as cirrhosis or cardiac disease.
3. **Is there ascites?** If there is ascites along with hepatomegaly, cirrhosis of the liver is the most likely cause of the edema. However, one should not forget constrictive pericarditis. If there is no ascites along with the hepatomegaly, then congestive heart failure should be considered.
4. **Is there jugular vein distention?** Jugular vein distention certainly would be most suggestive of congestive heart failure, but other causes of jugular vein distention include superior vena cava syndrome due to a mediastinal mass such as carcinoma of the lung and constrictive pericarditis. Right heart failure secondary to pulmonary emphysema and fibrosis can also cause jugular vein distention.
5. **Is there an abnormal urinary sediment?** If there is an abnormal urinary sediment, consider nephritis, whether it might be due to chronic glomerulonephritis or whether it is secondary to diabetes mellitus or a collagen disease.
6. **Is the patient taking any drugs that could cause the edema?** Among the drugs that should be considered are corticosteroids, progesterone, estrogen, anti-inflammatory drugs such as naproxen (Naprosyn®) and ibuprofen (Motrin®), antihypertensive drugs such as methyldopa (Aldomet®) and clonidine hydrochloride, calcium channel blockers, beta-adrenergic blockers, and antidepressants.

DIAGNOSTIC WORKUP

A CBC should be done to rule out significant anemia that may be the cause of the edema. If there is anemia, we need to determine its source (page 28). Liver function tests are done to rule out liver disease, and serum protein electrophoresis and tests for BUN and creatinine should be done to exclude renal disease. The urinalysis is very important both for the routine studies and also to examine the urinary sediment for diseases such as chronic glomerulonephritis and collagen disease. If there is significant loss of protein in the urine, one should be considering nephrosis. An EKG, chest x-ray, brain natriuretic peptide (BNP), and venous pressure and circulation time will be extremely helpful in diagnosing congestive heart failure, but pulmonary function tests can be done as the vital capacity is significantly reduced in this disease. When there is a strong suspicion of congestive heart failure, echocardiography or radionuclide-gated blood pool scintigraphy should be done to determine the left ventricular ejection fraction (LVEF). A value of less than 45% is considered abnormal. A thyroid profile should be done to diagnose myxedema. A CT scan of the chest will help diagnose constrictive pericarditis. Occasionally, the edema is due to an abdominal tumor. A CT scan of the abdomen and pelvis will be helpful in those cases. Contrast lymphangiography may be necessary to diagnose lymphedema.

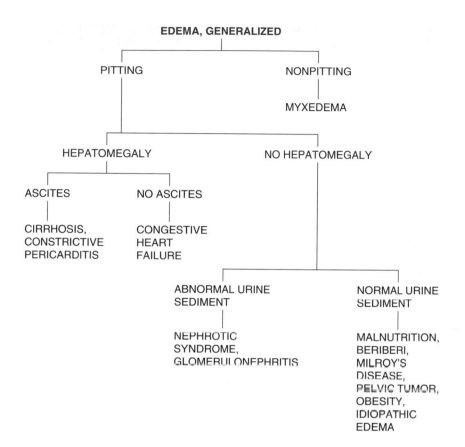

EDEMA, LOCALIZED

ASK THE FOLLOWING QUESTIONS:

1. **Is the edema acute or chronic?** Acute edema, if it is localized, should always bring to mind a deep vein thrombophlebitis. Look for a Baker's cyst obstructing the vein. It also should bring to mind acute lymphangitis, particularly if there is erythema in the area. Finally, it should also make one think of trauma or a focal infection such as cellulitis. Chronic localized edema, on the other hand, is more likely related to varicose veins or lymphedema.

2. **Is the edema pitting or nonpitting?** If the edema pits, it is more likely related to inflammation or venous incompetence. If it is nonpitting, it is more likely due to obstruction of the lymphatics, i.e., lymphedema.

3. **Is there erythema, a rash, or focal tenderness, or all three?** Erythema and focal tenderness would suggest cellulitis, lymphangitis, thrombophlebitis, angioneurotic edema, insect bite, or snake bite. It also would suggest a sprain or contusion. Focal tenderness alone with pitting edema and no significant erythema or rash would suggest a deep vein thrombophlebitis. When there is no erythema or tenderness in a case of pitting edema of a localized nature, one should consider varicose veins or, in the lower extremities, a popliteal cyst that might be obstructing the veins on a chronic basis.

4. **If the edema is of the lower extremities, is there a positive Homans' sign?** A positive Homans' sign should always be looked for because this would suggest a deep vein thrombophlebitis. Action must be taken immediately in such cases.

DIAGNOSTIC WORKUP

A venous ultrasound study, impedance plethysmography, and contrast venography are very useful in the diagnosis of deep vein thrombophlebitis. D-dimer testing is also a sensitive indicator of active deep vein thrombophlebitis and the need for anticoagulants. If a pelvic vein thrombosis is suspected, it is wise to do an MRI of the pelvis, diagnosing osteomyelitis and fractures. Lymphangiography will be helpful in the diagnosis of carcinomatosis or lymphedema from other causes. A CT scan of the abdomen or pelvis may also demonstrate the malignant lymph nodes. A thyroid profile will diagnose cases of pretibial myxedema due to thyrotoxicosis. Patients with upper extremity edema should have a chest x-ray and CT scan of the mediastinum to determine the causes of superior vena cava syndrome.

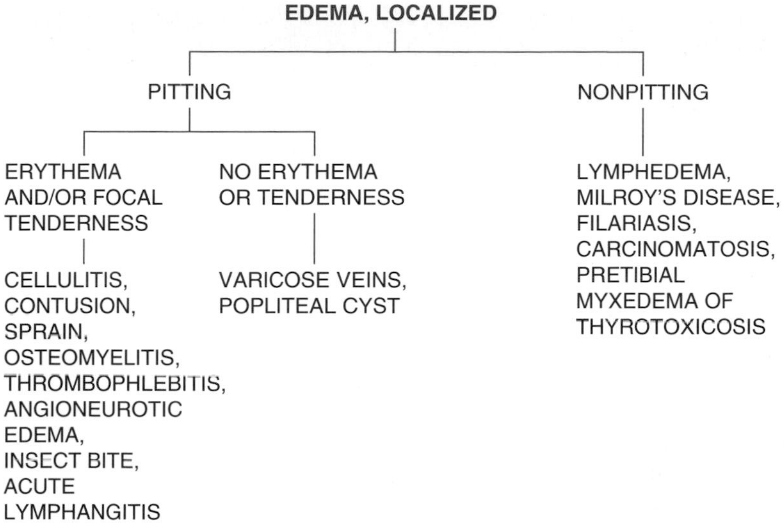

EDEMA, LOCALIZED

PITTING

ERYTHEMA AND/OR FOCAL TENDERNESS

CELLULITIS,
CONTUSION,
SPRAIN,
OSTEOMYELITIS,
THROMBOPHLEBITIS,
ANGIONEUROTIC
EDEMA,
INSECT BITE,
ACUTE
LYMPHANGITIS

NO ERYTHEMA OR TENDERNESS

VARICOSE VEINS,
POPLITEAL CYST

NONPITTING

LYMPHEDEMA,
MILROY'S DISEASE,
FILARIASIS,
CARCINOMATOSIS,
PRETIBIAL
MYXEDEMA OF
THYROTOXICOSIS

ENOPHTHALMOS

If the condition is unilateral, it is almost always due to paralysis of the cervical sympathetic ganglion and part of Horner's syndrome. Horner's syndrome includes enophthalmos, partial ptosis, constricted pupil, absence of sweating, and the presence of blushing on the side of the sympathetic paralysis. The various causes of Horner's syndrome can be found on page 237. Prolonged endophthalmitis may cause unilateral enophthalmos due to shrinkage of the eyeball.

Bilateral enophthalmos may be due to starvation or cachexia (in which case the cause should be obvious) or congenital.

ASK THE FOLLOWING QUESTIONS:

1. **Is the bed-wetting frequent or only occasional?** Frequent bed-wetting should signify pathology in the urogenital tract or endocrine system. If the bed-wetting is infrequent, one should consider epilepsy.

2. **Are there abnormalities found on the urogenital examination?** There are many causes of enuresis that can be found on a simple examination, such as phimosis, balanitis, meatal stricture, vulvitis, or intestinal worms.

3. **Are there abnormalities on the urinalysis?** Urinalysis alone is usually not adequate, and a urine culture should be done to rule out cystitis and pyelone-phritis. The simple examination of the urine sediment for bacteria is also helpful. Sugar in the urine may indicate diabetes mellitus, but it may also indicate Fanconi's syndrome.

4. **Is there polyuria?** Polyuria might indicate diabetes insipidus, diabetes mellitus, hyperthyroidism, and hypoparathyroidism.

5. **Are there abnormalities on the neurologic examination?** Here one would be looking for cerebral palsy and congenital anomalies of the spinal cord.

Finally, if the neurologic examination, urogenital examination, and urinalysis are normal, perhaps the patient has a simple neurosis or situational maladjustment.

DIAGNOSTIC WORKUP

Patients who are suspected of having a urologic condition as the cause of their enuresis should have a urinalysis, intravenous pyelogram, and voiding cystogram with a urine culture and colony count. Referral to a urologist for cystometric testing may be required. If there is polyuria, a glucose tolerance test, a thyroid profile, and tests for calcium, phosphorus, alkaline phosphatase, and parathyroid hormone level should be done. If epilepsy is suspected, an EEG should be ordered. If the neurologic examination is abnormal, referral to a neurologic specialist would be in order. If all the studies and examinations are within normal limits, a referral to a psychiatrist or psychologist may be in order. However, the child may have simple enuresis, in which case all that is required is to reassure the parents that the child will grow out of it by puberty. Enuresis that develops after a substantial period of dryness may indicate sexual abuse.

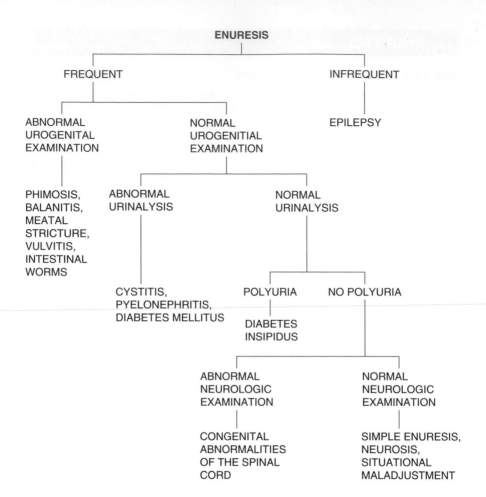

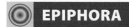

ASK THE FOLLOWING QUESTIONS:

1. **Is the epiphora unilateral or bilateral?** If it is bilateral, it is most likely due to emotional weeping or due to the effects of drugs such as bromides, arsenic, and mercury.
2. **Is the eye examination normal?** If the eye examination is abnormal, there are most likely obvious findings of conjunctivitis, foreign bodies, corneal ulcer, or other problems. A foreign body may be difficult to find, as may a corneal ulcer, and referral to an ophthalmologist would be in order. In any event, the conjunctiva will be red and inflamed. In addition, there may be lid problems, particularly in the elderly, and these may constitute ectropion or entropion. There is also the possibility of Bell's palsy causing incomplete closure of the eye, and therefore the eye will be chronically inflamed from constant exposure to air.

If the eye examination is normal, one must consider the possibility of obstruction of the nasolacrimal duct either due to trauma, congenital causes, a calculus, neoplasm, or due to dacryocystitis. Crocodile tears may occur when, due to aberrant nerve regeneration following facial paralysis, the lacrimal gland is stimulated to produce excessive tears while eating.

DIAGNOSTIC WORKUP

The first thing to do if the epiphora is bilateral is to determine if the patient has been on any particular drugs or has emotional problems. If the eye examination is abnormal or there are problems with the lids, referral to an ophthalmologist is in order. Even if the eye examination is normal, the referral to an ophthalmologist would be necessary to determine if obstruction of the nasolacrimal duct is the problem.

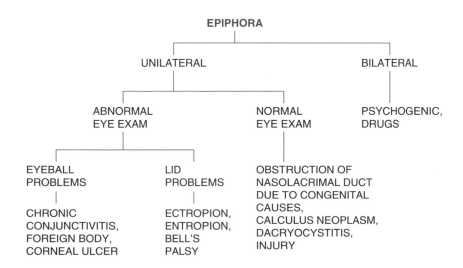

ASK THE FOLLOWING QUESTIONS:

1. **Is there hypertension?** The patient with hypertension could have either essential or symptomatic hypertension. Be sure to recheck the blood pressure, as other health professionals may miss the auscultatory gap. Next, treat the hypertension and examine the patient for symptomatic hypertension later (page 248).

2. **Is the bleeding from Little's area or is it farther up the nasal passageway?** Ninety percent of epistaxis results from bleeding in Little's area (Kiesselbach's plexus), and this area is most easily controlled. Be sure to ask about the use of cocaine or nasal sprays. Bleeding from this area is usually not a serious problem. However, when the bleeding is from the posterior nasal areas, one must always consider the possibility of carcinoma.

3. **Is there a history or are there clinical signs of a coagulation disorder?** There may be a history of hemophilia or leukemia. There may be splenomegaly. There may be bleeding sites elsewhere to indicate that there is a systemic disorder associated with the epistaxis. One can easily perform a Rumpel–Leede test to determine if there is a platelet deficiency or dysfunction.

4. **What drugs is the patient on?** Aspirin, warfarin sodium, and numerous other drugs can cause epistaxis.

DIAGNOSTIC WORKUP

The diagnostic workup of epistaxis should include a coagulation profile with prothrombin time, partial thromboplastin time (PTT), bleeding time, platelet count, Rumpel–Leede test, and CBC. If these tests suggest a coagulation disorder, referral to a hematologist can be done for further diagnostic workup.

A nasal smear should be done for eosinophils to determine if the patient has chronic allergic rhinitis.

When a carcinoma of the nasal pharynx or sinuses is suspected, x-rays of the paranasal sinuses can be done as well as nasopharyngoscopy. A CT scan of the sinuses is also of value in difficult diagnostic problems.

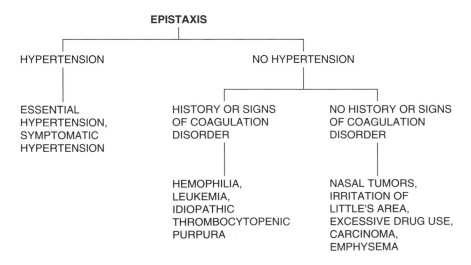

ASK THE FOLLOWING QUESTIONS:

1. **Is there a history of drug ingestion?** The patient will frequently not tell the truth about drug ingestion, but one should ask family and friends about whether the patient uses any illicit drugs such as LSD, marijuana, or cocaine. Other drugs that are prescribed by physicians may cause euphoria, such as corticosteroids and various narcotics.

2. **Is the neurologic examination abnormal?** The patient may demonstrate simple disorientation or disturbance in the thought process or excessive jocularity, as may be seen in witzelsucht. All these findings may suggest a frontal lobe tumor, a general paresis, or other forms of dementia. When there are long tract signs, such as posterior column or pyramidal tract involvement, one must consider the possibility of multiple sclerosis or a pontine glioma.

3. **Is there significant incoherence, delusions, or hallucinations?** These findings would most likely suggest schizophrenia.

4. **Is the euphoria sustained for long periods, or is it very short-lived?** If the euphoria is intermittent and very brief, one should consider temporal lobe epilepsy. If it is more sustained, one would consider manic-depressive psychosis.

DIAGNOSTIC WORKUP

A drug screen should be axiomatic on all patients, as the patient may lie. If this is negative, one may proceed with the more expensive testing, such as MRI, or at least a CT scan to rule out a brain tumor. If these tests are negative and the problem persists, the patient should be referred to a psychiatrist.

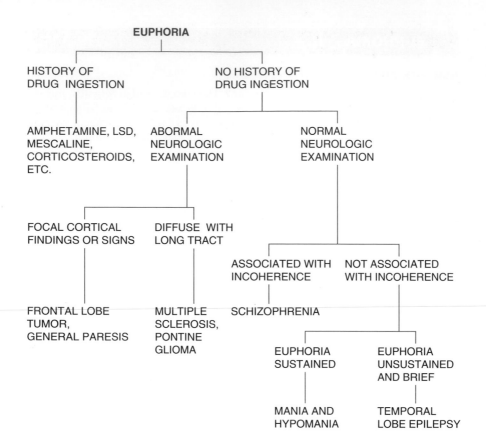

EUPHORIA

HISTORY OF
DRUG INGESTION

NO HISTORY OF
DRUG INGESTION

AMPHETAMINE, LSD,
MESCALINE,
CORTICOSTEROIDS,
ETC.

ABORMAL
NEUROLOGIC
EXAMINATION

NORMAL
NEUROLOGIC
EXAMINATION

FOCAL CORTICAL
FINDINGS OR SIGNS

DIFFUSE WITH
LONG TRACT

ASSOCIATED WITH
INCOHERENCE

NOT ASSOCIATED
WITH INCOHERENCE

FRONTAL LOBE
TUMOR,
GENERAL PARESIS

MULTIPLE
SCLEROSIS,
PONTINE
GLIOMA

SCHIZOPHRENIA

EUPHORIA
SUSTAINED

EUPHORIA
UNSUSTAINED
AND BRIEF

MANIA AND
HYPOMANIA

TEMPORAL
LOBE EPILEPSY

ASK THE FOLLOWING QUESTIONS:

1. **Is it bilateral or unilateral?** Bilateral exophthalmos would suggest hyperthyroidism. Unilateral exophthalmos suggests orbital tumor, abscess, or aneurysm.
2. **If it is bilateral, are there signs of hyperthyroidism?** If there are other indications of hyperthyroidism, Graves' disease would be the diagnosis.
3. **If it is unilateral, does the eyeball pulsate?** A pulsating eyeball would suggest an arteriovenous fistula, and there should be a loud blowing murmur over the orbit.
4. **Is there fever?** Fever would suggest acute cellulitis, acute sinusitis, periostitis, or a cavernous sinus thrombosis.
5. **Is there chemosis or ecchymosis?** These signs are suggestive of a cavernous sinus thrombosis.

DIAGNOSTIC WORKUP

In cases of bilateral exophthalmos, particularly if there is no fever or chemosis or ecchymosis, a thyroid profile is the most valuable test. Orbital MRI may also be done. However, Graves' disease may be present with normal thyroid function tests. Testing for thyrotropin receptor antibody and peroxidase antibodies should be done in these cases. Other endocrine studies may be necessary once hyperthyroidism has been excluded. In cases of unilateral exophthalmos, ultrasonography and plain films of the orbits and sinuses may be helpful, but a CT scan of the brain and sinuses is the most valuable diagnostic aid. Carotid angiography will need to be done to diagnose an arteriovenous fistula

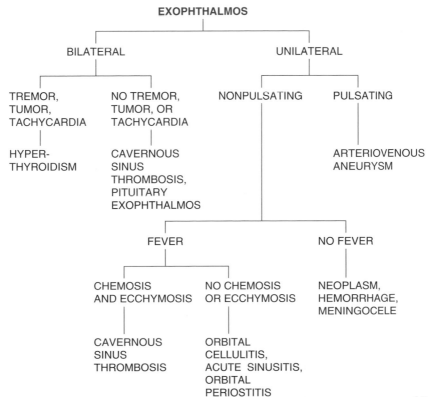

EXOPHTHALMOS

ASK THE FOLLOWING QUESTIONS:

1. **Is the extremity pain of acute or gradual onset?** Acute onset would suggest arterial embolism, deep vein thrombophlebitis, and cellulitis. If there is a history of trauma, it would suggest a fracture, sprain, or torn ligament.

2. **Is there limitation of motion of the joints?** A positive Patrick's test would indicate hip pathology, including greater trochanter bursitis. A positive McMurray test would indicate a torn meniscus.

3. **Are there positive neurologic findings?** A positive femoral stretch test would suggest a herniated disk at L2–3 or L3–4, whereas a positive Lasègue's sign would indicate a herniated disk at L4–5 or L5 to S1. Combined motor and sensory deficits may indicate radiculopathy or neuropathy.

4. **Is there a positive Homans' sign?** This is a very important examination, as one would not want to miss a deep vein thrombophlebitis.

5. **Is there diminished or absent peripheral pulses?** Diminished or absent pulses would suggest arterial embolism, peripheral arteriosclerosis, or Leriche's syndrome (thrombosis of the terminal aorta).

6. **Is there focal tenderness, swelling, or erythema of the extremity?** This would suggest cellulitis, superficial thrombophlebitis, osteomyelitis, lymphangitis, and other types of infections. Tenderness without significant swelling or erythema would be suggestive of bursitis or deep vein thrombophlebitis.

DIAGNOSTIC WORKUP

Often bursitis and myofascitis can be diagnosed by the dramatic relief obtained from a lidocaine injection. If there is clear-cut joint pathology, an x-ray of the joints, arthritis profile, and synovial fluid analysis will usually provide a diagnosis. MRI is useful in the diagnosis of a torn meniscus. If a deep vein thrombophlebitis is suspected, venous Doppler ultrasound, impedance plethysmography, or a contrast venogram may be done. Order a phospholipid antibody titer in patients with frequent episodes of thrombophlebitis. Frequently a D-dimer test will determine if thrombophlebitis is the problem. If the pelvis is suspected of being the embolic source, order an MRI. If an arterial embolism or chronic peripheral arterial disease is suspected, femoral angiography can be done. If a herniated disk or other pathology of the lumbar spine is suspected, plain films of the lumbar spine should be obtained. It might be wise at this point also to obtain a CBC, sedimentation rate, and chemistry panel to determine the alkaline phosphatase, calcium, and phosphorus. In older males, tests for acid phosphatase and PSA should be done.

If these tests are unrevealing, it is wise to refer the patient to a neurologic specialist before any more expensive tests are ordered. He will probably order a CT scan or MRI of the lumbar spine and may do nerve conduction velocity studies, EMG examinations, or dermatomal SSEP studies as indicated. In difficult neurologic problems, a combined myelography and CT scan is preferred over MRI. Bone scans will help diagnose obscure fractures and osteomyelitis, both of the lumbar spine and the lower extremities.

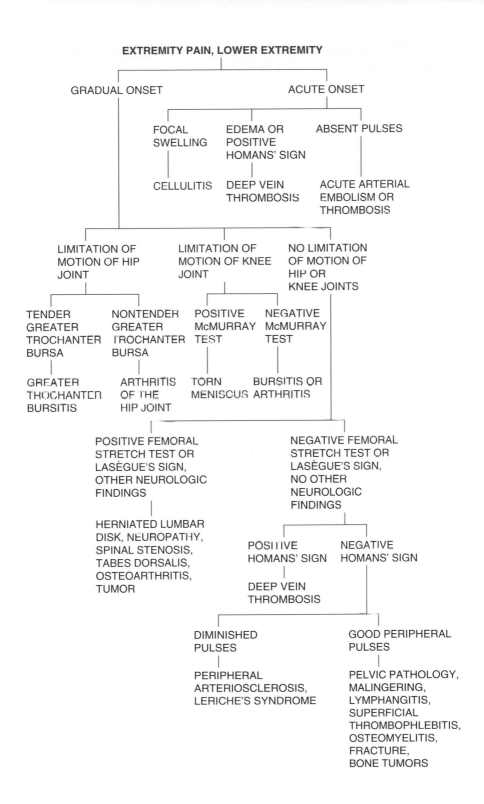

EXTREMITY PAIN, LOWER EXTREMITY

GRADUAL ONSET

ACUTE ONSET

FOCAL SWELLING

EDEMA OR POSITIVE HOMANS' SIGN

ABSENT PULSES

CELLULITIS

DEEP VEIN THROMBOSIS

ACUTE ARTERIAL EMBOLISM OR THROMBOSIS

LIMITATION OF MOTION OF HIP JOINT

LIMITATION OF MOTION OF KNEE JOINT

NO LIMITATION OF MOTION OF HIP OR KNEE JOINTS

TENDER GREATER TROCHANTER BURSA

NONTENDER GREATER TROCHANTER BURSA

POSITIVE McMURRAY TEST

NEGATIVE McMURRAY TEST

GREATER TROCHANTER BURSITIS

ARTHRITIS OF THE HIP JOINT

TORN MENISCUS

BURSITIS OR ARTHRITIS

POSITIVE FEMORAL STRETCH TEST OR LASÈGUE'S SIGN, OTHER NEUROLOGIC FINDINGS

NEGATIVE FEMORAL STRETCH TEST OR LASÈGUE'S SIGN, NO OTHER NEUROLOGIC FINDINGS

HERNIATED LUMBAR DISK, NEUROPATHY, SPINAL STENOSIS, TABES DORSALIS, OSTEOARTHRITIS, TUMOR

POSITIVE HOMANS' SIGN

NEGATIVE HOMANS' SIGN

DEEP VEIN THROMBOSIS

DIMINISHED PULSES

GOOD PERIPHERAL PULSES

PERIPHERAL ARTERIOSCLEROSIS, LERICHE'S SYNDROME

PELVIC PATHOLOGY, MALINGERING, LYMPHANGITIS, SUPERFICIAL THROMBOPHLEBITIS, OSTEOMYELITIS, FRACTURE, BONE TUMORS

ASK THE FOLLOWING QUESTIONS:

1. **Is there limitation of motion of the joints?** Limitation of motion of a joint would suggest not only various types of arthritis, fracture, or torn ligaments, but also inflammation of surrounding structures such as the bursa or tendons. For example, limitation of motion of the shoulder would suggest impingement syndrome, frozen shoulder, rheumatoid or osteoarthritis, subacromial bursitis, and a torn rotator cuff.

2. **Is the limitation of motion both active and passive, or active only?** If the limitation of motion is only active, one should suspect tendinitis or bursitis. If the limitation of motion is both active and passive, one should suspect the various forms of arthritis, as well as bone tumors, osteomyelitis, and adhesive capsulitis.

3. **Is there weakness or paresthesia?** Weakness and especially paresthesia suggest a neurologic origin for the pain, and one should be considering brachial plexus neuritis, carpal tunnel syndrome, ulnar entrapment, and radiculopathy.

4. **Are there vasomotor or trophic changes?** Vasomotor changes would suggest Raynaud's phenomena and sympathetic dystrophy. Trophic changes along with vasomotor changes would suggest a peripheral neuropathy also.

5. **Are there positive neurologic signs in the lower extremities?** Diffuse hypoactive reflexes with stocking deficits in the lower extremities would suggest a peripheral neuropathy, whereas hyperactive reflexes in the lower extremities would suggest a cervical cord tumor, cervical spondylosis, or multiple sclerosis.

6. **Is there a positive Tinel's sign at the wrist or elbow?** Tinel's sign at the wrist would suggest carpal tunnel syndrome, whereas Tinel's sign at the elbow would suggest ulnar entrapment if it is over the ulnar nerve or pronator syndrome if it is over the median nerve.

7. **Are Adson's tests positive?** Adson's tests are positive in thoracic outlet syndrome, whether it is due to a cervical rib, scalenus-anticus syndrome, Wright syndrome (pectoralis minor syndrome), or a costoclavicular compression.

DIAGNOSTIC WORKUP

X-rays of the affected joints need to be done if there is tenderness or limitation of motion. Further workup of joint pain can be found on page 289. When there are abnormal neurologic findings, an x-ray of the cervical spine (always with A-P, laterals, and obliques), nerve conduction velocity studies, and EMG examinations need to be done. Referral to a neurologist should be made for these tests. If there is a typical radicular pain and a herniated cervical disk is strongly suspected, MRI of the cervical spine should be done. This is an expensive test, but when there are obvious signs of radiculopathy, it is worthwhile. Perhaps dermatomal somatosensory studies should be done when there is confusion about whether a herniated disk is pathologic. If a vascular lesion is suspected, angiography and venography should be ordered. ANA and nailfold capillary loop dilation and dropout study may diagnose Raynaud's phenomena; a small injection of lidocaine and steroids locally may be diagnostic in cases of carpal tunnel syndrome.

When there is intermittent pain, an exercise tolerance test should be done to exclude coronary insufficiency. A stellate ganglion block may be helpful in diagnosing reflex sympathetic dystrophy. Remember that other nerve blocks may be done and one should not hesitate to call an anesthesiologist for help in this area. Various forms of bursitis may be diagnosed by a therapeutic trial of lidocaine and corticosteroid injections.

EXTREMITY PAIN, UPPER EXTREMITY

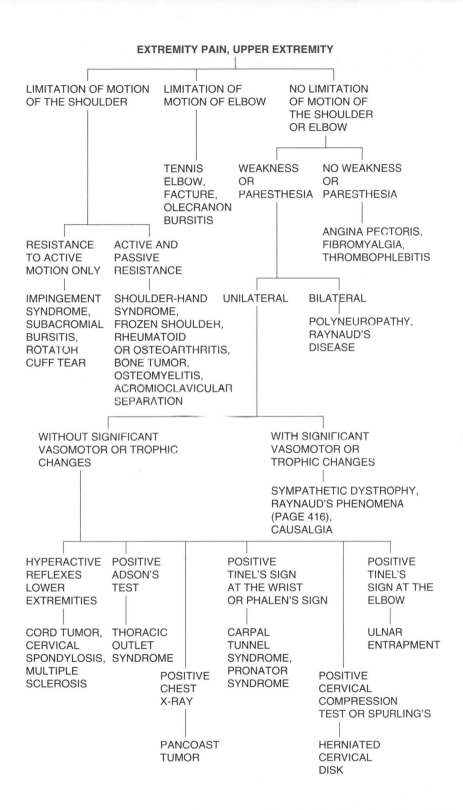

LIMITATION OF MOTION OF THE SHOULDER

LIMITATION OF MOTION OF ELBOW

NO LIMITATION OF MOTION OF THE SHOULDER OR ELBOW

TENNIS ELBOW, FACTURE, OLECRANON BURSITIS

WEAKNESS OR PARESTHESIA

NO WEAKNESS OR PARESTHESIA

ANGINA PECTORIS, FIBROMYALGIA, THROMBOPHLEBITIS

RESISTANCE TO ACTIVE MOTION ONLY

ACTIVE AND PASSIVE RESISTANCE

IMPINGEMENT SYNDROME, SUBACROMIAL BURSITIS, ROTATOR CUFF TEAR

SHOULDER-HAND SYNDROME, FROZEN SHOULDER, RHEUMATOID OR OSTEOARTHRITIS, BONE TUMOR, OSTEOMYELITIS, ACROMIOCLAVICULAR SEPARATION

UNILATERAL

BILATERAL

POLYNEUROPATHY, RAYNAUD'S DISEASE

WITHOUT SIGNIFICANT VASOMOTOR OR TROPHIC CHANGES

WITH SIGNIFICANT VASOMOTOR OR TROPHIC CHANGES

SYMPATHETIC DYSTROPHY, RAYNAUD'S PHENOMENA (PAGE 416), CAUSALGIA

HYPERACTIVE REFLEXES LOWER EXTREMITIES

POSITIVE ADSON'S TEST

POSITIVE TINEL'S SIGN AT THE WRIST OR PHALEN'S SIGN

POSITIVE TINEL'S SIGN AT THE ELBOW

CORD TUMOR, CERVICAL SPONDYLOSIS, MULTIPLE SCLEROSIS

THORACIC OUTLET SYNDROME

CARPAL TUNNEL SYNDROME, PRONATOR SYNDROME

ULNAR ENTRAPMENT

POSITIVE CHEST X-RAY

POSITIVE CERVICAL COMPRESSION TEST OR SPURLING'S

PANCOAST TUMOR

HERNIATED CERVICAL DISK

ASK THE FOLLOWING QUESTIONS:

1. **Is there redness of the eye?** Redness of the eye suggests definite eye pathology. Besides conjunctivitis and scleritis, be sure to look for closed angle glaucoma (dilated pupil) which is associated with nausea and vomiting and is a medical emergency. That is why visual acuity should always be checked. Without redness, one should suspect disease in the adjacent structures or retrobulbar neuritis. However, contact lens wearers may present with eye pain without redness, but there will be white spots on the cornea.

2. **If there is redness, is there periorbital edema as well?** Periorbital edema should suggest a cavernous sinus thrombosis or herpes zoster.

3. **If there is periorbital edema, is there a rash?** A rash, particularly vesicular rash, would suggest herpes zoster.

4. **In cases without redness of the eye, is there any abnormality on examination both with the naked eye and with the ophthalmoscope?** A dilated pupil would certainly suggest glaucoma; ophthalmoscopic examination may show optic neuritis or retinal detachment. A visual field examination may detect optic neuritis, retrobulbar neuritis, and retinal artery occlusion. A visual acuity check may pick up a refractive error.

5. **Finally, is there headache associated with the eye pain?** This would be suggestive of migraine or cluster headache.

6. **Is there fever?** In children with fever and conjunctivitis, look for measles and Kawasaki disease.

DIAGNOSTIC WORKUP

The primary care specialist may want to treat cases of obvious conjunctivitis without a culture and sensitivity. However, a smear and culture is useful especially if *Neisseria* is suspected. A smear may also reveal eosinophils suggesting allergic conjunctivitis. The primary care specialist may also use fluorescein dye to diagnose a foreign body. Most primary care physicians feel competent to use tonometry to diagnose glaucoma and may feel competent to use a slit lamp. If all tests are negative, a trial of sumatriptan orally or by nasal spray may help diagnose migraine or histamine headaches. However, when there is any doubt about the diagnosis, the most cost-effective approach is to refer the patient to an ophthalmologist.

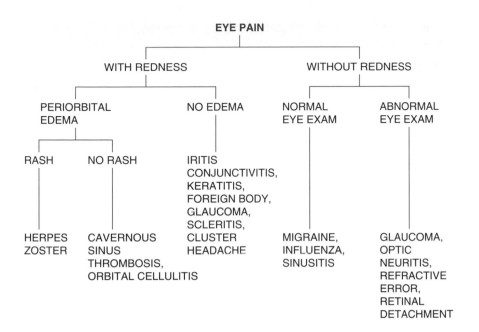

EYE PAIN

WITH REDNESS | WITHOUT REDNESS

PERIORBITAL EDEMA | NO EDEMA | NORMAL EYE EXAM | ABNORMAL EYE EXAM

RASH | NO RASH | IRITIS CONJUNCTIVITIS, KERATITIS, FOREIGN BODY, GLAUCOMA, SCLERITIS,

HERPES ZOSTER | CAVERNOUS SINUS THROMBOSIS, ORBITAL CELLULITIS | CLUSTER HEADACHE | MIGRAINE, INFLUENZA, SINUSITIS | GLAUCOMA, OPTIC NEURITIS, REFRACTIVE ERROR, RETINAL DETACHMENT

ASK THE FOLLOWING QUESTIONS:

1. **Is the pain constant or intermittent?** Intermittent pain would suggest trigeminal neuralgia, cluster headaches, or atypical migraine. Constant pain would suggest any local abnormalities in the structures underlying the face such as an abscessed sinus, an abscessed tooth, or a neoplasm in these areas.

2. **Is the pain increased by chewing?** Pain that is increased by chewing very often may be related to the temporomandibular joint syndrome, but it could be related to trigeminal neuralgia or dental caries. An elongated styloid process may cause face pain (Eagle's syndrome).

3. **Is there an associated nasal discharge?** An associated bloody nasal discharge would make one think of a nasopharyngeal carcinoma, but a purulent discharge would make one think of acute or chronic sinusitis. A watery nasal discharge often accompanies cluster headaches or atypical migraine.

4. **Are there abnormal neurologic findings?** Face pain sometimes accompanies multiple sclerosis, acute Wallenberg's syndrome, and advanced acoustic neuromas. The pain in the trigeminal distribution associated with multiple sclerosis often is intermittent and suggests trigeminal neuralgia.

DIAGNOSTIC WORKUP

The first thing to determine is whether there is an infectious or neoplastic process in the structures underlying the face. X-rays of the sinuses and teeth and CT scans of the sinuses and brain may be necessary to further elucidate this. An x-ray of the temporomandibular joint may be helpful. An MRI of the temporomandibular joint is the procedure of choice to rule out pathology of this joint. Referral to a dentist to evaluate the patient's teeth or to an ear, nose, and throat specialist to evaluate sinusitis may be necessary.

To rule out cluster headaches or atypical migraine, a histamine test may be done. It may be wise to see the patient during an attack so that superficial temporal artery compression can be done to rule out migraine and/or a shot of sumatriptan succinate can be given, which should provide immediate results in cluster headache and atypical migraine.

A trial of carbamazepine (Tegretol®) can be given in cases of suspected trigeminal neuralgia, but referral to a neurosurgeon for an alcoholic injection of the maxillary or mandibular branches of trigeminal nerve will more likely make the diagnosis and solve the patient's problem.

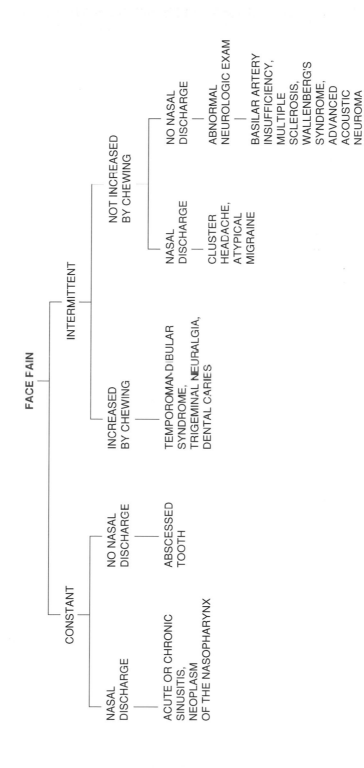

FACE PAIN

CONSTANT

NASAL DISCHARGE
- ACUTE OR CHRONIC SINUSITIS, NEOPLASM OF THE NASOPHARYNX

NO NASAL DISCHARGE
- ABSCESSED TOOTH

INTERMITTENT

INCREASED BY CHEWING
- TEMPOROMANDIBULAR SYNDROME, TRIGEMINAL NEURALGIA, DENTAL CARIES

NOT INCREASED BY CHEWING

NASAL DISCHARGE
- CLUSTER HEADACHE, ATYPICAL MIGRAINE

NO NASAL DISCHARGE

ABNORMAL NEUROLOGIC EXAM
- BASILAR ARTERY INSUFFICIENCY, MULTIPLE SCLEROSIS, WALLENBERG'S SYNDROME, ADVANCED ACOUSTIC NEUROMA

ASK THE FOLLOWING QUESTIONS:

1. **Is the flushing constant or intermittent?** Intermittent flushing suggests menopause, carcinoid syndrome, systemic mastocytosis, pheochromocytoma, and Zollinger–Ellison syndrome. Constant flushing might suggest alcoholism, polycythemia, or the malar flush of mitral stenosis.

2. **Is there associated obesity?** Associated obesity would certainly bring to mind Cushing's syndrome, but it may also be associated with alcoholism.

3. **Is there associated rash on the face or elsewhere?** A rash would most likely bring to mind rosacea if it is on the face, but if it is elsewhere, one might consider systemic mastocytosis or dermatomyositis.

4. **Are there associated systemic symptoms and signs?** Diarrhea would suggest carcinoid or Zollinger–Ellison syndrome. A headache along with the flushing would suggest a systemic mastocytosis. Fainting might suggest pheochromocytoma or epilepsy.

DIAGNOSTIC WORKUP

Urinalysis for 5-HIAA should be done if carcinoid syndrome is suspected. Urine samples may be taken for drug and alcohol screen in all cases in which there is any doubt about drug or alcohol history. Tests for serum FSH and estradiol should be done in patients suspected of having menopause. A 24-hr urine collection for catecholamines should be done for patients suspected of having pheochromocytoma. Serum gastrin tests should be done for patients suspected of having Zollinger–Ellison syndrome. In patients with systemic mastocytosis or dermatomyositis, a skin biopsy or muscle biopsy can be done. In patients with suspected Cushing's disease, a serum cortisol and cortisol suppression test can be done.

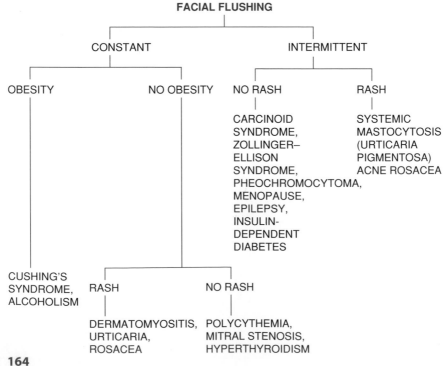

FACIAL FLUSHING

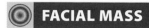

A facial mass may come from the skin, the subcutaneous tissue, the teeth, the sinuses, the bones, or the salivary glands. In the skin there may be moles, simple nevi, sebaceous cysts, papillomas, carcinoma, comedones, and urticaria. In the subcutaneous tissue there may be angioneurotic edema, trauma, and erysipelas and actinomycosis.

Swelling coming from the teeth includes dental abscess or dental cyst. The sinuses may become infected and cause swelling over the surface. The bones may develop an odontoma, a sarcoma, or a dermoid cyst. The bones may be fractured and there may be bruising with considerable swelling. If the bones of the sinuses are broken, there may be subcutaneous emphysema.

Mumps and uveoparotid fever may cause swelling of the salivary glands. Mixed tumors of the parotid gland cause unilateral swelling of the face. A stone may obstruct Stensen's or Wharton's ducts, causing intermittent swelling. Nonspecific inflammation of the parotid glands occurs in the elderly and malnourished individuals.

DIAGNOSTIC WORKUP

Most of the skin lesions will be obvious, but a skin biopsy can be performed when in doubt. Smears and cultures should be done when infection is suspected. A therapeutic trial of epinephrine or antihistamines can be tried in angioneurotic edema or urticaria. X-rays of the skull, jaw, and sinuses may be necessary. A CT scan may be needed to identify some fractures and sinus infections. Referral to an oral surgeon or otolaryngologist should be made early in confusing cases.

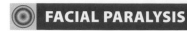

ASK THE FOLLOWING QUESTIONS:

1. **Is it acute or gradual onset?** If it is acute onset, Bell's palsy, diabetic neuropathy, and cerebral vascular accident must be considered. If it is gradual onset, one must consider an acoustic neuroma, advancing petrositis, or a brain tumor or abscess.

2. **Is there associated hemiplegia or hemiparesis?** If there is associated hemiplegia or hemiparesis and it is acute onset, one should consider cerebral vascular accident or extradural or subdural hematoma. If the hemiparesis, however, is contralateral, one should consider a brain stem thrombosis or hemorrhage. There are two clinical syndromes that are due to basilar artery lesions: Foville's syndrome and Millard–Gubler syndrome. If the hemiparesis is gradual onset, one should consider brain tumor or abscess or degenerative disease.

3. **Is there earache or hearing loss?** Associated earache or hearing loss should make one think of acoustic neuroma, petrositis, mastoiditis, herpes zoster, and cholesteatoma.

DIAGNOSTIC WORKUP

Immediate referral to a neurologist is indicated. One should do a complete examination of the ear, nose, and throat to determine if there is any rupture of the drum, discharge, evidence of otitis media, etc. Then x-rays of the mastoids and petrous bones should be done along with tomography. A CT scan of the brain with emphasis on the internal auditory foramina should be done if acoustic neuroma is suspected. Culture of the discharge from the ears and blood culture should be done if there are associated signs of an infectious process. Testing for Lyme disease may be indicated. Spinal fluid analysis should be done to look for Guillain–Barré syndrome. If myasthenia gravis is suspected, a Tensilon test may be done. Spinal fluid culture should be done in cases of brain abscess. Carotid scans and a workup for an embolic source should be done in cases of cerebral vascular accident. Of course, when there is a brain tumor or abscess or a cerebral vascular accident is suspected, CT scans of the brain should be done. If these are not helpful or are inconclusive, MRI of the brain can be done. Glucose tolerance testing should be done to rule out diabetic neuropathy. If lead poisoning is suspected, a blood level for lead should be done.

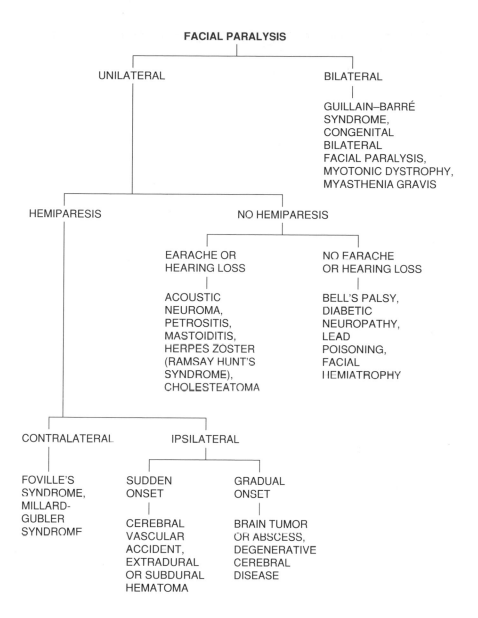

FACIAL PARALYSIS

UNILATERAL

BILATERAL

GUILLAIN–BARRÉ
SYNDROME,
CONGENITAL
BILATERAL
FACIAL PARALYSIS,
MYOTONIC DYSTROPHY,
MYASTHENIA GRAVIS

HEMIPARESIS

NO HEMIPARESIS

EARACHE OR
HEARING LOSS

ACOUSTIC
NEUROMA,
PETROSITIS,
MASTOIDITIS,
HERPES ZOSTER
(RAMSAY HUNT'S
SYNDROME),
CHOLESTEATOMA

NO EARACHE
OR HEARING LOSS

BELL'S PALSY,
DIABETIC
NEUROPATHY,
LEAD
POISONING,
FACIAL
HEMIATROPHY

CONTRALATERAL

IPSILATERAL

FOVILLE'S
SYNDROME,
MILLARD-
GUBLER
SYNDROME

SUDDEN
ONSET

CEREBRAL
VASCULAR
ACCIDENT,
EXTRADURAL
OR SUBDURAL
HEMATOMA

GRADUAL
ONSET

BRAIN TUMOR
OR ABSCESS,
DEGENERATIVE
CEREBRAL
DISEASE

FACIAL SWELLING

ASK THE FOLLOWING QUESTIONS:

1. **Is the facial swelling focal or diffuse?** If it is focal, one should consider a local condition in the structures underlying the face such as the salivary glands, the teeth, or the sinuses. Mumps is a common condition, of course, especially in children. If it is diffuse facial swelling, one should consider a systemic disease such as glomerulonephritis, myxedema, or Cushing's disease.

2. **Is the swelling associated with generalized edema?** If there is generalized edema, one must consider acute glomerulonephritis, nephrotic syndrome, congestive heart failure, or cirrhosis. If the generalized edema is nonpitting, one would consider myxedema and cretinism. If there is no generalized edema, one must consider conditions such as Cushing's syndrome, dermatomyositis, acromegaly, mongolism, and Paget's disease.

3. **If the edema is generalized, is it pitting edema or nonpitting edema?** Nonpitting edema would suggest myxedema and cretinism.

4. **Is there associated flushing?** With flushing one would consider Cushing's syndrome, dermatomyositis, and a superior vena cava syndrome. If there is no flushing, one should consider acromegaly, mongolism, or Paget's disease.

5. **Is there associated fever?** If there is associated fever, look for infections in the structures underlying the skin such as mumps, abscess of the salivary gland, an abscessed tooth, sinusitis, or syphilis.

DIAGNOSTIC WORKUP

Cases of focal swelling should have a routine CBC and sedimentation rate. X-rays of the sinuses and teeth should be done. If mumps is suspected, a mumps skin test or antibody titer may be done. If all these tests are negative and there is a focal swelling, referral to an oral surgeon may be wise at this point.

If the swelling is diffuse, the basic workup is a CBC, chemistry panel, and urinalysis. A streptozyme test or ASO titer can be done if glomerulonephritis is suspected, but a microscopic examination of the urine is extremely important in this condition. If congestive heart failure is suspected, a chest x-ray, EKG, arm-to-tongue circulation time, and pulmonary function testing should be done. In cases of Cushing's disease, a 24-hr urine-free cortisol and cortisol suppression test may be done. X-rays of the skull and long bones should be done in suspected cases of acromegaly or Paget's disease.

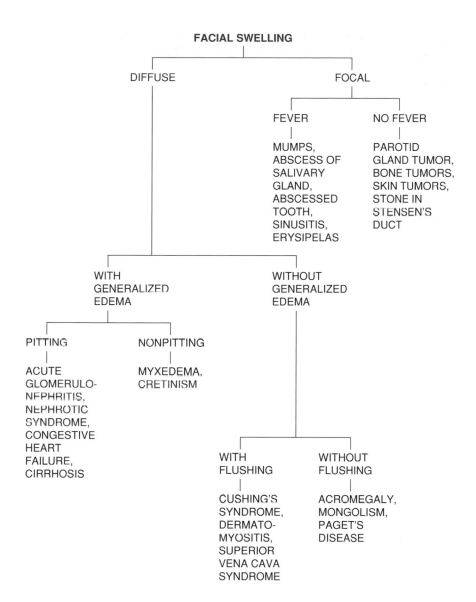

FACIAL SWELLING

DIFFUSE

FOCAL

FEVER

MUMPS,
ABSCESS OF
SALIVARY
GLAND,
ABSCESSED
TOOTH,
SINUSITIS,
ERYSIPELAS

NO FEVER

PAROTID
GLAND TUMOR,
BONE TUMORS,
SKIN TUMORS,
STONE IN
STENSEN'S
DUCT

WITH
GENERALIZED
EDEMA

WITHOUT
GENERALIZED
EDEMA

PITTING

ACUTE
GLOMERULO-
NEPHRITIS,
NEPHROTIC
SYNDROME,
CONGESTIVE
HEART
FAILURE,
CIRRHOSIS

NONPITTING

MYXEDEMA,
CRETINISM

WITH
FLUSHING

CUSHING'S
SYNDROME,
DERMATO-
MYOSITIS,
SUPERIOR
VENA CAVA
SYNDROME

WITHOUT
FLUSHING

ACROMEGALY,
MONGOLISM,
PAGET'S
DISEASE

⊚ FACIES, ABNORMAL

Perhaps every clinician has at one time or another experienced the joy of seeing a patient's face and making the diagnosis. The round flushed face of Cushing's disease, the pop-eyes of hyperthyroidism, or the expressionless face of Parkinson's disease quickly come to mind. There are many other abnormal facies you will want to remember. Let's enumerate them.

1. In glomerulonephritis, the face is pale and puffy with edematous bags under the eyes.
2. In myxedema, the facial features become coarse; consequently, the nostrils are broad, and the lips are thick. The face is expressionless and puffy.
3. In mongolism, there is epicanthus, and the face is Oriental in appearance with the tongue protruding.
4. In mental retardation, the face is often dull and expressionless.
5. In tetanus, we see the sarcastic smile of risus sardonicus.
6. In myasthenia gravis, the face is also expressionless, but the variable degree of ptosis should be a warning.
7. In mitral stenosis, the malar flush is very helpful in making the diagnosis.
8. The flushing of the face in alcoholism, carcinoid syndrome, and menopause is also helpful.
9. In acromegaly, the features are coarse, but the brows are enlarged and the jaw protrudes. The spaces between the lower teeth widen.
10. In myotonic dystrophy, the face is hatchet-shaped due to the facial wasting and weakness, and there is bilateral partial ptosis.
11. In bulbar and pseudobulbar palsy, regardless of the cause, the face is expressionless, the mouth remains open most of the time, and there is drooling.
12. In Bell's palsy, the mouth is drawn to the unaffected side during a smile, and the nasolabial fold is flat. The eye does not close completely.
13. In Paget's disease, the forehead protrudes, and the face appears disproportionately small.
14. In scleroderma, there is smoothing out of all the wrinkles of the face along with thinning of the skin, giving a waxy appearance.
15. In cachectic states, the face begins to appear like a skull with skin over it.
16. In hypertelorism, the eyes are wide apart.
17. In Wilson's disease, the face looks like it is ready to crack a smile, and the mouth is open with frequent drooling.
18. The cyanosis of congenital heart disease would hardly be missed.

There are many other rare facies that, once seen, won't be forgotten.

ASK THE FOLLOWING QUESTIONS:

1. **Is there a history of an abnormal gestation?** There may be a history that the mother was a chronic alcoholic or ingested such drugs as phenytoin, trimethadione, or narcotics. The mother may have had toxoplasmosis, rubella, herpes simplex, or other diseases during her gestation.
2. **Is the child's environment abnormal?** Careful investigation may disclose that the child has been neglected or that there are economic circumstances to indicate that the child is not getting enough food. Investigation may also indicate that the child is not getting adequate love or practicing good hygiene.
3. **Are there abnormalities found on the neurologic examination?** Neurologic examination may reveal findings to suggest microcephaly, muscular atrophy, hydrocephalus, spastic diplegia, and other neurologic causes of mental retardation.
4. **Are there endocrine abnormalities?** Cretinism, pituitary tumors, and genital abnormalities may be suggested from the endocrine examination
5. **Are there findings to suggest a GI disorder?** Wasting and a distended abdomen may suggest a malabsorption syndrome. The history of frequent pneumonia may indicate fibrocystic disease. Cataracts may suggest galactosemia.

DIAGNOSTIC WORKUP

The routine diagnostic workup should include a CBC, sedimentation rate, urinalysis, urine culture, chemistry panel, thyroid profile, sweat test, stool for quantitative fat, chest x-ray, and an EKG. Bone age x-rays are often helpful in indicating a growth delay.

If there are focal neurologic signs or a pituitary tumor is suspected, a CT scan of the brain may be necessary. Additional endocrinologic tests include serum growth hormone level before and after exercise, somatomedin-C level, and overnight dexamethasone suppression test. However, an endocrinologist, pediatrician, or orthopedic surgeon should be consulted before ordering expensive diagnostic tests. When the workup fails to yield a diagnosis, consider constitutional growth delay.

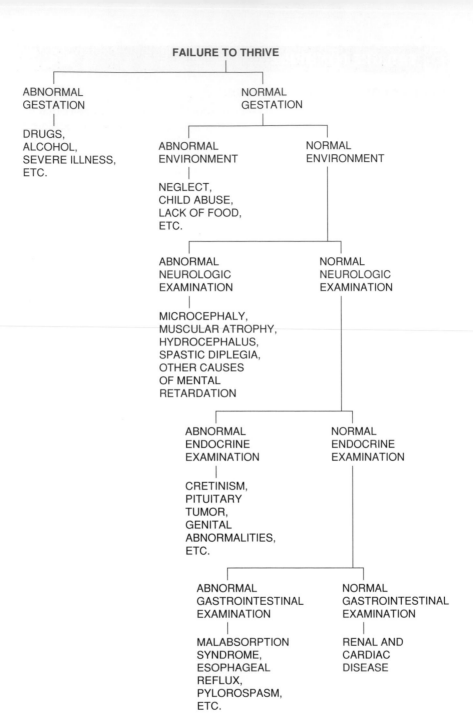

ASK THE FOLLOWING QUESTIONS:

1. **Is there weight loss?** If there is weight loss, one must consider a neoplasm, endocrine disorders such as hyperthyroidism or diabetes mellitus, malnutrition or malabsorption, and chronic infectious diseases such as tuberculosis or subacute bacterial endocarditis.
2. **Is there fever?** If there is fever, one should consider an infectious disease such as tuberculosis, subacute bacterial endocarditis, toxoplasmosis, infectious mononucleosis, or brucellosis.
3. **Is there pallor?** If there is pallor, the most likely cause is a type of anemia such as that associated with malabsorption syndrome or iron deficiency anemia, pernicious anemia, or anemia blood loss.
4. **Is the fatigue intermittent or constant?** Intermittent fatigue would make one suspect myasthenia gravis or Eaton–Lambert syndrome. Constant fatigue would be related to any of the conditions we have already discussed. Constant fatigue, however, with no weight loss would make one consider a psychiatric disorder.
5. **Is there a positive drug or alcohol history?** Alcoholism, cocaine abuse, and chronic aspirin ingestion are just a few of the disorders that can be associated with chronic fatigue. Statins may cause myalgia and frank rhabdomyolysis. Don't forget caffeine abuse!
6. **Are there associated neurologic findings?** Many neurologic disorders are associated with fatigue, and they include muscular dystrophy, amyotrophic lateral sclerosis, and Parkinson's disease.
7. **Is there polyuria?** Polyuria would make one think of hyperthyroidism, diabetes mellitus, hyperparathyroidism, and chronic renal failure.

DIAGNOSTIC WORKUP

All patients should have routine laboratory studies, including CBC, sedimentation rate, chemistry panel, venereal disease research laboratory (VDRL) test, and a urinalysis including analysis for myoglobin. CPK, LDH, aspartate aminotransferase (AST), and urine creatine and creatinine should be done to rule out muscle disease. A thyroid profile should be done to rule out hyperthyroidism. Further endocrine workup including serum cortisol will help differentiate Addison's disease and hypopituitarism. Because fatigue is associated with aldosteronism, a 24-hr urine aldosterone determination should be done.

Tests for chronic infectious disease, such as febrile agglutinins, brucellin antibody titer, heterophile antibody titer or Monospot test, sputum for AFB, and various skin tests for tuberculosis and fungi, can be done. HIV testing may be appropriate if there is a history of high-risk sexual behavior. Serial blood cultures also would be of value if there is significant fever. Tests for chronic organ failure such as BUN, creatinine, serum electrolytes, and liver function tests should be done. A workup of anemia including a workup of malabsorption syndrome may be necessary. Consequently, stool analysis for fat content as well as D-xylose absorption testing may be done.

A search for neoplasm will include chest x-rays, x-rays of the skull and long bones, a bone scan, an upper GI series, and small bowel follow-through as well as a barium enema and intravenous pyelogram. A muscle biopsy will help differentiate certain collagen diseases, muscular dystrophy, and trichinosis. An ANA test and serum complement to screen for collagen disease should be done. A Tensilon test or acetylcholine receptor antibody titer may be necessary to differentiate myasthenia gravis. If a neurologic disease is suspected, referral to a neurologist would be in order. Consider EMG also. If sleep apnea is a possibility, overnight polysomnography is indicated. An MRI of the brain or spinal cord may be indicated to rule out multiple sclerosis.

If all the tests prove negative, referral to a psychiatrist would be appropriate. On the other hand, it may be appropriate to refer the patient to a psychiatrist earlier in the course of the workup. The diagnosis of chronic fatigue syndrome is sometimes made when all the diagnostic tests are negative, but whether it is truly a disease is questionable.

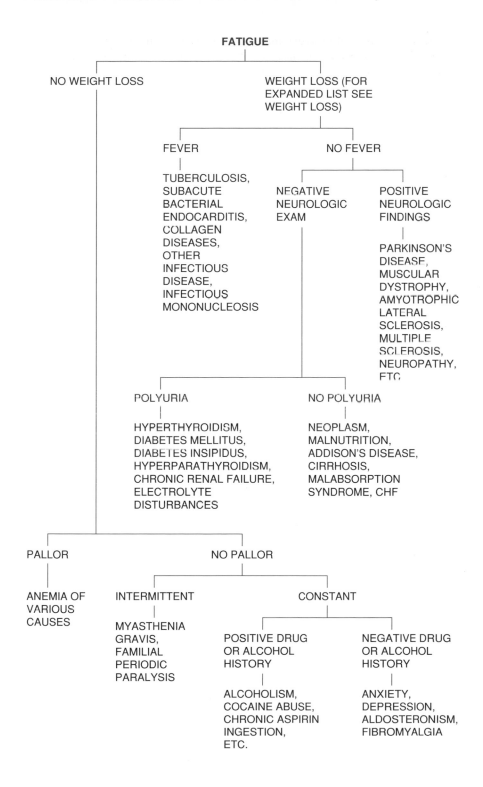

FATIGUE

NO WEIGHT LOSS

WEIGHT LOSS (FOR EXPANDED LIST SEE WEIGHT LOSS)

FEVER

TUBERCULOSIS, SUBACUTE BACTERIAL ENDOCARDITIS, COLLAGEN DISEASES, OTHER INFECTIOUS DISEASE, INFECTIOUS MONONUCLEOSIS

NO FEVER

NEGATIVE NEUROLOGIC EXAM

POSITIVE NEUROLOGIC FINDINGS

PARKINSON'S DISEASE, MUSCULAR DYSTROPHY, AMYOTROPHIC LATERAL SCLEROSIS, MULTIPLE SCLEROSIS, NEUROPATHY, ETC.

POLYURIA

HYPERTHYROIDISM, DIABETES MELLITUS, DIABETES INSIPIDUS, HYPERPARATHYROIDISM, CHRONIC RENAL FAILURE, ELECTROLYTE DISTURBANCES

NO POLYURIA

NEOPLASM, MALNUTRITION, ADDISON'S DISEASE, CIRRHOSIS, MALABSORPTION SYNDROME, CHF

PALLOR

ANEMIA OF VARIOUS CAUSES

NO PALLOR

INTERMITTENT

MYASTHENIA GRAVIS, FAMILIAL PERIODIC PARALYSIS

CONSTANT

POSITIVE DRUG OR ALCOHOL HISTORY

ALCOHOLISM, COCAINE ABUSE, CHRONIC ASPIRIN INGESTION, ETC.

NEGATIVE DRUG OR ALCOHOL HISTORY

ANXIETY, DEPRESSION, ALDOSTERONISM, FIBROMYALGIA

FEMORAL MASS OR SWELLING

ASK THE FOLLOWING QUESTIONS:

1. **Is it reducible?** If the mass is reducible, it is most likely a femoral hernia or saphenous varix.
2. **Is there an associated kyphotic curvature of the spine?** The findings of a kyphotic curvature of the spine suggest a psoas abscess, which is usually tuberculous.
3. **Is the mass firm and ovoid?** A firm, ovoid mass suggests an enlarged lymph node or an ectopic testis.
4. **Is there resonance or bowel sounds over the mass?** These findings suggest a femoral hernia.
5. **Is the corresponding half of the scrotum empty?** These findings suggest an ectopic testis.

DIAGNOSTIC WORKUP

Surgical consultation may be wise at the outset. A reducible mass would suggest a femoral hernia, but an upper GI series with a small bowel follow-through would confirm this diagnosis. Of course, if it is felt that the femoral hernia is irreducible, this study would not be done, and exploratory surgery would be indicated. If the mass is suspected to be a lymph node, a biopsy should be done. If the mass is suspected to be an abscess, an incision and drainage should be done. If tuberculosis is suspected, a tuberculin test as well as an AFB smear and culture should be done. If the mass is suspected to be a saphenous varix, venography will confirm the diagnosis. Exploratory surgery of the groin will clarify the diagnosis in confusing cases.

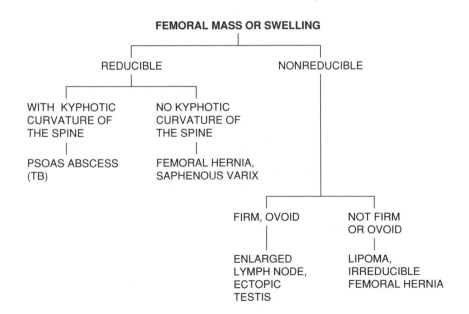

ASK THE FOLLOWING QUESTIONS:

1. **Is there a history of drug ingestion or injection?** This will help diagnose drug reactions and serum sickness, which are common and easily discovered in the history. Patients with glucose-6-phosphate dehydrogenase deficiency may develop fever after receiving certain drugs.

2. **Is there a rash?** The presence of a rash should make one think of a drug reaction, meningococcemia, the various exanthems, and subacute bacterial endocarditis.

3. **Is there localized pain?** If there is a sore throat, obviously streptococcal pharyngitis or a viral URI is likely. If there is headache, meningitis or encephalitis must be considered. If there is chest pain, one should consider a pulmonary infarct, myocardial infarction, or Bornholm disease. If there is abdominal pain, one would consider pyelonephritis, cholecystitis, and appendicitis among the various conditions. If there is joint pain, one should consider rheumatic fever, rheumatoid arthritis, or septic arthritis.

4. **Is there a focal discharge?** A productive cough would make one consider pneumonia. A rectal discharge would make one consider a perirectal abscess. A urethral discharge should make one think of gonorrhea.

5. **Are there other localizing signs?** Frequency of urination should make one think of pyelonephritis. A productive cough should make one think of pneumonia, whereas jaundice would make one think of hepatitis.

DIAGNOSTIC WORKUP

Routine studies include a CBC, sedimentation rate, chemistry panel, urinalysis, chest x-rays, VDRL test, and tuberculin skin test. A normal sedimentation rate suggests factitious fever. Serial blood cultures should be done on all patients. Febrile agglutinins usually should be done. An ASO titer or streptozyme test should be done to exclude rheumatic fever. RNA, ANA, and DNA tests should be done to look for lupus and other connective tissue disease. An HIV antibody titer may need to be ordered. Serologic tests for Lyme disease may be indicated. A serum procalcitonin will often distinguish bacterial infections from viral infections.

The next step is to culture any discharge or various body fluids that might be suspect. Thus, a urinalysis and urine culture should be done. A nose and throat culture should be done. A sputum smear and culture may need to be done. The next consideration is to do various serologic tests. A heterophile antibody titer should be done in teenagers. Febrile agglutinin tests may need to be done. Acute and convalescent phase sera for viral studies may need to be done. Do a urine test for legionella antigen in persistent fever associated with cough.

Next one should do skin testing. Thus, histoplasmin, coccidioidin, and blastomycin skin testing should be done on patients with a cough. *Trichinella* skin testing may need to be done, as well as brucellin skin testing. A Kveim test might need to be done for suspected sarcoidosis.

The next step is to do plain x-rays of suspected areas. For instance, x-rays of the teeth may disclose an abscessed tooth. X-rays of the long bones may disclose a metastatic carcinoma.

The next step is contrast x-ray studies of various organ systems. An intravenous pyelogram may show a hypernephroma. A cholecystogram may show gallstones. An upper GI series and barium enema may show chronic pancreatitis or diverticulitis. Angiography may disclose periarteritis nodosa, aortitis, or giant cell arteritis.

The next step is to do a CT scan of the abdomen and pelvis. If this is negative, consider a CT scan of the chest and mediastinum. Echocardiography may disclose valvular vegetations or an atrial myxoma.

Next, consider biopsying various organ systems. For instances, a lymph node biopsy may disclose a lymphoma or sarcoidosis. A muscle biopsy may disclose periarteritis nodosa, polymyositis, or trichinella.

Next one should do bone scans and gallium scans for possible metastasis, osteomyelitis, or localized abscesses.

If all these procedures fail to turn up a lesion, then an exploratory laparotomy may need to be done. A fibrin test may indicate Mediterranean fever, or urine for etiocholanolone may also indicate a relapsing type of fever. A urine test for porphobilinogen may diagnose porphyria.

The wisest move is to conduct this investigation with the help of an infectious disease specialist or a specialist in the body organ system most likely suspected of harboring the infection.

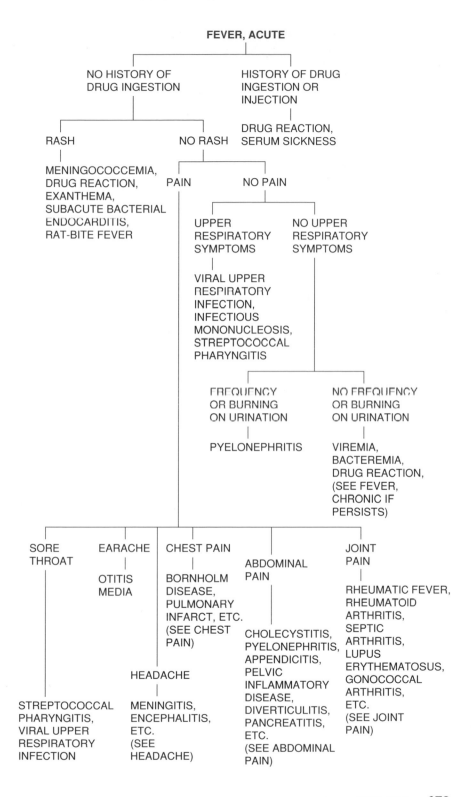

FEVER, ACUTE

NO HISTORY OF DRUG INGESTION

HISTORY OF DRUG INGESTION OR INJECTION

DRUG REACTION, SERUM SICKNESS

RASH

MENINGOCOCCEMIA, DRUG REACTION, EXANTHEMA, SUBACUTE BACTERIAL ENDOCARDITIS, RAT-BITE FEVER

NO RASH

PAIN

NO PAIN

UPPER RESPIRATORY SYMPTOMS

VIRAL UPPER RESPIRATORY INFECTION, INFECTIOUS MONONUCLEOSIS, STREPTOCOCCAL PHARYNGITIS

NO UPPER RESPIRATORY SYMPTOMS

FREQUENCY OR BURNING ON URINATION

PYELONEPHRITIS

NO FREQUENCY OR BURNING ON URINATION

VIREMIA, BACTEREMIA, DRUG REACTION, (SEE FEVER, CHRONIC IF PERSISTS)

SORE THROAT

EARACHE

OTITIS MEDIA

CHEST PAIN

BORNHOLM DISEASE, PULMONARY INFARCT, ETC. (SEE CHEST PAIN)

ABDOMINAL PAIN

JOINT PAIN

RHEUMATIC FEVER, RHEUMATOID ARTHRITIS, SEPTIC ARTHRITIS, LUPUS ERYTHEMATOSUS, GONOCOCCAL ARTHRITIS, ETC. (SEE JOINT PAIN)

HEADACHE

STREPTOCOCCAL PHARYNGITIS, VIRAL UPPER RESPIRATORY INFECTION

MENINGITIS, ENCEPHALITIS, ETC. (SEE HEADACHE)

CHOLECYSTITIS, PYELONEPHRITIS, APPENDICITIS, PELVIC INFLAMMATORY DISEASE, DIVERTICULITIS, PANCREATITIS, ETC. (SEE ABDOMINAL PAIN)

FEVER, CHRONIC

ASK THE FOLLOWING QUESTIONS:

1. **Is there a history of drug ingestion or injection?** Of course, the history should reveal that the patient has been on a certain drug or has received certain antitoxins, serums, or vaccines.
2. **Is there a rash?** If there is a rash, one should suspect subacute bacterial endocarditis, Rocky Mountain spotted fever, secondary syphilis, rat-bite fever, pemphigus, a drug reaction, lupus erythematosus, dermatomyositis, or typhoid fever. There are other conditions associated with a rash also.
3. **Is there a characteristic pattern to the fever?** The various forms of malaria give a characteristic pattern of the fever, as well as undulant fever in Hodgkin's disease.
4. **Is there localized pain?** Abdominal pain should suggest a cholecystitis, hepatic abscess, diverticulitis, etc. A sore throat should suggest infectious mononucleosis, leukemia, and subacute thyroiditis. Joint pain should suggest rheumatoid arthritis, rheumatic fever, or gonococcal arthritis. Earache should suggest otitis media or mastoiditis. Chest pain should suggest tuberculosis, pleurisy, or empyema.
5. **Is there a localized discharge?** Purulent sputum should suggest pneumonia, tuberculosis, or chronic fungal disease in the lung. A urethral discharge would suggest gonorrhea or Reiter's disease.
6. **Is there a localized mass or swelling?** An abdominal mass would suggest hepatic abscess, pancreatic cyst, or diverticular abscess. A flank mass might suggest hypernephroma or perinephric abscess.

DIAGNOSTIC WORKUP

The diagnostic workup is similar to that for acute fever on page 177.

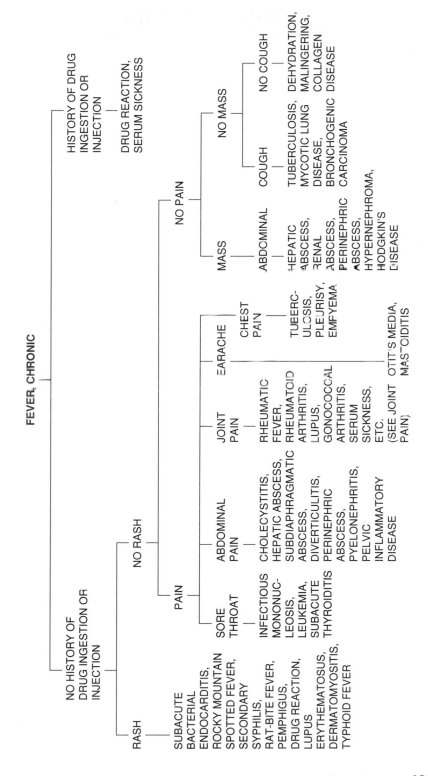

FEVER, CHRONIC

HISTORY OF DRUG INGESTION OR INJECTION
- DRUG REACTION, SERUM SICKNESS

NO HISTORY OF DRUG INGESTION OR INJECTION
- RASH
  - SUBACUTE BACTERIAL ENDOCARDITIS, ROCKY MOUNTAIN SPOTTED FEVER, SECONDARY SYPHILIS, RAT-BITE FEVER, PEMPHIGUS, DRUG REACTION, LUPUS ERYTHEMATOSUS, DERMATOMYOSITIS, TYPHOID FEVER
- NO RASH
  - PAIN
    - SORE THROAT
      - INFECTIOUS MONONUCLEOSIS, LEUKEMIA, SUBACUTE THYROIDITIS
    - ABDOMINAL PAIN
      - CHOLECYSTITIS, HEPATIC ABSCESS, SUBDIAPHRAGMATIC ABSCESS, DIVERTICULITIS, PERINEPHRIC ABSCESS, PYELONEPHRITIS, PELVIC INFLAMMATORY DISEASE
    - JOINT PAIN
      - RHEUMATIC FEVER, RHEUMATOID ARTHRITIS, LUPUS, GONOCOCCAL ARTHRITIS, SERUM SICKNESS, ETC. (SEE JOINT PAIN)
    - EARACHE
      - OTITIS MEDIA, MASTOIDITIS
    - CHEST PAIN
      - TUBERCULOSIS, PLEURISY, EMPYEMA
  - NO PAIN
    - MASS
      - ABDOMINAL
        - HEPATIC ABSCESS, RENAL ABSCESS, PERINEPHRIC ABSCESS, HYPERNEPHROMA, HODGKIN'S DISEASE
    - NO MASS
      - COUGH
        - TUBERCULOSIS, MYCOTIC LUNG DISEASE, BRONCHOGENIC CARCINOMA
      - NO COUGH
        - DEHYDRATION, MALINGERING, COLLAGEN DISEASE

FLANK MASS

ASK THE FOLLOWING QUESTIONS:

1. **Are there bilateral flank masses?** If the masses are bilateral, one should consider polycystic kidney or early bilateral hydronephrosis.
2. **Is there associated hypertension?** If there is hypertension, one should consider polycystic kidneys, hypernephroma, pheochromocytoma, or adrenocortical carcinoma.
3. **Is the mass painful?** A painful flank mass should make one think of perinephric abscess, hydronephrosis with partial obstruction, or tuberculosis.
4. **Is there blood in the urine?** Hematuria should make one think of hypernephroma, a Wilms' tumor, tuberculosis, renal calculus, or polycystic kidneys.

DIAGNOSTIC WORKUP

If the mass is unilateral, the most cost-effective approach would be to refer the patient to a urologist at the outset. If the urologist is not available or if the mass is bilateral, one might proceed with a workup. This should include a CBC, chemistry panel, VDRL test, urinalysis or urine culture, and a flat plate of the abdomen. Catheterization for residual urine may be done to determine if there is bladder neck obstruction with associated hydronephrosis. An intravenous pyelogram would be the next step.

If these tests fail to make a definitive diagnosis, perhaps abdominal ultrasound may help with the diagnosis of a renal cyst. A CT scan of the abdomen would be the next logical step in confusing cases. Renal angiography and cystoscopy with retrograde pyelography are not usually necessary.

FLANK MASS

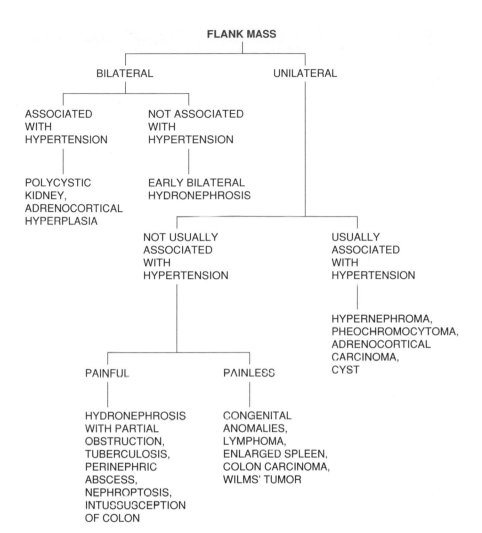

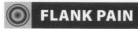
ASK THE FOLLOWING QUESTIONS:

1. **Is there associated fever?** The presence of fever along with chest pain should make one think of a perinephric abscess or pyelonephritis. Occasionally, however, hypernephroma can cause fever and flank pain, as can bilateral hydronephrosis.

2. **Is there a flank mass?** The presence of flank pain along with a flank mass should make one think of a hypernephroma, hydronephrosis, polycystic kidneys, or perinephric abscess.

3. **Is there hematuria?** The presence of pain and hematuria should make one think of renal calculus first, but the possibility of a renal infarction, polycystic kidneys, and tuberculosis of the kidneys must be considered also. Hematuria is also found in a hypernephroma.

DIAGNOSTIC WORKUP

Routine tests include a CBC, sedimentation rate, chemistry panel, urinalysis, and urine culture. A non-contrast helical CT scan of the abdomen is the next logical step. If these fail to make a definitive diagnosis, one should consider ordering an abdominal ultrasound of the abdomen. Alternatively, a trial of antibiotic may be indicated. If a renal infarction is suspected, aortography and renal angiography may be ordered. When the above tests are all negative, one should consider x-rays of the lumbosacral spine and MRI of the thoracic and lumbar spine. Consulting a urologist is prudent before ordering expensive diagnostic tests.

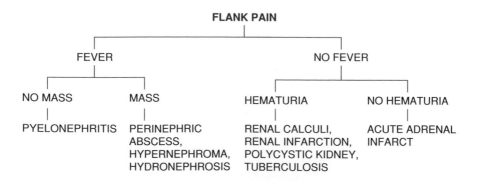

FLATULENCE

ASK THE FOLLOWING QUESTIONS:

1. **Is the flatulence associated with heartburn or regurgitation?** The presence of flatulence with heartburn or regurgitation should suggest reflux esophagitis, gastric or duodenal ulcer, or chronic cholecystitis.
2. **Is there a history of a gastrectomy?** History of a gastrectomy may indicate that there is gastric dilatation due to the fact that the stomach fails to drain adequately.
3. **Is there abdominal pain or distention?** The presence of abdominal pain or distention would indicate the possibility of partial intestinal obstruction, steatorrhea, or diverticulitis.
4. **Are there other signs of a nervous disorder?** If there is a history of emotional trauma or there is hyperkinesis, increased sweating, insomnia, loss of appetite, or other signs of a nervous disorder, aerophagia should be considered.

DIAGNOSTIC WORKUP

If the gas is eructated, stools for occult blood and an upper GI series and esophagogram should be ordered. These may disclose a hiatal hernia and esophagitis, a gastric or duodenal ulcer, and other upper intestinal disorders. A gallbladder series may be done if the upper GI series is unremarkable. Gastroscopy and esophagoscopy may be necessary, as well as a gastric analysis.

If the excessive gas is passed rectally, stools for occult blood, stools for ovum and parasite, and stool cultures should be done. A flat plate of the abdomen may disclose evidence of intestinal obstruction. If these are negative, a barium enema may be done and that may be followed with a small bowel series. Colonoscopy may be indicated. Analysis of flatus for volume and composition of intestinal gases may be helpful. A quantitative stool-fat analysis should be done to determine if there is steatorrhea, and if so, the workup would proceed (page 457). A lactose tolerance test can be done in cases suspected of lactase deficiency. Hydrogen breath testing is useful in detecting lactase deficiency and other carbohydrate intolerance and bacterial overgrowth. A trial of proton pump inhibitors may be all that is needed. When extensive testing is negative, a psychiatrist may need to be consulted.

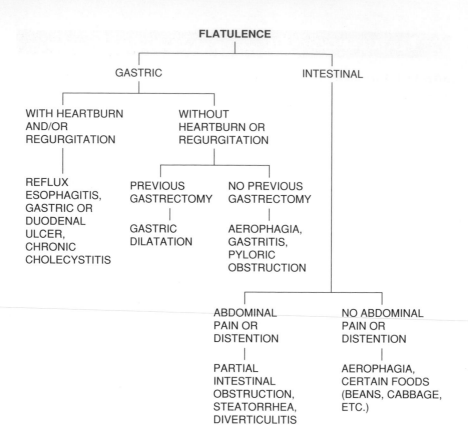

FLATULENCE

GASTRIC

INTESTINAL

WITH HEARTBURN AND/OR REGURGITATION

WITHOUT HEARTBURN OR REGURGITATION

REFLUX ESOPHAGITIS, GASTRIC OR DUODENAL ULCER, CHRONIC CHOLECYSTITIS

PREVIOUS GASTRECTOMY

NO PREVIOUS GASTRECTOMY

GASTRIC DILATATION

AEROPHAGIA, GASTRITIS, PYLORIC OBSTRUCTION

ABDOMINAL PAIN OR DISTENTION

NO ABDOMINAL PAIN OR DISTENTION

PARTIAL INTESTINAL OBSTRUCTION, STEATORRHEA, DIVERTICULITIS

AEROPHAGIA, CERTAIN FOODS (BEANS, CABBAGE, ETC.)

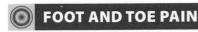

ASK THE FOLLOWING QUESTIONS:

1. **Is there fever or localized erythema?** Localized erythema would suggest phlebitis, gout, osteomyelitis, cellulitis, ingrown toenail, and paronychia. Achilles bursitis and tendonitis may be associated with Reiter's syndrome and ankylosing spondylitis. The presence of fever would make one suspect osteomyelitis and cellulitis.

2. **Is there associated deformity of the foot?** Hallux valgus, hammertoe, hallux rigidus, arthritis, and displaced fracture are the main causes of a deformity of the foot.

3. **Are the peripheral pulses palpable?** Diminished arterial pulses would make one think of arterial embolism, peripheral arteriosclerosis, and diabetes.

4. **Are there associated neurologic findings?** The presence of loss of sensation to touch and pain should make one think of peripheral neuropathy and tarsal tunnel syndrome. Numbness or loss of sensation in the third and fourth toes is often associated with a Morton's neuroma.

DIAGNOSTIC WORKUP

Routine diagnostic tests include a CBC, sedimentation rate, chemistry panel, VDRL test, and an x-ray of the foot. If the peripheral pulses are diminished, Doppler studies and angiography should be considered. If there is diffuse swelling and erythema, venography may need to be done. If there are neurologic findings, nerve conduction velocity studies and electromyograms (EMGs) may be helpful. Consider bone scans, CT scans, and arthroscopy if the above tests are negative. An MRI may be needed to diagnose stress fractures. Stress fractures, Achilles tendonitis, and tarsal tunnel syndrome are common in runners. Abnormal weight distribution is diagnosed by quantitative scintigraphs. It is wise to refer the patient to an orthopedic surgeon or podiatrist before ordering expensive diagnostic tests.

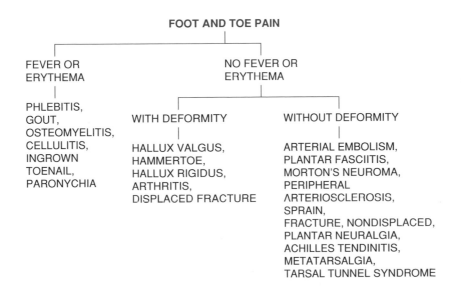

ASK THE FOLLOWING QUESTION:

1. **Are there signs of a neurologic disease?** Many foot deformities are associated with neurologic disease. For example, a pes cavus may be associated with a peroneal muscular atrophy, poliomyelitis, and Friedreich's ataxia. Muscular dystrophy produces an equinovarus deformity. Friedreich's ataxia may produce a talipes equinovarus. Amyotrophic lateral sclerosis and progressive muscular atrophy may also cause foot deformities.

DIAGNOSTIC WORKUP

Rather than undertaking an extensive diagnostic workup, it is wise to refer the patient to the appropriate specialist. If there are neurologic signs, the patient should be referred to a neurologist. Otherwise, the patient should be referred to an orthopedic surgeon or podiatrist.

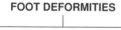

FOOT DEFORMITIES

WITH NEUROLOGIC DISEASE	WITHOUT NEUROLOGIC DISEASE
CHARCOT-MARIE-TOOTH DISEASE, FRIEDREICH'S ATAXIA, VOLKMANN'S CONTRACTURE, REITER'S DISEASE, MUSCULAR DYSTROPHY, AMYOTONIA CONGENITA POLIOMYELITIS, OTHER DISEASES OF BRAIN AND SPINAL CORD	TALIPES EQUINOVARUS, TALIPES VARUS, TALIPES CALCANEOVALGUS, CONGENITAL METATARSUS VARUS, PES VALGUS, PES CAVUS

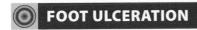

FOOT ULCERATION

ASK THE FOLLOWING QUESTIONS:

1. **Are there diminished or absent peripheral pulses?** The finding of poor peripheral pulses would suggest that the lesion is secondary to ischemia from arteriosclerosis, Buerger's disease, diabetic arteriolar sclerosis, familial hyperlipidemia, and cryoproteinemia.

2. **Are there abnormalities on neurologic examination?** The presence of good peripheral pulses should make one look for a neurologic explanation for the ulcer, and if there is diminished sensation to touch and pain in the periphery, peripheral neuropathy is very likely. Ulcers may also form in paraplegia of any cause, leprosy, and tabes dorsalis.

3. **Is there a history of diabetes?** A history of diabetes makes the diagnosis of diabetic arteriolar sclerosis very likely. Remember, the pulses may be normal in this condition.

4. **Is there a positive smear or culture?** The presence of good peripheral pulses should prompt one to do a smear and culture of material from the lesion, and if this is positive, then the diagnosis is made. We would consider, in addition to the normal bacteria, blastomycosis, sporotrichosis, maduromycosis, and syphilis.

DIAGNOSTIC WORKUP

Diminished pulses is a clear indication for Doppler ultrasound studies. Routine tests include a CBC, sedimentation rate, urinalysis, chemistry panel, VDRL test, and glucose tolerance test. An x-ray of the involved foot should be done to rule out osteomyelitis. A bone scan or CT scan is even more sensitive to osteomyelitis and other disorders of the bone that may be causing the ulcer. A smear should be made of the ulcer material and a culture done also, not just for the common pathogens, but for AFB and fungi. A dark field preparation may be necessary. Skin testing for blastomycosis and other fungi should be done. A nerve conduction velocity study of the lower extremities will be helpful in differentiating neurologic causes. Femoral angiography may be valuable in determining the exact level of the lesion and whether it can be approached surgically.

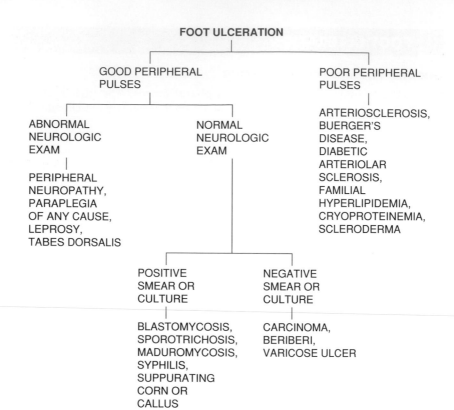

FOOT ULCERATION

GOOD PERIPHERAL PULSES

POOR PERIPHERAL PULSES

ARTERIOSCLEROSIS, BUERGER'S DISEASE, DIABETIC ARTERIOLAR SCLEROSIS, FAMILIAL HYPERLIPIDEMIA, CRYOPROTEINEMIA, SCLERODERMA

ABNORMAL NEUROLOGIC EXAM

PERIPHERAL NEUROPATHY, PARAPLEGIA OF ANY CAUSE, LEPROSY, TABES DORSALIS

NORMAL NEUROLOGIC EXAM

POSITIVE SMEAR OR CULTURE

BLASTOMYCOSIS, SPOROTRICHOSIS, MADUROMYCOSIS, SYPHILIS, SUPPURATING CORN OR CALLUS

NEGATIVE SMEAR OR CULTURE

CARCINOMA, BERIBERI, VARICOSE ULCER

In adults, forehead enlargement is seen in Paget's disease, fibrous dysplasia, leontiasis ossea, and acromegaly. It may also be a normal process as the frontal air sinuses develop over the years. In children, forehead enlargement may be due to hydrocephalus, rickets, congenital syphilis, and a large hematoma.

DIAGNOSTIC WORKUP

X-ray of the skull; tests for calcium, phosphorus, and acid alkaline phosphatase; and a VDRL test should be performed in all cases. When other signs of acromegaly are present, serum growth hormone level should be measured. Children may need a referral to a pediatrician.

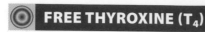

FREE THYROXINE (T₄)

INCREASED

ASK THE FOLLOWING QUESTIONS:

1. **Is there an elevated sedimentation rate?** An elevated sedimentation rate coupled with an increased Free T_4 suggests subacute thyroiditis.
2. **Is the radioactive iodine (RAI) uptake increased?** This would indicate Grave's disease or toxic nodular goiter. If the RAI uptake is normal or decreased, look for iatrogenic hyperthyroidism.

DECREASED

ASK THE FOLLOWING QUESTIONS:

1. **What is the TSH level?** If the TSH is elevated, the patient has myxedema (hypothyroidism).
2. **What are the results of a thyroid releasing factor (TRF) stimulation test?**

If there is no response to this test, the patient has pituitary insufficiency. If there is a response, the patient probably has tertiary hypothyroidism (a lesion in the hypothalamus) or T3 thyrotoxicosis.

DIAGNOSTIC WORKUP

To further evaluate an increased Free thyroxine, it would be wise to order a CT Scan of the brain and thyroid as well as an endocrinology consult or a trial of therapy. The same holds true for a low Free thyroxine except, in addition, one may need to order ultrasonography of the thyroid, a needle biopsy, or exploratory surgery.

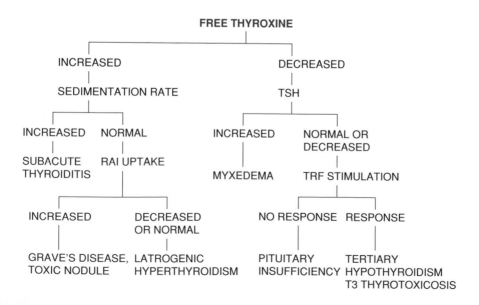

ASK THE FOLLOWING QUESTIONS:

1. **Is the 24-hr urine volume increased?** If the 24-hr urine volume is increased, then one has identified polyuria. The differential diagnosis of this condition is found on page 379.
2. **Is there dysuria?** If there is dysuria, one should consider cystitis, urethritis, prostatitis, bladder calculi, and tuberculosis of the bladder. If there is no dysuria, then a bladder neck obstruction from conditions such as prostatic hypertrophy or urethral stricture might be considered. One should also consider a spastic neurogenic bladder.
3. **Is there fever?** If there is fever along with frequency of urination, this could be due to a systemic condition, but it is more important to look for pyelonephritis.

DIAGNOSTIC WORKUP

The first thing to do is a urinalysis and examine the urinary sediment. This will help determine if there is a UTI and if there is diabetes or one of the other causes of polyuria. A sterile sample of the urine should be sent to the lab for culture regardless of whether the urinalysis is normal.

If these studies are unremarkable, a 24-hr urine volume is determined. If the urine volume is substantially increased, the workup may proceed for polyuria (see page 379). If the 24-hr urine volume is normal, a pelvic and rectal examination must be done for a mass that might be pressing on the bladder. Even if the pelvic and rectal examination is negative, pelvic ultrasound may disclose a pelvic mass.

The next step would be to catheterize for residual urine. If the residual urine is large, bladder neck obstruction is probably the problem, and prostatic hypertrophy, median bar hypertrophy, and urethral stricture must be considered.

Further studies include an intravenous pyelogram, cystogram, cystoscopy, and retrograde pyelography, but these should be done in consultation with a urologist. If a spastic neurogenic bladder is suspected, order cystometric tests and a neurology consult.

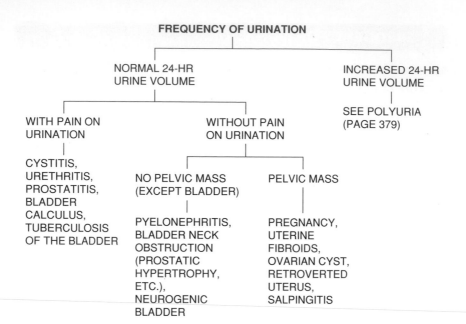

FREQUENCY OF URINATION

NORMAL 24-HR URINE VOLUME

INCREASED 24-HR URINE VOLUME

SEE POLYURIA (PAGE 379)

WITH PAIN ON URINATION

CYSTITIS, URETHRITIS, PROSTATITIS, BLADDER CALCULUS, TUBERCULOSIS OF THE BLADDER

WITHOUT PAIN ON URINATION

NO PELVIC MASS (EXCEPT BLADDER)

PYELONEPHRITIS, BLADDER NECK OBSTRUCTION (PROSTATIC HYPERTROPHY, ETC.), NEUROGENIC BLADDER

PELVIC MASS

PREGNANCY, UTERINE FIBROIDS, OVARIAN CYST, RETROVERTED UTERUS, SALPINGITIS

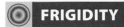

ASK THE FOLLOWING QUESTIONS:

1. **Are there abnormalities on the vaginal examination?** Imperforated hymen, a mass in the cul-de-sac, a retroverted uterus, pregnancy, pelvic inflammatory disease, and cystitis are just a few of the conditions that might be found.
2. **Are there abnormalities on the rectal examination?** The rectal examination may disclose anal fissures, hemorrhoids, or perirectal abscess.
3. **Are there abnormalities of the secondary sexual characteristics?** Turner's syndrome and testicular feminization are two of the conditions that may be associated with these abnormalities.
4. **Is there a history of emotional trauma?** Childhood sexual molestations and marital difficulties are among the conditions that may be found on a careful history.

DIAGNOSTIC WORKUP

First, one should do a good pelvic and rectal examination. If abnormalities are found on these examinations, referral to a gynecologist or a proctologist can be made. If the pelvic and rectal examinations are normal, the patient should probably be referred to a psychiatrist or psychologist for treatment. If there are abnormalities of the secondary sexual characteristics, the clinician may undertake studies of these disorders, but referral to an endocrinologist is probably more cost-effective.

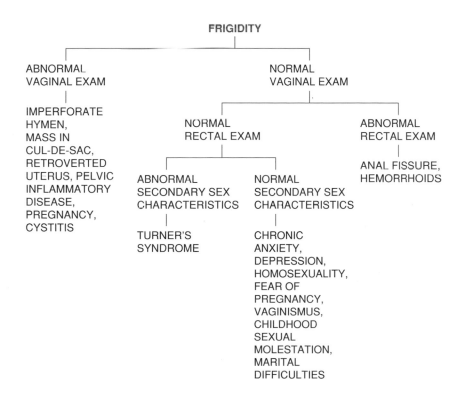

ASK THE FOLLOWING QUESTIONS:

1. **Are there abnormalities on neurologic examination?** An abnormal neurologic examination should make one think of multiple sclerosis, peripheral neuropathy, muscular dystrophy, Parkinson's disease, Huntington's chorea, and a host of degenerative neurologic conditions.
2. **Is there a painful limp?** The findings of a painful limp should make one suspect hip, knee, or ankle joint pathology. In children, consider child abuse. A herniated lumbar disk may also cause a characteristic antalgic gait.
3. **Is the gait characteristic of a particular type?** Characteristic gaits include the short-stepped shuffling gait of Parkinson's disease, the ataxic gait of multiple sclerosis and cerebellar disorders, the reeling, clownish gait of Huntington's chorea, the pelvic tilt of muscular dystrophy, and the steppage gait of peripheral neuropathy.
4. **Could the gait disturbance be due to malingering or hysteria?** The gait of conversion hysteria is quite remarkable. The patient has a normal neurologic examination and has no difficulty maintaining balance while sitting down, but there is total inability to walk or stand without reeling about.

DIAGNOSTIC WORKUP

Routine orders would include a CBC, sedimentation rate, chemistry panel, VDRL test, and urinalysis. If there is a painful limp, x-rays of the hip, knee, or ankle on the affected side should be performed. An x-ray of the lumbar spine will not usually be of great assistance, however. If plain x-rays are negative, a CT scan or MRI of the lumbar spine, hip, knee, or ankle may be of assistance in the diagnosis. A bone scan may pick up obscure fractures and other pathology.

If there are abnormalities on the neurologic examination, MRI or CT scan of the appropriate level of suspected pathology will be done. A spastic gait with abnormal cranial nerve findings would suggest a cerebral tumor or other brain disease, and a CT scan or MRI of the brain should be done. Keep in mind that the MRI is almost double the cost of a CT scan, and the diagnostic yield is not that much greater in many cases.

A spastic gait without cranial nerve signs or papilledema would suggest a spinal cord disorder, and an MRI or CT scan of the appropriate level of the spinal cord should be done. A CT scan of the cervical spine, however, is not very useful and MRI is preferred.

If multiple sclerosis is suspected, a spinal tap for myelin basic protein or gamma-globulin levels should be done. A VEP study, a BSEP study, or a SSEP study will also be useful in diagnosing multiple sclerosis.

If there is an ataxic gait, cerebellar disorder should be suspected, and a CT scan of the brain may be done. However, an ataxic gait may also suggest multiple sclerosis, pernicious anemia, and tabes dorsalis. If the VDRL test is negative, a FTA-ABS test should be done. Blood levels for vitamin B_{12} and folic acid will help diagnose pernicious anemia. A Schilling test, however, is sometimes necessary to facilitate this diagnosis. If muscular dystrophy is suspected, electromyographic examination and muscle biopsy will help confirm the diagnosis. If the patient has a steppage gait, the workup of peripheral neuropathy should be done, as noted on page 356.

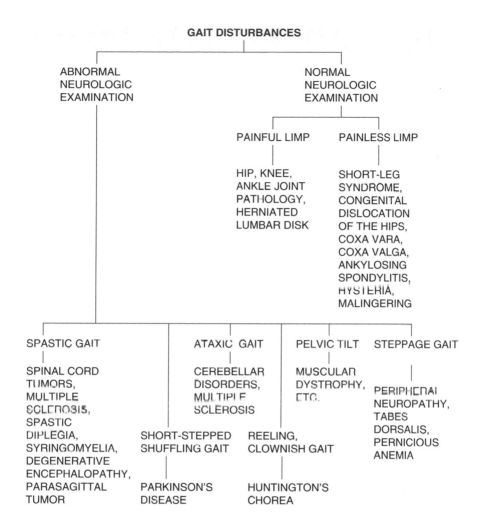

GAIT DISTURBANCES

ABNORMAL NEUROLOGIC EXAMINATION

NORMAL NEUROLOGIC EXAMINATION

PAINFUL LIMP

HIP, KNEE, ANKLE JOINT PATHOLOGY, HERNIATED LUMBAR DISK

PAINLESS LIMP

SHORT-LEG SYNDROME, CONGENITAL DISLOCATION OF THE HIPS, COXA VARA, COXA VALGA, ANKYLOSING SPONDYLITIS, HYSTERIA, MALINGERING

SPASTIC GAIT

SPINAL CORD TUMORS, MULTIPLE SCLEROSIS, SPASTIC DIPLEGIA, SYRINGOMYELIA, DEGENERATIVE ENCEPHALOPATHY, PARASAGITTAL TUMOR

ATAXIC GAIT

CEREBELLAR DISORDERS, MULTIPLE SCLEROSIS

SHORT-STEPPED SHUFFLING GAIT

PARKINSON'S DISEASE

REELING, CLOWNISH GAIT

HUNTINGTON'S CHOREA

PELVIC TILT

MUSCULAR DYSTROPHY, ETC.

STEPPAGE GAIT

PERIPHERAL NEUROPATHY, TABES DORSALIS, PERNICIOUS ANEMIA

GANGRENE

ASK THE FOLLOWING QUESTIONS:

1. **Does it involve the upper or lower extremity?** Involvement of the upper extremities should suggest Raynaud's disease, scleroderma, and other collagen diseases. The Allen test will be helpful in diagnosing Raynaud's disease.
2. **Are there good peripheral pulses?** The complete absence of a peripheral pulse, particularly if it is sudden onset, should suggest an arterial embolism. If it is gradual onset, suspect arteriosclerosis or diabetic ulcer.
3. **Are there signs of systemic disease?** If there are other signs of systemic disease, collagen disease, macroglobulinemia, and cryoglobulinemia should be suspected.
4. **Is the gangrene sudden in onset?** A sudden onset of the gangrene should make one suspect clostridia infections or arterial embolism.
5. **Is there a positive culture?** The culture will be positive in clostridia infections, anthrax, and cancrum oris.

DIAGNOSTIC WORKUP

Routine orders include a CBC, sedimentation rate, chemistry panel, VDRL test, serum protein electrophoresis, ANA titer, and glucose tolerance test. The gangrenous area should be cultured. Plain x-rays of the area sometimes are helpful. If there are diminished pulses, especially if the onset is acute, angiography will be useful. A muscle biopsy or skin biopsy will be useful in diagnosing collagen diseases. The Sia water test and serum immunoelectrophoresis will be useful in diagnosing macroglobulinemia and cryoglobulinemia.

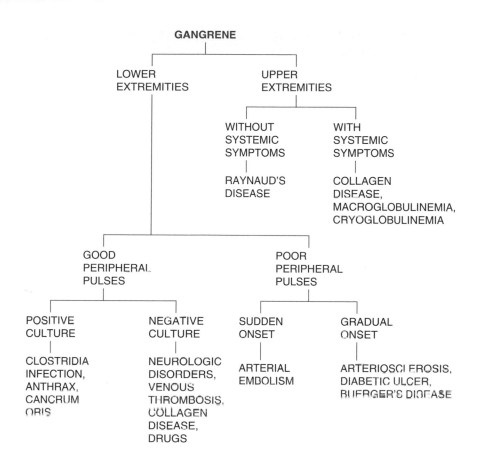

GANGRENE

LOWER
EXTREMITIES

UPPER
EXTREMITIES

WITHOUT
SYSTEMIC
SYMPTOMS

RAYNAUD'S
DISEASE

WITH
SYSTEMIC
SYMPTOMS

COLLAGEN
DISEASE,
MACROGLOBULINEMIA,
CRYOGLOBULINEMIA

GOOD
PERIPHERAL
PULSES

POOR
PERIPHERAL
PULSES

POSITIVE
CULTURE

CLOSTRIDIA
INFECTION,
ANTHRAX,
CANCRUM
ORIS

NEGATIVE
CULTURE

NEUROLOGIC
DISORDERS,
VENOUS
THROMBOSIS,
COLLAGEN
DISEASE,
DRUGS

SUDDEN
ONSET

ARTERIAL
EMBOLISM

GRADUAL
ONSET

ARTERIOSCLEROSIS,
DIABETIC ULCER,
BUERGER'S DISEASE

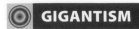

GIGANTISM

ASK THE FOLLOWING QUESTIONS:

1. **Are there abnormal secondary sex characteristics?** Patients with Klinefelter's syndrome, supermale, superfemale, sexual precocity, and virilism have abnormal secondary sex characteristics and a tall stature.
2. **Is there arachnodactyly?** Arachnodactyly is associated with Marfan's syndrome and homocystinuria.
3. **Is there a family history?** Patients with a family history of tall stature often have constitutional tall stature and not pituitary gigantism.

DIAGNOSTIC WORKUP

X-rays of the skull and a CT scan will help identify a pituitary eosinophilic adenoma, but serum growth hormone will also be elevated early, and FSH and LH may be depressed later. An MRI will be necessary to pick up microadenomas. Serum FSH and LH will be elevated in Klinefelter's syndrome. A chromosome study should be done to identify Klinefelter's syndrome, supermale, and superfemale. A serum testosterone, dihydrotestosterone, and dehydroepiandrosterone sulfate will be helpful in diagnosing sexual precocity and virilism caused by tumors and hyperplasia of the adrenal gland. Echocardiography and urinary hydroxyproline will help identify Marfan's syndrome, whereas a urine for homocystine will help diagnose homocystinuria. A thyroid profile should be done to rule out thyrotoxicosis.

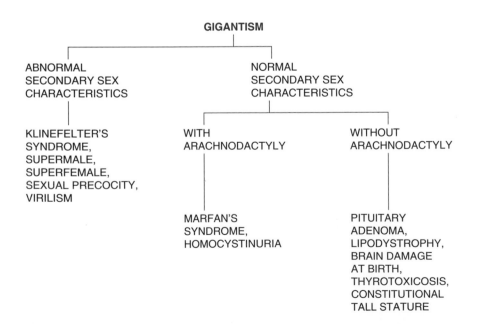

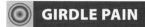

ASK THE FOLLOWING QUESTIONS:

1. **Is there an associated rash?** Presence of a rash, whether it is macular or vesicular, especially if it is in a dermatomal distribution, would suggest herpes zoster. Occasionally, herpes zoster occurs without a rash and should still be considered in the differential diagnosis.

2. **Are there pyramidal tract or other long tract signs?** The findings of long tract signs would indicate compression, degeneration, or inflammation of the spinal cord, and conditions such as multiple sclerosis, acute transverse myelitis, spinal cord tumor, herniated disk, and pernicious anemia should be considered. If there are no long tract signs and no rash, one should consider early spinal cord tumor or herniated disk, intercostal neuralgia, fractured ribs, and sometimes a compression fracture of the vertebra.

DIAGNOSTIC WORKUP

Patients with a rash, particularly if it is vesicular and in a dermatomal distribution, may be treated for herpes zoster before doing an extensive diagnostic workup. However, one should remember that herpes zoster may be associated with an underlying neoplasm, particularly Hodgkin's disease.

If a patient does not have a rash, routine laboratory tests include a CBC, chemistry panel, sedimentation rate, VDRL test, serum B_{12}, and folic acid. In addition, x-rays of the chest, ribs, and thoracic spine should be done. If these are normal and the diagnosis remains in doubt, one should consult a neurologist. If none is available, MRI of the thoracic spine may be ordered. A spinal tap may be done to help rule out multiple sclerosis and tabes dorsalis. SSEP studies can be done to diagnose multiple sclerosis. A thoracic myelogram is occasionally necessary in confusing cases.

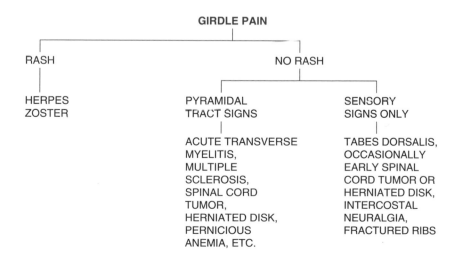

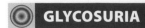
GLYCOSURIA

ASK THE FOLLOWING QUESTIONS:

1. **Was the test used specific for glucose?** Glucose oxidase tests (Clinistix, etc.) are specific for glucose, whereas other tests (Benedict's, etc.) are not. Thus, the latter will give false positives for lactose, fructose, galactose, and salicylates.
2. **What is the blood sugar?** If the blood sugar is elevated or a glucose tolerance test is positive, one should suspect diabetes mellitus. If these tests are normal, one should suspect renal glycosuria, pregnancy, or renal tubular acidosis.

DIAGNOSTIC WORKUP

The investigation of glycosuria should include a glucose tolerance test, chemistry panel, and electrolyte panel. If there are clinical features of an endocrine disorder, the various tests for these disorders should be ordered.

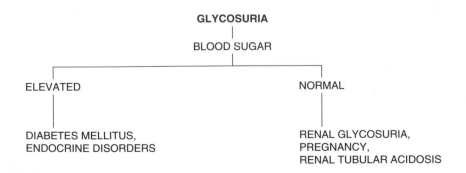

GYNECOMASTIA

ASK THE FOLLOWING QUESTIONS:

1. **Is there a history of drug or alcohol ingestion?** Digitalis, phenothiazine, amphetamine, marijuana, and many other drugs may cause gynecomastia.
2. **Is there a testicular mass?** Leydig's cell and Sertoli's cell tumors of the testicle may cause gynecomastia.
3. **Are there abnormal secondary sex characteristics?** Klinefelter's syndrome, male pseudohermaphroditism, and testicular feminization syndrome may cause gynecomastia.
4. **Is there a bronze skin?** If there is a bronze skin, one should consider hemochromatosis, as this may be associated with gynecomastia.
5. **Are there other endocrine abnormalities?** Cushing's syndrome, Addison's disease, and hyperthyroidism may cause gynecomastia.
6. **Are there abnormalities on neurologic examination?** Myotonic dystrophy, paraplegias of various types, and Friedreich's ataxia are among the many neurologic disorders that may be associated with gynecomastia.

DIAGNOSTIC WORKUP

A urine drug screen and thyroid profile should be done at the outset. Liver function studies, liver biopsy, and serum iron and iron-binding capacity will help rule out hemochromatosis and cirrhosis of the liver. A serum FSH, LH, IICG, and estradiol will help diagnose testicular tumors, Klinefelter's syndrome, and testicular feminization syndrome. Further evidence of Klinefelter's syndrome is obtained by a buccal smear (Barr bodies). Normal gonadotropin and sex hormone levels make serious pathology unlikely. A serum cortisol, cortisol suppression test, and rapid adrenocorticotropic hormone (ACTH) test will help diagnose Cushing's syndrome and Addison's disease. There is a specific beta-HCG assay that can be done to rule out an HCG-secreting tumor such as carcinoma of the lung.

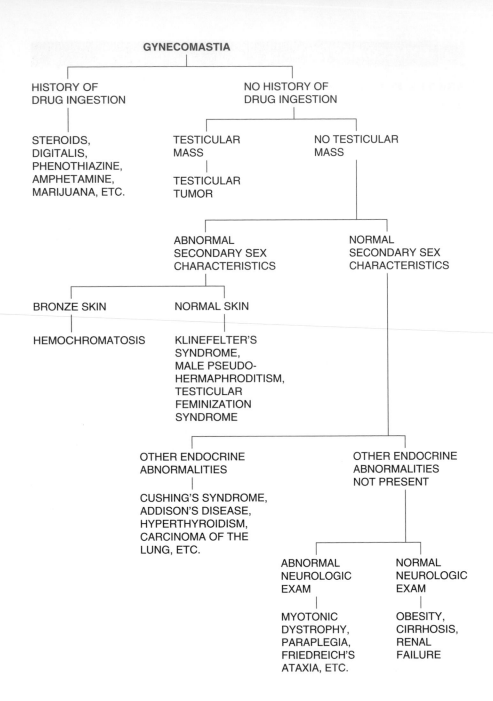

GYNECOMASTIA

HISTORY OF
DRUG INGESTION

STEROIDS,
DIGITALIS,
PHENOTHIAZINE,
AMPHETAMINE,
MARIJUANA, ETC.

NO HISTORY OF
DRUG INGESTION

TESTICULAR
MASS

TESTICULAR
TUMOR

NO TESTICULAR
MASS

ABNORMAL
SECONDARY SEX
CHARACTERISTICS

NORMAL
SECONDARY SEX
CHARACTERISTICS

BRONZE SKIN

HEMOCHROMATOSIS

NORMAL SKIN

KLINEFELTER'S
SYNDROME,
MALE PSEUDO-
HERMAPHRODITISM,
TESTICULAR
FEMINIZATION
SYNDROME

OTHER ENDOCRINE
ABNORMALITIES

CUSHING'S SYNDROME,
ADDISON'S DISEASE,
HYPERTHYROIDISM,
CARCINOMA OF THE
LUNG, ETC.

OTHER ENDOCRINE
ABNORMALITIES
NOT PRESENT

ABNORMAL
NEUROLOGIC
EXAM

MYOTONIC
DYSTROPHY,
PARAPLEGIA,
FRIEDREICH'S
ATAXIA, ETC.

NORMAL
NEUROLOGIC
EXAM

OBESITY,
CIRRHOSIS,
RENAL
FAILURE

ASK THE FOLLOWING QUESTIONS:

1. **Is there a history of ingestion or use of a foul substance?** Such a history may suggest that the cause is onions, garlic, alcohol, tobacco, paraldehyde, mercury, or other substances. A garlic odor to the breath is common to many poisonings (arsenic, organophosphates, etc.).

2. **Are there abnormalities of examination of the mouth, nose, and throat?** Abnormalities that may be found on examination of the mouth, nose, and throat include gingivitis, carious teeth, pyorrhea, stomatitis, sinusitis, pharyngitis, and tonsillitis.

3. **Is there a chronic productive cough?** The presence of a chronic productive cough should suggest bronchiectasis, lung abscess, gangrene of the lungs, tuberculosis, and other lung infections.

4. **Is there esophageal regurgitation?** The history of esophageal regurgitation should suggest reflux esophagitis, peptic ulcer, partial intestinal obstruction, and esophageal diverticula. If there are none of these findings, one should look for uremia or cirrhosis.

DIAGNOSTIC WORKUP

Routine tests include a CBC and sedimentation rate to rule out chronic inflammation; a chemistry panel to rule out uremia and cirrhosis; and sputum, nose, and throat cultures to rule out chronic infections of the sinuses, nose, throat, and lungs. Cultures of any suspicious area of inflammation in the mouth, nose, and throat should be done. X-rays of the teeth, sinuses, and chest should also be done. An upper GI series and esophagogram will help diagnose reflux esophagitis, peptic ulcer, partial intestinal obstruction, and esophageal diverticula.

A 24-hr sputum collection may help differentiate bronchiectasis and lung abscesses. A tuberculin test and sputum for AFB smear, culture, and possible guinea pig inoculation may identify tuberculosis.

HALITOSIS

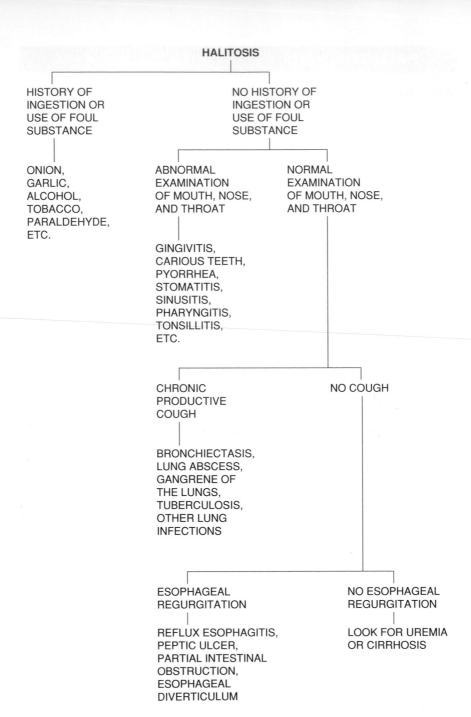

HISTORY OF
INGESTION OR
USE OF FOUL
SUBSTANCE

NO HISTORY OF
INGESTION OR
USE OF FOUL
SUBSTANCE

ONION,
GARLIC,
ALCOHOL,
TOBACCO,
PARALDEHYDE,
ETC.

ABNORMAL
EXAMINATION
OF MOUTH, NOSE,
AND THROAT

NORMAL
EXAMINATION
OF MOUTH, NOSE,
AND THROAT

GINGIVITIS,
CARIOUS TEETH,
PYORRHEA,
STOMATITIS,
SINUSITIS,
PHARYNGITIS,
TONSILLITIS,
ETC.

CHRONIC
PRODUCTIVE
COUGH

NO COUGH

BRONCHIECTASIS,
LUNG ABSCESS,
GANGRENE OF
THE LUNGS,
TUBERCULOSIS,
OTHER LUNG
INFECTIONS

ESOPHAGEAL
REGURGITATION

NO ESOPHAGEAL
REGURGITATION

REFLUX ESOPHAGITIS,
PEPTIC ULCER,
PARTIAL INTESTINAL
OBSTRUCTION,
ESOPHAGEAL
DIVERTICULUM

LOOK FOR UREMIA
OR CIRRHOSIS

HALLUCINATIONS

ASK THE FOLLOWING QUESTIONS:

1. **Is there a history of drug or alcohol ingestion?** Hallucinations are common during alcohol withdrawal but also may be noted in cocaine addiction, marijuana addiction, LSD intoxication, and PCP intoxication.

2. **Are the hallucinations primarily visual in nature?** This would suggest an organic cause such as organic brain syndrome, epilepsy, brain tumor, etc.

3. **Are the hallucinations episodic?** If the hallucinations occur in episodes with normal behavior in between, one should consider epilepsy or narcolepsy.

4. **Are the hallucinations associated with early stages of falling asleep or awakening?** These types of hallucinations are called *hypnogogic* and are common in narcolepsy but may also be seen in normal people.

5. **Are the hallucinations primarily auditory in nature?** This is the type of hallucination most commonly associated with schizophrenia.

DIAGNOSTIC WORKUP

A blood alcohol level and urine drug screen are essential at the outset. A therapeutic trial of IV thiamine should be tried if Wernickes encephalopathy or Korsakoff's psychosis is suspected. Most physicians will want to refer the patient to a psychiatrist if these studies are negative. However, the interested physician may proceed further with a wake-and-sleep EEG to identify psychomotor epilepsy, or a CT scan and MRI to identify brain tumors and other causes of organic brain syndrome. Remember, the MRI costs twice as much as a CT scan. A spinal tap will be helpful in diagnosing central nervous system lues. A sleep study will help diagnose narcolepsy. Psychometric testing will help identify schizophrenia and other psychiatric disorders.

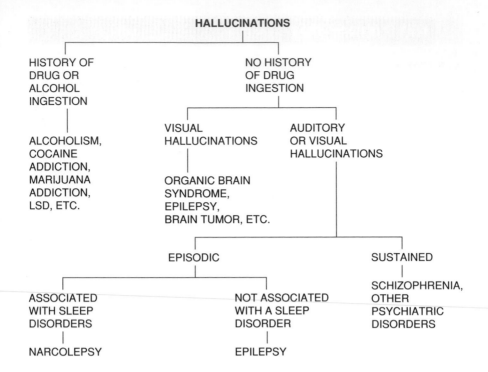

HALLUCINATIONS

HISTORY OF
DRUG OR
ALCOHOL
INGESTION

NO HISTORY
OF DRUG
INGESTION

ALCOHOLISM,
COCAINE
ADDICTION,
MARIJUANA
ADDICTION,
LSD, ETC.

VISUAL
HALLUCINATIONS

AUDITORY
OR VISUAL
HALLUCINATIONS

ORGANIC BRAIN
SYNDROME,
EPILEPSY,
BRAIN TUMOR, ETC.

EPISODIC

SUSTAINED

SCHIZOPHRENIA,
OTHER
PSYCHIATRIC
DISORDERS

ASSOCIATED
WITH SLEEP
DISORDERS

NOT ASSOCIATED
WITH A SLEEP
DISORDER

NARCOLEPSY

EPILEPSY

Smaller localized, freely movable masses are the sebaceous cysts, hematomas, lipomas, and lymph nodes. Masses that seem to be attached to the skull are osteomas, dermoid cysts, and sarcomas. Brain tumor tissue may occasionally protrude out beneath the scalp through a craniotomy defect. Mastoiditis may spread to the subcutaneous tissues also. In the newborn, there may be edema of the scalp (called *caput succedaneum*) following a vertex delivery due to molding or a large hematoma over one or both parietal bones (called *cephalhematoma*) due to the trauma of delivery. There may be meningoceles or encephalomeningoceles due to imperfect closure of the skull (cranium bifidum). Vascular abnormalities of the skin may be found and include angiomas, arteriovenous fistulas, and telangiectasis.

DIAGNOSTIC WORKUP

A skull x-ray will help distinguish the bone lesions, whereas aspiration or biopsy will help distinguish the others. Referral to the appropriate specialist would be the most cost-effective approach.

CASE HISTORY

A 29-year-old obese Hispanic female, gravid ii, para ii, complains of generalized headache for the past 3 months. It is usually worse in the morning and occasionally is associated with nausea but no vomiting. She also complains of blurred vision for the past 6 weeks. Following the algorithm, you ask about a history of drugs, caffeine, or alcohol ingestion with negative results. She denies a history of trauma. There is no nuchal rigidity or focal neurologic signs, but funduscopic examination reveals papilledema and a visual field examination reveals an inferior nasal quadranopsia and enlarged blind spot. You suspect pseudotumor cerebri and an MRI confirms your suspicion.

ASK THE FOLLOWING QUESTIONS:

1. **Is there a history of drug, caffeine, or alcohol ingestion?** The hangover headache is well known and should not present a problem in diagnosis. Caffeine withdrawal headaches are also common because of the large amount of caffeine consumed in coffee, various soft drinks, and chocolate. Drugs that may induce headache include the nonsteroidal anti-inflammatory drugs such as indomethacin (Indocin®) and the antihypertensives such as clonidine, aspirin, quinidine, and bromides.

2. **Is there a history of trauma?** Trauma may cause concussion and postconcussion headaches, intracranial neoplasms such as subdural hematoma, and cervical sprain, all of which can induce headaches.

3. **Is the headache acute or chronic?** An acute onset of a headache can be a serious problem. It should be taken seriously because it may mean a subarachnoid hemorrhage or meningitis. This can be easily confirmed by checking for nuchal rigidity. Whenever there is an acute onset of a headache, this must be done. Chronic headaches, on the other hand, are most likely due either to migraine if they occur in exacerbations or remissions, or to tension headaches if they are fairly constant, mild, and chronic. The headache of a brain tumor is rarely severe and is rarely the presenting symptom of a brain tumor. Headaches that occur in clusters almost daily for 6 to 8 weeks with interruptions of several months must make one consider cluster headaches. Unilateral headaches in the elderly with acute onset should make one think of temporal arteritis.

4. **Is there nuchal rigidity?** The presence of nuchal rigidity should make one think of a subarachnoid hemorrhage or meningitis, but it may also be due to cerebral hemorrhage or cerebral abscess.

5. **Is there fever?** If the headache is associated with fever, the possibility of acute sinusitis should be considered, and the sinuses should be transilluminated. Other sources of the fever should be looked for, and meningitis or encephalitis should be considered.

6. **Is there papilledema or are there focal neurologic signs?** With acute headache and focal neurologic signs and/or papilledema, one should consider cerebral abscess or cerebral hemorrhage. With a chronic headache and papilledema or focal neurologic signs, one should consider a space-occupying lesion such as a primary brain tumor or metastatic neoplasm.

7. **Do the sinuses transilluminate well?** A sinus transilluminator should be in the armamentarium of every physician who expects to diagnose headache. If the sinuses fail to transilluminate, one should consider acute sinusitis as the diagnosis.

8. **Is there tenderness of the superficial temporal artery?** The presence of a tender superficial temporal artery should make one think of temporal arteritis, particularly in the elderly, but it may also be related to a long-standing migraine attack.

9. **Is the headache relieved by superficial temporal artery compression?** Relief of the headache on superficial temporal artery compression should suggest classical or common migraine. If one can relieve the headache by compression of the occipital artery, occipital migraine should be considered. When there is no relief on compression of the superficial temporal artery, one should consider tension headaches, occipital neuralgia, cervical spondylosis, and cluster headaches as the cause.

DIAGNOSTIC WORKUP

Routine diagnostic tests include a CBC to rule out severe anemia, a sedimentation rate to rule out temporal arteritis, a chemistry panel to rule out liver and kidney disease, a VDRL test to rule out central nervous system syphilis, an x-ray of the sinuses to rule out sinusitis, and an x-ray of the cervical spine to exclude cervical spondylosis. A chest x-ray should also be done to rule out the possibility of metastatic neoplasm. A tonometry study may be done if glaucoma is suspected. X-rays or SPECT scans of the temporomandibular joints and referral to an oral surgeon should be done if T-M joint syndrome is suspected.

If there are focal neurologic signs, referral should be made to a neurologist or neurosurgeon as soon as possible. If one is not readily available, a CT scan or MRI may be done, the CT scan being the preferred procedure if the expense is a consideration.

If there is nuchal rigidity, a CT scan should be done to rule out a space-occupying lesion before proceeding with a spinal tap. If the CT scan is negative, a spinal tap can be done, and this will ascertain whether there is intracranial bleeding or meningitis. It is usually best to refer the patient to a neurologist or neurosurgeon if there is nuchal rigidity.

If the headaches are chronic and episodic, and there are no focal neurologic signs, papilledema, or nuchal rigidity, an imaging study can be postponed for a while until the response to treatment is evaluated. However, if the response to treatment is poor, one should not hesitate to order a CT scan or MRI.

Difficult cases of headache should also be studied with 24-hr blood pressure monitoring, a 24-hr urine for catecholamines, and lumbar puncture to diagnose central nervous system lues. Histamine phosphate 0.5 cc subcutaneously may help diagnose cluster headaches. If the patient presents with an acute headache, it is wise to assess the response to sumatriptan orally or by nasal spray. Relief will usually be achieved in patients with migraine or histamine headaches. Response to beta-blockers may help diagnose migraine. Cerebral angiography may be necessary to diagnose aneurysms and arteriovenous malformations. Patients with chronic headache, unresponsive to therapy, should be referred to a psychiatrist.

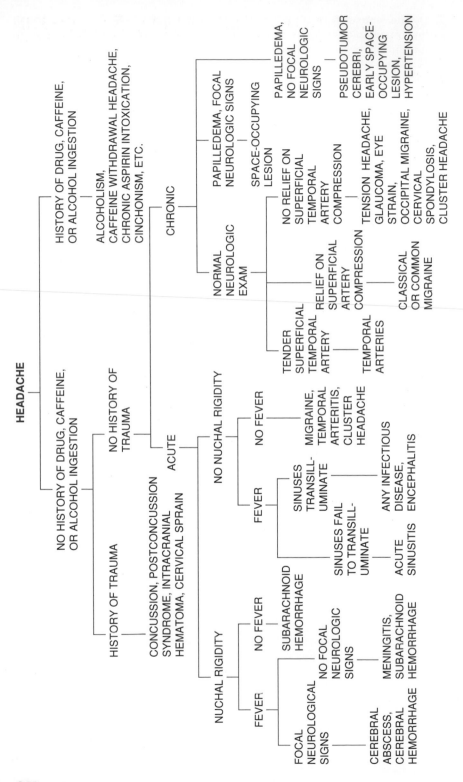

HEADACHE

- HISTORY OF DRUG, CAFFEINE, OR ALCOHOL INGESTION
  - ALCOHOLISM, CAFFEINE WITHDRAWAL HEADACHE, CHRONIC ASPIRIN INTOXICATION, CINCHONISM, ETC.

- NO HISTORY OF DRUG, CAFFEINE, OR ALCOHOL INGESTION
  - HISTORY OF TRAUMA
    - CONCUSSION, POSTCONCUSSION SYNDROME, INTRACRANIAL HEMATOMA, CERVICAL SPRAIN
  - NO HISTORY OF TRAUMA
    - ACUTE
      - NUCHAL RIGIDITY
        - FEVER
          - FOCAL NEUROLOGICAL SIGNS
            - CEREBRAL ABSCESS, CEREBRAL HEMORRHAGE
          - NO FOCAL NEUROLOGIC SIGNS
            - MENINGITIS, SUBARACHNOID HEMORRHAGE
        - NO FEVER
          - SUBARACHNOID HEMORRHAGE
      - NO NUCHAL RIGIDITY
        - FEVER
          - SINUSES TRANSILL-UMINATE
            - ANY INFECTIOUS DISEASE, ENCEPHALITIS
          - SINUSES FAIL TO TRANSILL-UMINATE
            - ACUTE SINUSITIS
        - NO FEVER
          - MIGRAINE, TEMPORAL ARTERITIS, CLUSTER HEADACHE
    - CHRONIC
      - NORMAL NEUROLOGIC EXAM
        - TEMPORAL ARTERIES
          - TENDER SUPERFICIAL TEMPORAL ARTERY
            - RELIEF ON SUPERFICIAL ARTERY COMPRESSION
              - CLASSICAL OR COMMON MIGRAINE
            - NO RELIEF ON SUPERFICIAL TEMPORAL ARTERY COMPRESSION
              - TENSION HEADACHE, GLAUCOMA, EYE STRAIN, OCCIPITAL MIGRAINE, CERVICAL SPONDYLOSIS, CLUSTER HEADACHE
      - PAPILLEDEMA, FOCAL NEUROLOGIC SIGNS
        - SPACE-OCCUPYING LESION
        - PAPILLEDEMA, NO FOCAL NEUROLOGIC SIGNS
          - PSEUDOTUMOR CEREBRI, EARLY SPACE-OCCUPYING LESION, HYPERTENSION

CASE HISTORY

A 52-year-old white male laboratory technician is brought to the emergency room with acute chest pain and pain on swallowing. He gives a long history of heartburn relieved by antacids. Following the algorithm, you administer nitroglycerin without relief. The heartburn is associated with regurgitation, so you administer a GI "cocktail" which includes lidocaine viscus and his pain is relieved. You suspect reflux esophagitis and your diagnosis is confirmed by esophageal pH monitoring and esophagoscopy.

ASK THE FOLLOWING QUESTIONS:

1. **Is there frequent regurgitation?** If there is frequent regurgitation, the most likely diagnosis is reflux esophagitis and hiatal hernia. Gastritis and a previous gastrectomy will also cause frequent regurgitation.
2. **Is there recurrent nausea or vomiting?** If there is recurrent nausea or vomiting, the most likely diagnosis is cholecystitis and cholelithiasis. Chronic pancreatitis can cause the same symptoms, however.
3. **Is the heartburn precipitated by exercise and/or relieved by nitroglycerin?** These findings suggest coronary insufficiency.
4. **Is there associated hematemesis or recurrent black stool?** The presence of hematemesis or recurrent black stools should suggest a peptic ulcer.
5. **Is there relief with lidocaine hydrochloride (Xylocaine® Viscous Solution)?** The relief of the pain on viscous lidocaine suggests reflux esophagitis, hiatal hernia, and previous gastrectomy with bile esophagitis. Gastritis is not usually relieved by viscous Xylocaine®.

DIAGNOSTIC WORKUP

The workup begins with an upper GI series and esophagogram and stools for occult blood. If these studies are negative, it may be prudent to give the patient a trial of proton pump inhibitors. If there is recurrent vomiting and right upper quadrant pain, a gallbladder ultrasound or cholecystogram should be done. If these are negative, it is best to refer the patient to a gastroenterologist for esophagoscopy and gastroscopy. The gastroenterologist may do a Bernstein test, which will reproduce symptoms by an infusion of dilute hydrochloric acid into the distal esophagus, or perform esophageal manometry or pH monitoring of the distal esophagus. An exercise tolerance test and coronary angiography also have their place in the diagnostic armamentarium. A breath test or a stool for *Helicobacter pylori* antigen should be ordered in persistent cases.

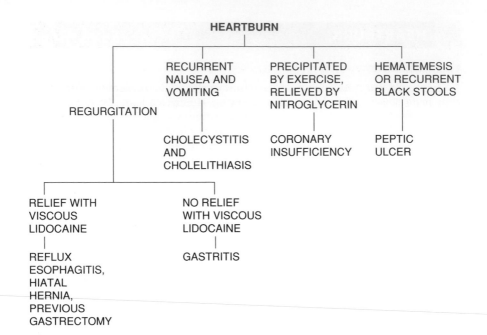

ASK THE FOLLOWING QUESTIONS:

1. **Are there abnormalities on inspection of the heel?** Inspection of the heel may disclose an ulcer, foreign body, cellulitis, plantar wart, and other disorders.
2. **Is the patient a child?** Children often have Sever's disease (osteochondritis of the heel).
3. **Is there tenderness or deformity of the Achilles tendon?** Tenderness or deformity of the Achilles tendon should suggest Achilles tendinitis, rupture, or bursitis.
4. **Are there abnormalities on x-ray examination?** An x-ray may disclose a calcaneal fracture, osteomyelitis, a tumor, or calcaneal spur. If the x-ray is negative, plantar fasciitis is the most likely diagnosis, but one should also consider gout.

DIAGNOSTIC WORKUP

In addition to a plain x-ray of the foot, a CBC, sedimentation rate, chemistry panel, and arthritis panel should be done. A bone scan may disclose an occult fracture. Response to a trigger point injection should be evaluated. If the diagnosis is still in doubt, referral to an orthopedic surgeon or podiatrist should be made before ordering expensive diagnostic tests such as a CT scan or MRI.

HEEL PAIN

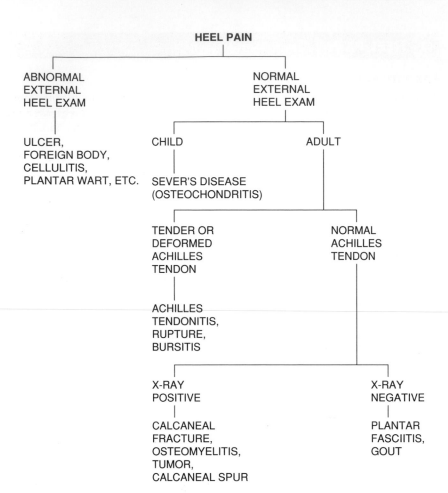

HEMATEMESIS

CASE HISTORY

A 44-year-old white female is brought in the middle of the night to the emergency room with a history of vomiting bright red blood. Following the algorithm, you look for a history of fever and chills, and find none. Her temperature is 97.8° F. There is no history of drug or alcohol ingestion, but she ate out the evening prior to admission and the food did not agree with her. There is no abdominal pain. On further questioning, you find out that there was no blood in the initial episodes of vomiting. You suspect a Mallory–Weiss Syndrome, and esophagoscopy confirms your suspicion.

ASK THE FOLLOWING QUESTIONS:

1. **Is there fever?** The presence of fever should suggest scarlet fever, measles, malaria, leptospirosis, yellow fever, and other acute and chronic infectious diseases.
2. **Is there a history of ingestion of poison, drugs, or alcohol?** Poison, many drugs, and alcohol may cause acute gastritis, gastric ulcer, and corrosive esophagitis.
3. **Is there associated abdominal pain?** Abdominal pain associated with the hematemesis suggests the possibility of gastric or duodenal ulcer, a hiatal hernia, and esophagitis or carcinoma of the stomach. Of course, any of these conditions may occur without abdominal pain.
4. **Was the hematemesis preceded by blood-free vomitus?** If in the initial stages of vomiting the vomitus was blood-free, one should consider Mallory–Weiss syndrome, which is a tear of the distal esophagus due to severe vomiting.
5. **Is there hepatomegaly or splenomegaly?** Hepatomegaly would suggest cirrhosis of the liver, whereas a portal vein thrombosis may occur without hepatomegaly but almost certainly is associated with splenomegaly. Splenomegaly should suggest Banti's syndrome with depression of platelets, leukocytes, and anemia. Splenomegaly also suggests other blood dyscrasias.
6. **Is there a positive tourniquet test or Ivy skin bleeding time?** These tests may indicate thrombocytopenia and other blood dyscrasias. If these tests are negative and there is no hepatomegaly, splenomegaly, or abdominal pain, one should consider hereditary hemorrhagic telangiectasia, an aortic aneurysm, and pseudoxanthoma elasticum.

DIAGNOSTIC WORKUP

Hematemesis, no matter how small, is a clear indication for immediate consultation with a gastroenterologist and esophagoscopy, gastroscopy, and duodenoscopy. To delay this while ordering an upper GI series and other diagnostic tests may place the patient in serious jeopardy. The clinician would be prudent to order a CBC and coagulation profile, type, and cross-match of several units of blood while waiting for the gastroenterologist to see the patient. If endoscopy fails to locate the site of bleeding, arteriography may do so. A technetium-99m bleeding scan may be ordered to detect suspected bleeding but will not locate the exact site of bleeding. Liver function tests should be ordered to rule out cirrhosis in all cases.

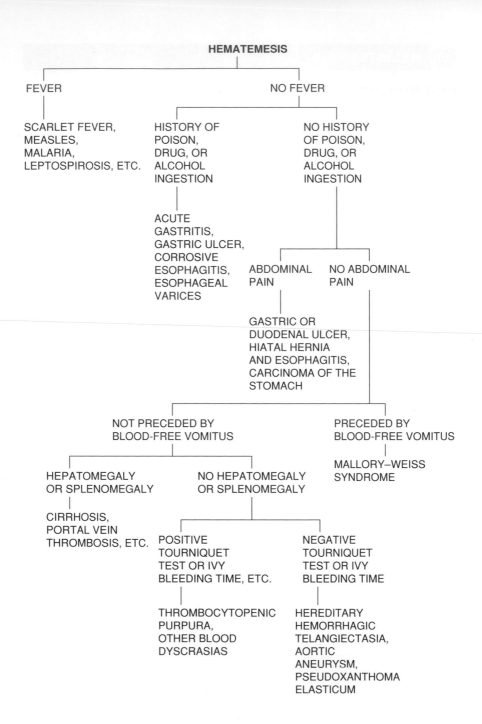

HEMATEMESIS

FEVER

SCARLET FEVER,
MEASLES,
MALARIA,
LEPTOSPIROSIS, ETC.

NO FEVER

HISTORY OF
POISON,
DRUG, OR
ALCOHOL
INGESTION

ACUTE
GASTRITIS,
GASTRIC ULCER,
CORROSIVE
ESOPHAGITIS,
ESOPHAGEAL
VARICES

NO HISTORY
OF POISON,
DRUG, OR
ALCOHOL
INGESTION

ABDOMINAL
PAIN

NO ABDOMINAL
PAIN

GASTRIC OR
DUODENAL ULCER,
HIATAL HERNIA
AND ESOPHAGITIS,
CARCINOMA OF THE
STOMACH

NOT PRECEDED BY
BLOOD-FREE VOMITUS

PRECEDED BY
BLOOD-FREE VOMITUS

MALLORY–WEISS
SYNDROME

HEPATOMEGALY
OR SPLENOMEGALY

CIRRHOSIS,
PORTAL VEIN
THROMBOSIS, ETC.

NO HEPATOMEGALY
OR SPLENOMEGALY

POSITIVE
TOURNIQUET
TEST OR IVY
BLEEDING TIME, ETC.

THROMBOCYTOPENIC
PURPURA,
OTHER BLOOD
DYSCRASIAS

NEGATIVE
TOURNIQUET
TEST OR IVY
BLEEDING TIME

HEREDITARY
HEMORRHAGIC
TELANGIECTASIA,
AORTIC
ANEURYSM,
PSEUDOXANTHOMA
ELASTICUM

HEMATURIA

CASE HISTORY

A 28-year-old white male is found to have blood in his urine on a routine physical examination. Your investigation follows the algorithm. He denies a history of abdominal pain or dysuria, but you order a urine culture anyway. There is no history of fever or chills.

Your examination reveals bilateral flank masses and hypertension. You suspect polycystic kidney disease and you would be correct.

ASK THE FOLLOWING QUESTIONS:

1. **Is there abdominal pain?** The presence of abdominal pain with hematuria should first suggest renal calculus, but other causes, such as renal embolism, renal contusion, or laceration, must be considered.
2. **Is there dysuria or frequency of micturition associated with the hematuria?** The presence of dysuria and frequency with the hematuria should suggest a bladder stone, prostatic disease, or a UTI.
3. **Is there fever?** The presence of fever with the hematuria would suggest pyelonephritis.
4. **Is there a flank mass?** The presence of bilateral flank masses with hematuria should suggest polycystic kidneys and hydronephrosis, whereas a unilateral flank mass would suggest a hypernephroma or unilateral hydronephrosis. A solitary cyst or renal vein thrombosis may also present with a flank mass and hematuria.
5. **Is there hypertension?** The presence of hypertension with the hematuria suggests glomerulonephritis, polycystic kidneys, and collagen diseases.
6. **Are there other systemic signs and symptoms?** If there are other systemic signs and symptoms, one should be looking for collagen disease, coagulation disorders, leukemia, and sickle cell anemia. When there is no hypertension or other signs and symptoms of systemic diseases, one should be looking for a benign or malignant tumor of the bladder, tuberculosis, or parasitic infection.

DIAGNOSTIC WORKUP

The workup begins with a urinalysis and microscopic examination of the urinary sediment. The physician can easily do this in his office. If there is proteinuria, granular cast, and red cell cast, glomerulonephritis or collagen disease should be suspected. A culture and sensitivity and colony count should be done if a UTI is suspected. A three-glass test may be done. If there is blood in the initial specimen, the cause is most likely in the urethra or male genitalia. If it is in the final specimen, the cause is most likely a bladder lesion. Phase-contrast microscopy may also be helpful in identifying hematuria from a glomerular lesion. If this is negative, an anaerobic culture should be done also and then an AFB smear and culture and guinea pig inoculation to rule out tuberculosis. Instead of doing an IVP a spiral CT scan of the abdomen is done at this point because it yields much more information. A CBC, sedimentation rate, chemistry panel, coagulation profile, and ANA test will help rule out blood dyscrasias, collagen diseases, and other systemic diseases. Ultrasonography may help diagnose a renal cyst.

If the above are not revealing, referral to a urologist is indicated. He will probably do a cystoscopy and retrograde pyelography. He may also want to order a renal biopsy. Renal angiography and aortography may be necessary to evaluate renovascular hypertension and renal embolism.

HEMATURIA

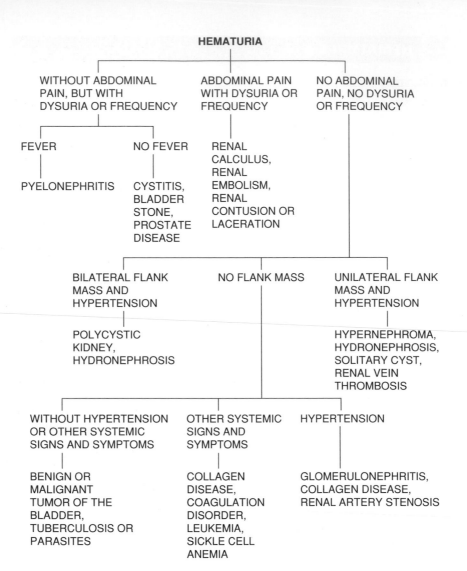

WITHOUT ABDOMINAL PAIN, BUT WITH DYSURIA OR FREQUENCY

ABDOMINAL PAIN WITH DYSURIA OR FREQUENCY

NO ABDOMINAL PAIN, NO DYSURIA OR FREQUENCY

FEVER

NO FEVER

RENAL CALCULUS, RENAL EMBOLISM, RENAL CONTUSION OR LACERATION

PYELONEPHRITIS

CYSTITIS, BLADDER STONE, PROSTATE DISEASE

BILATERAL FLANK MASS AND HYPERTENSION

NO FLANK MASS

UNILATERAL FLANK MASS AND HYPERTENSION

POLYCYSTIC KIDNEY, HYDRONEPHROSIS

HYPERNEPHROMA, HYDRONEPHROSIS, SOLITARY CYST, RENAL VEIN THROMBOSIS

WITHOUT HYPERTENSION OR OTHER SYSTEMIC SIGNS AND SYMPTOMS

OTHER SYSTEMIC SIGNS AND SYMPTOMS

HYPERTENSION

BENIGN OR MALIGNANT TUMOR OF THE BLADDER, TUBERCULOSIS OR PARASITES

COLLAGEN DISEASE, COAGULATION DISORDER, LEUKEMIA, SICKLE CELL ANEMIA

GLOMERULONEPHRITIS, COLLAGEN DISEASE, RENAL ARTERY STENOSIS

HEMIANOPSIA

ASK THE FOLLOWING QUESTIONS:

1. **Is it intermittent?** Intermittent hemianopsia, whether it is bitemporal or homonymous in type, would suggest migraine, carotid artery insufficiency, or vertebral basilar artery insufficiency.

2. **Is the hemianopsia of sudden or gradual onset?** Sudden onset of hemianopsia would suggest a vascular disorder such as cerebral thrombosis, embolism, or hemorrhage, but it may also suggest multiple sclerosis or a ruptured aneurysm. Gradual onset of hemianopsia would suggest a space-occupying lesion.

3. **What type of hemianopsia is it?** A bitemporal hemianopsia often suggests a pituitary tumor, especially if there are endocrine changes, but it may also be due to an aneurysm compressing the optic chiasm. Homonymous hemianopsia suggests involvement of the optic tract or occipital cortex. This may be by a space-occupying lesion, an aneurysm, arterial thrombosis, an embolism, or a hemorrhage.

4. **Are there long tract signs?** Neurologic signs of pyramidal tract involvement or posterior column involvement would suggest anterior or middle cerebral artery occlusion, epidural hematoma, or multiple sclerosis if it is acute, and compression of the cortex by a subdural hematoma or brain tumor if it is chronic.

5. **Are there endocrine changes?** The presence of weight loss, hair loss, or diabetes insipidus would suggest a chromophobe adenoma of the pituitary. On the other hand, a protruding jaw, enlargement of the hands and fingers, and hypertrophy of the other tissues suggest acromegaly.

6. **Is there macular sparing?** The presence of macular sparing suggests that the lesion is in the optic cortex. This is most often a space-occupying lesion.

DIAGNOSTIC WORKUP

Referral to an ophthalmologist for a thorough visual field examination is suggested at the outset. A neurology consultation also needs to be obtained. The neurologist will probably order a CT scan of the brain to rule out a space-occupying lesion unless multiple sclerosis is suspected.

If multiple sclerosis is suspected, MRI would be the study of choice, even though it is more expensive. In addition, VEP studies and spinal fluid analysis may be ordered to rule out multiple sclerosis.

A carotid duplex scan will help diagnose carotid vascular insufficiency, but four-vessel cerebral angiography or an MRA will most likely be done so that both carotid and vertebral basilar artery diseases can be evaluated. If there are endocrine changes, an endocrinologist should be consulted.

If a cerebral embolism is suspected, a source for the embolism should be sought. A cardiologist can best determine what tests to order to search for an embolic source.

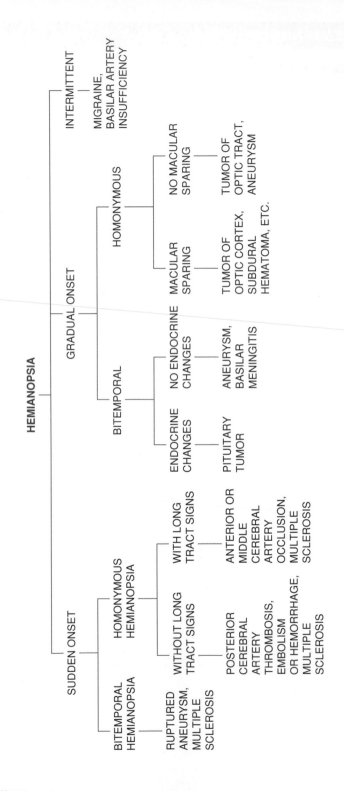

ASK THE FOLLOWING QUESTIONS:

1. **Is it intermittent?** Intermittent hemiparesis or hemiplegia would suggest migraine or transient ischemic attacks from basilar artery or carotid artery disease.

2. **Is it sudden or gradual in onset?** Sudden onset of hemiparesis would suggest a cerebral thrombosis, hemorrhage, or embolism. However, contusion or concussion of the spinal cord can occasionally produce a sudden onset of hemiparesis or hemiplegia. If there is a history of trauma, a subdural or epidural hematoma must be suspected. Gradual onset of hemiparesis or hemiplegia would suggest a space-occupying lesion.

3. **Is there facial paralysis or other cranial nerve signs?** If there is a central facial palsy or other cranial nerve signs, one would look for a lesion above the foramen magnum (i.e., in the brain). If there are no cranial nerve signs, a spinal cord lesion should be suspected.

4. **Is there a fever?** The presence of fever should suggest a cerebral abscess, venous sinus thrombosis, or encephalitis.

5. **Is there a history of trauma?** The history of trauma with hemiparesis or hemiplegia would suggest a subdural or epidural hematoma or a hemorrhage in the brain itself.

6. **Is there a history of hypertension?** The history of hypertension along with hemiparesis or hemiplegia suggests a cerebral hemorrhage. However, a cerebral thrombosis or cerebral aneurysm may also occur with a history of hypertension.

7. **Is there auricular fibrillation or another embolic source?** The presence of auricular fibrillation, cardiac murmur, or other signs of an embolic source would suggest a cerebral embolism.

DIAGNOSTIC WORKUP

A neurologist should be consulted at the outset because he can best determine what type of imaging study should be done and whether thrombolytic therapy is indicated. A spinal tap is no longer done without first doing an imaging study. It may pick up a subarachnoid hemorrhage when the CT scan is negative. Carotid scans can be done to rule out carotid artery insufficiency. Four-vessel cerebral angiography may be indicated, especially in transient ischemic attacks. Magnetic resonance angiography has become an acceptable noninvasive technique for evaluating the cerebral blood flow, especially in the vertebral-basilar arteries. EKG, echocardiography, and blood cultures will help identify an embolic source, but a cardiologist should be consulted to investigate this further. SSEP, BSEP, and VEP studies along with a spinal tap will help diagnose multiple sclerosis.

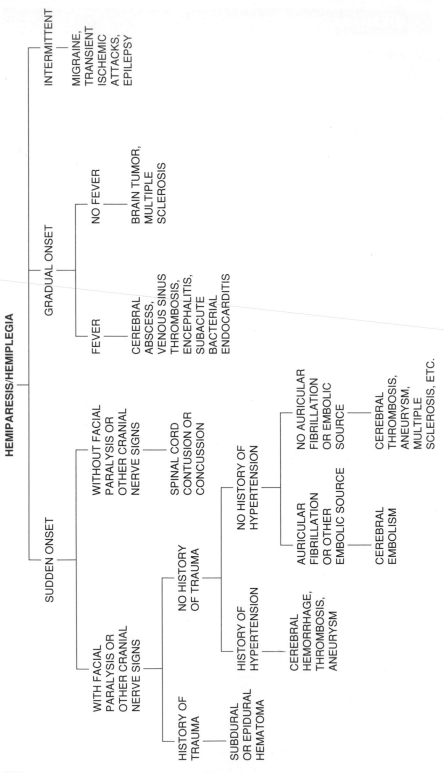

HEMOPTYSIS

CASE HISTORY

A 32-year-old black female complains of a recurrent cough which has recently been productive of blood tinged sputum. She did not complain of chest pain. She denies fever and chills and your nurse recorded a temperature of 97.9°F making pneumonia, lung abscess, or tuberculosis unlikely. She is, however, experiencing exertional dyspnea.

Your examination reveals bilateral crepitant rales at both bases and a presystolic murmur with a sharp first heart sound. You suspect mitral stenosis and congestive heart failure. Further studies confirm your suspicion.

ASK THE FOLLOWING QUESTIONS:

1. **Is there chest pain?** If there is chest pain along with the hemoptysis, one should suspect a pulmonary embolism.
2. **Is there fever and/or purulent sputum?** The presence of fever and purulent sputum suggests pneumonia, lung abscess, tuberculosis, and bronchiectasis. However, bronchiectasis does not usually occur with fever.
3. **Is there dyspnea, cardiomegaly, or a heart murmur?** These findings suggest congestive heart failure or mitral stenosis.
4. **Is there copious sputum?** The presence of copious sputum should suggest bronchiectasis or lung abscess. If there is fever along with it, lung abscess is more likely. Copious foamy sputum suggests congestive heart failure.

DIAGNOSTIC WORKUP

Routine diagnostic tests include a CBC, sedimentation rate, chemistry panel, coagulation profile, sputum smear, culture and sensitivity, a chest x-ray, and an EKG.

If a pulmonary embolism or infarction is suspected, arterial blood gases, D-Dimer and a ventilation-perfusion scan or helical CT scan of the chest should be ordered. In some cases, a pulmonary angiogram may be necessary. Objective testing for deep vein thrombosis with ultrasonography or impedance plethysmography may help confirm suspicion of a pulmonary embolism.

If tuberculosis is suspected, one should order a sputum or gastric washings for AFB smear, culture, and guinea pig inoculation. A tuberculin test should also be done. Apical lordotic views of the lung as well as lateral and oblique views may help identify a tuberculous cavity. There are serologic tests for antibodies against specific mycobacterial antigens.

Sputum cultures for fungi and skin tests for various fungi may need to be done. If congestive heart failure is suspected, venous pressure and circulation time should be measured, and a pulmonary function test should be done. Echocardiography will help diagnose mitral stenosis.

A consultation with a pulmonologist and bronchoscopy need to be done if bronchogenic carcinoma or bronchiectasis is suspected. Other studies that are helpful in diagnosing bronchogenic carcinoma are sputa for pap smear, transbronchial needle biopsy, and CT. MRI may confirm vascular etiologies for the bleeding such as pulmonary aneurysm. Serologic studies [ANA, antineutrophil cytoplasmic antibody (ANCA), etc.] may be useful in detecting collagen diseases. A bronchogram will be helpful in diagnosing bronchiectasis and foreign bodies.

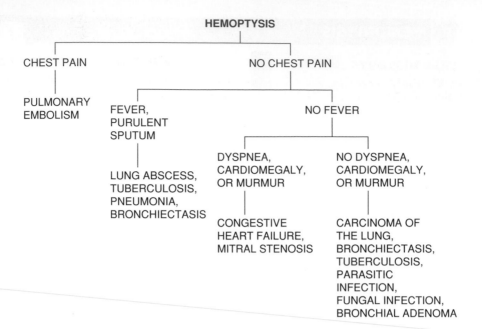

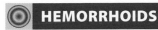
HEMORRHOIDS

Hemorrhoids are dilated perianal veins that become thrombosed or can rupture, producing subcutaneous or submucosal hematomas. They are usually due to chronic constipation but may be the cause of constipation also. Although they are usually considered to be a disease, it is important to remember that they may be a sign of cirrhosis of the liver and other conditions associated with portal hypertension. As such, they may point to the diagnosis of esophageal varices in cases of hematemesis, and their absence would make this diagnosis unlikely.

HEPATOMEGALY

ASK THE FOLLOWING QUESTIONS:

1. **Is there jaundice?** Hepatomegaly with jaundice may make one think of hemolytic anemias; toxic or infectious hepatitis; bile duct obstruction due to stones, carcinoma of the pancreas, or ampulla of Vater; and biliary cirrhosis.
2. **Is there fever?** Hepatomegaly with fever should make one think of viral hepatitis, infectious mononucleosis, ascending cholangitis, and other infectious diseases.
3. **Is there splenomegaly?** Hepatomegaly and splenomegaly should make one think of alcoholic cirrhosis, amyloidosis, reticuloendotheliosis, various hemolytic anemias, biliary cirrhosis, and myeloid metaplasia. It should also make one think of various parasitic diseases.
4. **Is there an enlarged gallbladder?** The presence of hepatomegaly with jaundice and enlarged gallbladder is characteristic of bile duct obstruction due to carcinoma of the pancreas, bile ducts, or ampulla of Vater. The clinician should remember that hydrops of the gallbladder with a common duct stone can mimic the same clinical presentation.
5. **Is the splenomegaly massive?** Massive splenomegaly is characteristic of Gaucher's disease, kala azar, and myeloid metaplasia. Occasionally, other forms of reticuloendotheliosis may also be associated with massive splenomegaly.
6. **Is there another abdominal mass?** The presence of another abdominal mass suggests metastatic carcinoma.
7. **Is the liver tender?** Tenderness of the liver is seen with viral or toxic hepatitis, congestive heart failure, and ascending cholangitis.

DIAGNOSTIC WORKUP

Routine diagnostic studies include a CBC, sedimentation rate, ANA test, Monospot test, chemistry panel, chest x-ray, EKG, and flat plate of the abdomen.

If viral hepatitis is suspected, a hepatitis profile should be ordered. If congestive heart failure is suspected, a venous pressure and circulation time or BNP and pulmonary function tests should be done. A CT scan of the abdomen will assist in the diagnosis of metastatic carcinoma and often find a primary source for the metastasis. Metastatic neoplasms and the various forms of cirrhosis may be diagnosed by liver biopsy, but one should keep in mind that it is dangerous to do a liver biopsy if biliary cirrhosis is suspected. Gallbladder ultrasound or cholecystography should be done if cholecystitis and cholelithiasis are suspected. Transhepatic cholangiography or endoscopic retrograde cholangiopancreatography (ERCP) may need to be done. Exploratory surgery may be the only way to get a diagnosis, especially in obstructive jaundice.

The various infectious diseases will need antibody titers and skin tests to pin down the diagnosis. For example, a brucellin antibody titer or a Monospot test can be done. Skin tests for the various fungi and tuberculosis can be done.

The various hemolytic anemias may be diagnosed by blood smears, a sickle cell preparation, serum haptoglobin, and hemoglobin electrophoresis. The reticuloendothelioses require liver biopsy. Hemochromatosis is also diagnosed by liver biopsy, but a test for serum iron and iron-binding capacity should also be done. Wilson's disease is diagnosed by serum copper and ceruloplasmin tests. Venography will diagnose hepatic vein thrombosis.

Most physicians prefer to refer the patient with hepatomegaly to a gastroenterologist once the preliminary studies have been done. This would be the most cost-effective approach.

HEPATOMEGALY

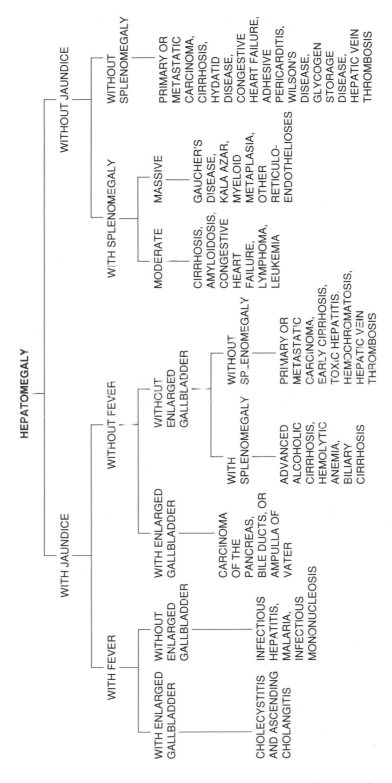

⊚ HICCUPS

ASK THE FOLLOWING QUESTIONS:

1. **Is there a history of alcoholism?** Alcoholic gastritis is a frequent cause of hiccups.
2. **Is there a fever?** The presence of fever should make one think of pneumonia with pleurisy, pericarditis, subdiaphragmatic abscess, and peritonitis. It should also make one think of epidemic hiccups.
3. **Is there heartburn or regurgitation?** The presence of heartburn and regurgitation should make one think of a hiatal hernia and esophagitis.
4. **Is there a mediastinal mass?** Because they irritate the phrenic nerve, mediastinal masses such as Hodgkin's disease, bronchogenic carcinoma, and esophageal carcinoma may cause hiccups.
5. **Are there abnormalities on neurologic examination?** Hiccups may occur in tabes dorsalis, syringomyelia, encephalitis, chorea, and cerebral hemorrhage.

DIAGNOSTIC WORKUP

The basic workup includes a CBC, sedimentation rate, chemistry panel, a VDRL test, tuberculin test, EKG, chest x-ray, and a fiat plate of the abdomen. If these are negative, an upper GI series and esophagogram should be done. If these are negative, it may be wise to evaluate the response to Pepto-Bismol or lidocaine viscus. If there is relief from one of these, the patient may well have a reflux esophagitis.

If there is still confusion at this point, a gastroenterologist should be consulted before ordering other expensive diagnostic tests. The gastroenterologist will probably do an esophagoscopy, gastroscopy, and duodenoscopy, and may order a CT scan of the abdomen and mediastinum. A Bernstein test may help diagnose reflux esophagitis. Esophageal manometry and pH monitoring of the distal esophagus may also help in this regard.

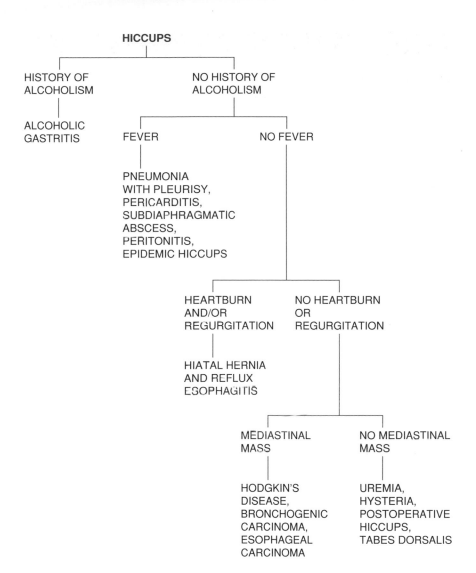

HICCUPS

HISTORY OF
ALCOHOLISM

ALCOHOLIC
GASTRITIS

NO HISTORY OF
ALCOHOLISM

FEVER

PNEUMONIA
WITH PLEURISY,
PERICARDITIS,
SUBDIAPHRAGMATIC
ABSCESS,
PERITONITIS,
EPIDEMIC HICCUPS

NO FEVER

HEARTBURN
AND/OR
REGURGITATION

HIATAL HERNIA
AND REFLUX
ESOPHAGITIS

NO HEARTBURN
OR
REGURGITATION

MEDIASTINAL
MASS

HODGKIN'S
DISEASE,
BRONCHOGENIC
CARCINOMA,
ESOPHAGEAL
CARCINOMA

NO MEDIASTINAL
MASS

UREMIA,
HYSTERIA,
POSTOPERATIVE
HICCUPS,
TABES DORSALIS

CASE HISTORY

A 62-year-old Hispanic female complains of low back and hip pain of 6 weeks duration. She has curtailed her activities and uses a cane. Following the algorithm, you do a neurologic examination and perform a straight-leg raising test with negative results. In fact, you find that all of the tenderness is confined to her right hip. She has a positive Patrick's sign and exquisite tenderness over the greater trochanter. You diagnose greater trochanter bursitis and infiltrate the bursa with 1% lidocaine which relieves her pain and restores her range of motion of the right hip.

ASK THE FOLLOWING QUESTIONS:

1. **Is there a positive straight-leg raising test or other neurologic signs?** The presence of positive straight-leg raising tests or other neurologic signs would suggest a herniated disk, a cauda equina tumor, or other neurologic disorders of the lumbar spine. Meralgia paresthetica will cause characteristic loss of sensation in the distribution of the lateral femoral cutaneous nerve.

2. **Is there a positive Patrick's test or limitation of the range of motion of the hip?** These findings suggest a greater trochanter bursitis or hip joint pathology such as fracture, osteoarthritis, rheumatoid arthritis, metastasis, slipped femoral epiphysis, Legg–Perthes disease, rheumatic fever, or transient synovitis. Iliotibial band syndrome is a common cause of hip pain in runners.

3. **Is there tenderness of the greater trochanter bursa?** Tenderness of the greater trochanter bursa will help differentiate greater trochanter bursitis. It is also seen in hysteria.

4. **Is the patient a child or an adult?** If the patient is a child, transient synovitis, slipped femoral epiphysis, Legg–Perthes disease, and rheumatic fever should be considered. If the patient is an adult, it is more likely that the problem is osteoarthritis, a fracture, rheumatoid arthritis, metastasis, or avascular necrosis.

5. **Is there a history of trauma?** A history of trauma would suggest that there is a fracture or a sprain of the hip joint, but the clinician should remember that a fracture in the elderly often occurs with no history of trauma.

DIAGNOSTIC WORKUP

A CBC, sedimentation rate, chemistry panel, arthritis panel, tuberculin test, and x-rays of the lumbosacral spine and hip will diagnose 90% of the cases. These are relatively in expensive in comparison to MRI. A bone scan may be necessary to diagnose occult fractures. A serum protein electrophoresis will help diagnose multiple myeloma. A trigger point injection of the greater trochanter bursa or ischiogluteal bursa will assist in the diagnosis of these conditions. An orthopedic surgeon should be consulted before ordering MRI of the lumbar spine or hip. However, MRI is especially important if the diagnosis of avascular necrosis is suspected.

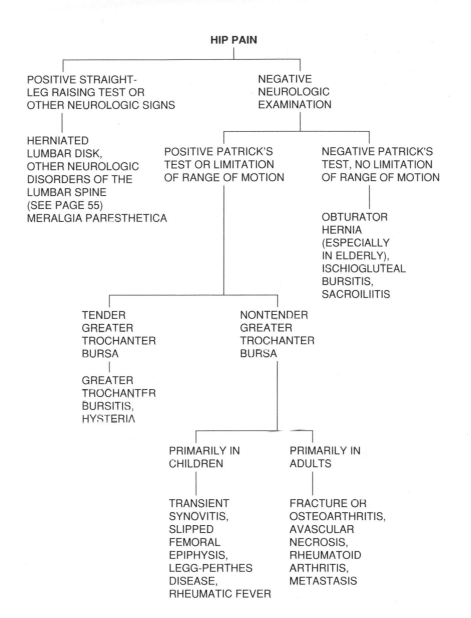

HIP PAIN

POSITIVE STRAIGHT-LEG RAISING TEST OR OTHER NEUROLOGIC SIGNS

HERNIATED LUMBAR DISK, OTHER NEUROLOGIC DISORDERS OF THE LUMBAR SPINE (SEE PAGE 55) MERALGIA PARESTHETICA

NEGATIVE NEUROLOGIC EXAMINATION

POSITIVE PATRICK'S TEST OR LIMITATION OF RANGE OF MOTION

NEGATIVE PATRICK'S TEST, NO LIMITATION OF RANGE OF MOTION

OBTURATOR HERNIA (ESPECIALLY IN ELDERLY), ISCHIOGLUTEAL BURSITIS, SACROILIITIS

TENDER GREATER TROCHANTER BURSA

GREATER TROCHANTER BURSITIS, HYSTERIA

NONTENDER GREATER TROCHANTER BURSA

PRIMARILY IN CHILDREN

TRANSIENT SYNOVITIS, SLIPPED FEMORAL EPIPHYSIS, LEGG-PERTHES DISEASE, RHEUMATIC FEVER

PRIMARILY IN ADULTS

FRACTURE OR OSTEOARTHRITIS, AVASCULAR NECROSIS, RHEUMATOID ARTHRITIS, METASTASIS

ASK THE FOLLOWING QUESTIONS:

1. **Is there clitoral enlargement or other signs of virilism?** These findings would suggest an ovarian tumor, an adrenal tumor or hyperplasia, chromosome mosaicism, and true hermaphroditism, which is rare.
2. **Is there obesity?** The presence of obesity and hirsutism should bring to mind Cushing's syndrome. However, it is also a sign of polycystic ovaries.
3. **Is there a history of the use of the steroids or other drugs?** Adrenocortical steroids, testosterone, phenytoin, minoxidil, and diazoxide are just a few of the drugs that may cause hirsutism.
4. **Is there an ovarian mass?** The presence of an ovarian mass should make one think of polycystic ovaries, an arrhenoblastoma, or granulosis cell tumor. Remember, there may be no ovarian mass in polycystic ovary syndrome (Stein–Leventhal syndrome).

DIAGNOSTIC WORKUP

The routine diagnostic workup includes a serum-free testosterone, free cortisol, prolactin, a skull x-ray (much more economical than a CT scan or MRI of the brain), and a urinary gonadotropin assay. If a pituitary tumor or lesion is strongly suspected, an FSH and LH should be done regardless of results of routine tests. An overnight dexamethasone suppression test is more accurate than a routine free cortisol in diagnosing Cushing's syndrome. A 24-hr urine-free cortisol may also be used. Pelvic ultrasound and CT scan of the abdomen would complete the workup, but why order these expensive diagnostic tests before consulting a gynecologist or endocrinologist?

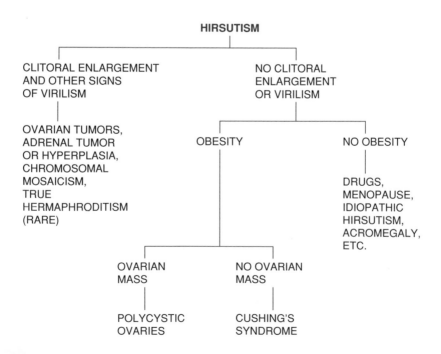

ASK THE FOLLOWING QUESTIONS:

1. **Is it acute?** Acute hoarseness is usually due to a viral URI, but acute simple laryngitis and acute subglottic laryngitis or rarely laryngeal diphtheria may be responsible. Simple strain may be responsible due to the patient's occupation.
2. **Is it intermittent?** Intermittent hoarseness would suggest myasthenia gravis, urticaria, occupational causes, reflux esophagitis, tobacco, and alcoholism.
3. **Are there abnormalities on the neurologic examination?** If there are other abnormalities on the neurologic examination, one should consider peripheral neuropathy, poliomyelitis, Guillain–Barré syndrome, brain stem tumors, and cerebrovascular disease.
4. **Are there abnormalities on the laryngoscopic examination?** Laryngoscopy will identify many intrinsic lesions of the vocal cords such as carcinoma, singer's nodes, polyps, tuberculosis, or syphilis. It will also identify vocal cord paralysis due to carcinoma of the lung, aortic aneurysm, cardiac enlargement, or other mediastinal tumors.

A normal laryngoscopic examination would suggest hysteria, myxedema, or acromegaly.

DIAGNOSTIC WORKUP

Acute hoarseness will require only a CBC, sedimentation rate, nose and throat culture, and sputum culture if sputum is available. A chest x-ray may also be ordered. Laryngoscopic examination is rarely necessary unless the acute hoarseness becomes chronic.

The laryngoscopic examination is the single most important test for chronic hoarseness. It will identify most intrinsic lesions. If vocal cord paralysis is found, a chest x-ray and possibly a CT scan of the mediastinum may be ordered. However, an ear, nose, and throat specialist should be consulted before ordering these expensive tests. If the chords are edematous, hypothyroidism or angioneurotic edema may be the cause. The latter may be excluded by ordering a C1-esterase inhibitor level. A barium swallow or esophagoscopy can be done to exclude a hiatal hernia or reflux esophagitis. If there are other neurologic abnormalities, a referral to a neurologist should be made before ordering a CT scan or MRI of the brain. In cases of intermittent hoarseness, a Tensilon test or acetylcholine receptor antibody titer should be done.

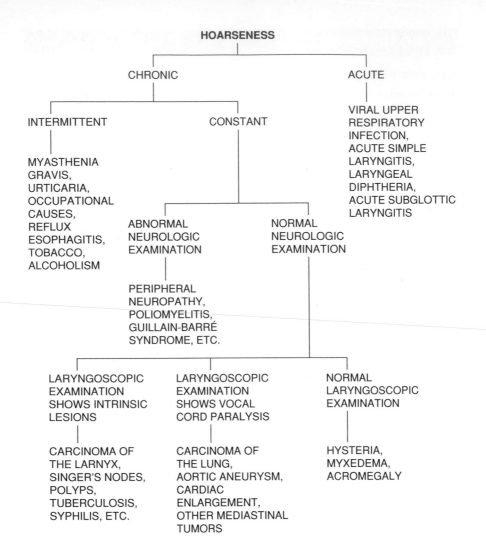

ASK THE FOLLOWING QUESTIONS:

1. **Is there pain in the ipsilateral upper extremity?** If there is pain in the ipsilateral upper extremity, one should consider brachial plexus neuritis, thoracic outlet syndrome, Pancoast's tumor, and spinal cord tumor.
2. **Is there hemiplegia or other long tract neurologic signs?** If there is hemiplegia or other long tract signs, one should consider carotid artery thrombosis, Wallenberg's syndrome, or syringomyelia.
3. **Is there a mediastinal mass?** A chest x-ray or an imaging study may be necessary to disclose a mediastinal mass, but this will establish the diagnosis of Horner's syndrome and carcinoma of the lung, lymphoma, aortic aneurysms, and mediastinitis. If there is no pain in the extremities, the neurologic examination is normal, and there is no mediastinal mass, one should consider the possibility of migraine and histamine headaches.

DIAGNOSTIC WORKUP

A neurologist should probably be consulted at the outset. If there is pain in the upper extremities along with the Horner's syndrome, x-rays of the chest should be done to rule out a Pancoast's tumor, and x-rays of the cervical spine should be done to rule out a cervical rib. Nerve conduction velocity studies, SSEP studies, and EMGs of the upper extremities may help diagnose a brachial plexus neuralgia. MRI will be necessary to diagnose a tumor of the cervical spinal cord.

If there is hemiplegia or other long tract neurologic signs, a CT scan or MRI of the brain or cervical spinal cord needs to be done. If these tests are negative and there is an isolated Horner's syndrome, a CT scan of the mediastinum should be ordered. Esophagograms, aortography, and mediastinoscopy may all be necessary to establish the diagnosis in difficult cases.

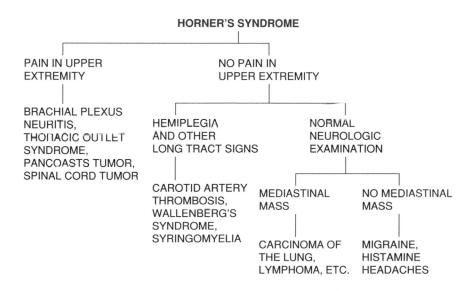

ASK THE FOLLOWING QUESTIONS:

1. **Are they intermittent or persistent?** If the hyperactive reflexes are intermittent, one should consider multiple sclerosis and cerebral vascular insufficiency.
2. **Are they focal?** If the hyperactive reflexes are focal, and especially if they are unilateral, one should consider vascular diseases, space-occupying lesions, or multiple sclerosis. Certain degenerative diseases such as amyotrophic lateral sclerosis may also present with focal hyperactive reflexes.
3. **If the hyperactive reflexes are focal, are they unilateral?** Unilateral hyperactive reflexes are characteristic of hemiplegia. Hemiplegia is usually associated with a cerebral vascular disease or space-occupying lesion of the brain, especially if there are cranial nerve signs. However, early spinal cord tumors may present with unilateral hyperactive reflexes.
4. **Are there cranial nerve signs?** The presence of cranial nerve signs suggests that the lesion is above the foramen magnum, and a cerebral or brain stem tumor is the first thing to be considered. A cerebral vascular lesion or multiple sclerosis must also be considered.
5. **Is there dementia?** The presence of dementia along with the hyperactive reflexes, especially if they are diffuse, suggests Alzheimer's disease, Pick's disease, general paresis, and Korsakoff's syndrome. There are many other causes of dementia to consider.
6. **Are there other long tract signs?** The presence of hyperactive reflexes with sensory changes should suggest pernicious anemia, syringomyelia, and Friedreich's ataxia. It may also indicate multiple sclerosis, a spinal cord tumor, a brain stem tumor, or basilar artery insufficiency.

DIAGNOSTIC WORKUP

Hyperactive reflexes, especially if they are unilateral, are a clear indication for an imaging study. It is wise to consult a neurologist or neurosurgeon before determining which imaging study to order. If there are cranial nerve findings and dementia, a CT scan or MRI of the brain should be ordered.

If there are hyperactive reflexes of all four extremities without dementia or cranial nerve signs, MRI of the cervical spine would probably be the most appropriate procedure. It may, however, be necessary to get a CT scan or MRI of the brain anyway.

If only the lower extremities are involved, MRI of the thoracic cord would probably be most appropriate, but then MRI of the cervical spine should be done if the thoracic MRI is negative. Spinal fluid analysis will help diagnose multiple sclerosis, central nervous system syphilis, cerebral hemorrhages, or abscess. A CBC, serum B_{12} and folic acid, and Schilling test will help diagnose pernicious anemia. Plain films of the appropriate level of the spine are necessary in trauma cases. An EEG and psychometric testing should be done in cases of dementia. SSEP, VEP, and BSEP studies are helpful in diagnosing multiple sclerosis. Carotid duplex scans and four-vessel angiography may be necessary for diagnosing cerebral vascular disease.

HYPERACTIVE REFLEXES

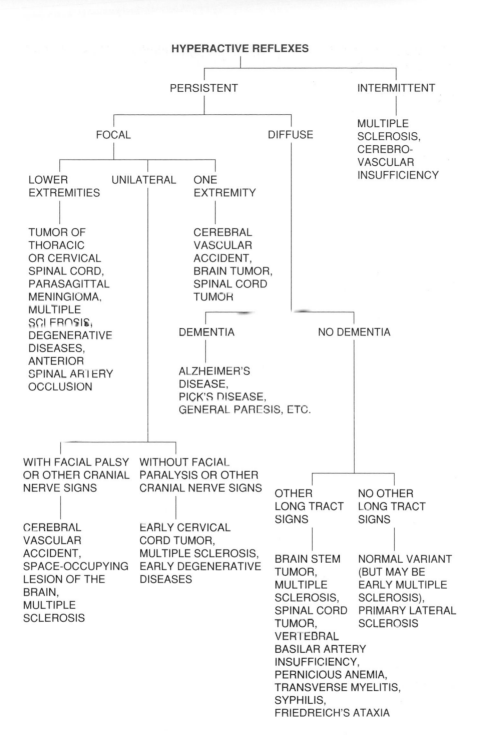

PERSISTENT

INTERMITTENT

MULTIPLE SCLEROSIS, CEREBRO-VASCULAR INSUFFICIENCY

FOCAL

DIFFUSE

LOWER EXTREMITIES

UNILATERAL

ONE EXTREMITY

TUMOR OF THORACIC OR CERVICAL SPINAL CORD, PARASAGITTAL MENINGIOMA, MULTIPLE SCLEROSIS, DEGENERATIVE DISEASES, ANTERIOR SPINAL ARTERY OCCLUSION

CEREBRAL VASCULAR ACCIDENT, BRAIN TUMOR, SPINAL CORD TUMOR

DEMENTIA

NO DEMENTIA

ALZHEIMER'S DISEASE, PICK'S DISEASE, GENERAL PARESIS, ETC.

WITH FACIAL PALSY OR OTHER CRANIAL NERVE SIGNS

WITHOUT FACIAL PARALYSIS OR OTHER CRANIAL NERVE SIGNS

OTHER LONG TRACT SIGNS

NO OTHER LONG TRACT SIGNS

CEREBRAL VASCULAR ACCIDENT, SPACE-OCCUPYING LESION OF THE BRAIN, MULTIPLE SCLEROSIS

EARLY CERVICAL CORD TUMOR, MULTIPLE SCLEROSIS, EARLY DEGENERATIVE DISEASES

BRAIN STEM TUMOR, MULTIPLE SCLEROSIS, SPINAL CORD TUMOR, VERTEBRAL BASILAR ARTERY INSUFFICIENCY, PERNICIOUS ANEMIA, TRANSVERSE MYELITIS, SYPHILIS, FRIEDREICH'S ATAXIA

NORMAL VARIANT (BUT MAY BE EARLY MULTIPLE SCLEROSIS), PRIMARY LATERAL SCLEROSIS

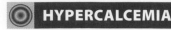

ASK THE FOLLOWING QUESTIONS:

1. **Is the parathyroid hormone (PTH) assay increased?** This would point to a parathyroid tumor or hyperplasia and ectopic PTH secretion. In any case of elevated PTH, look for type I or type II multiple endocrine neoplasm syndrome.

2. **Is the alkaline phosphatase elevated?** Hypercalcemia and an increased alkaline phosphatase without an increase in PTH assay suggests metastatic carcinoma of the bone, Paget's disease, and other bone tumors. Hypercalcemia without an elevated alkaline phosphatase is suggestive of multiple myeloma and hyperproteinemia due to other causes. A serum protein electrophoresis will help define this further.

DIAGNOSTIC WORKUP

A CBC, chemistry panel, 24-hr urine calcium, PTH assay, serum 25(OH) vitamin D_3, free tetraiodothyronine (thyroxine) (T_4), serum protein electrophoresis, skeletal survey, bone scan, and endocrinology consult may be part of any workup of hypercalcemia.

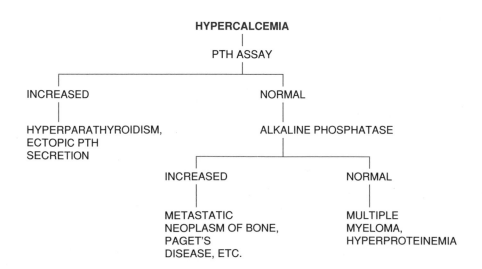

HYPERCHOLESTEROLEMIA

ASK THE FOLLOWING QUESTIONS:

1. **What is the serum albumin?** A decreased serum albumin associated with an increased cholesterol strongly suggests the nephrotic syndrome or liver disease. These two conditions may be further differentiated by the finding of proteinuria in the nephrotic syndrome.
2. **What is the free T_4?** Hypercholesterolemia associated with a low T_4 suggests myxedema.
3. **What is the triglyceride level?** An elevated cholesterol coupled with a marked increase in the triglyceride is typical of type I and type II lipoproteinemia. Type IIB, type III, and type IV lipoproteinemias are associated with a high cholesterol but only mild increase of triglyceride. Oral contraceptive use, atherosclerosis, and xanthomatosis may present the same picture. These may be further differentiated by lipoprotein electrophoresis.

DIAGNOSTIC WORKUP

A workup of hypercholesterolemia should include a CBC, urinalysis, chemistry panel, overnight refrigeration of plasma, free T_4, TSH, and lipoprotein electrophoresis. If these tests suggest liver disease, liver function tests and liver biopsy may be indicated. If these tests suggest kidney disease, a nephrologist should be consulted for consideration of renal function tests or renal biopsy. A metabolic disease specialist or an endocrinologist may need to be consulted for further diagnostic evaluation and management.

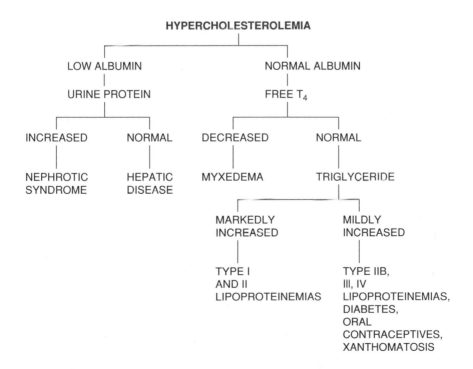

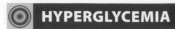

ASK THE FOLLOWING QUESTIONS:

1. **What is the free T$_4$?** If this is elevated, think of hyperthyroidism.
2. **What is the plasma cortisol?** If this is elevated, think of Cushing's syndrome.
3. **What is the plasma growth hormone?** If this is elevated, think of acromegaly or gigantism.
4. **What is the 24-hr urine catecholamine level?** If this is high, think of a pheochromocytoma.

If all of the above tests are normal, diabetes mellitus is usually the diagnosis, although some of these patients could have a glucagonoma or pancreatic disease. Certain drugs can cause a spurious hyperglycemia also.

DIAGNOSTIC WORKUP

Further workup may include a CBC, urinalysis, chemistry panel, glucose tolerance test, plasma cortisol, free T$_4$, TSH, plasma and urine catecholamines, skull x-ray, 24 hour urine vanillylmandelic acid (VMA), and endocrinology consult.

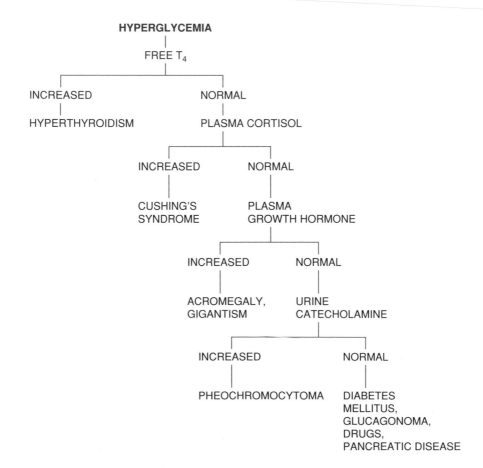

ASK THE FOLLOWING QUESTIONS:

1. **Is there hemolysis in the test tube?** This is just one of the spurious causes of hyperkalemia. Leucocytosis, thrombocytosis, and the use of an excessively tight tourniquet to draw blood may also be the cause.
2. **What is the BUN?** An increased potassium is most often due to renal failure, especially acute renal failure. Hyperkalemia can occur in some renal diseases even without an elevated BUN.
3. **What is the plasma cortisol?** Hyperkalemia with a low plasma cortisol suggests Addison's disease is the cause. Adrenogenital syndrome and chronic renal disease may be associated with a defect in aldosterone synthesis causing the same picture.
4. **What is the bicarbonate level?** Metabolic acidosis, especially diabetic acidosis, is often associated with hyperkalemia.

DIAGNOSTIC WORKUP

Additional tests to order include a CBC, urinalysis, chemistry panel, serial electrolytes, plasma cortisol, plasma renin, 24-hr urine aldosterone, renal function tests, and endocrinology and nephrology consults. As a precaution, it may be wise to hold all unnecessary drugs until the diagnosis is certain.

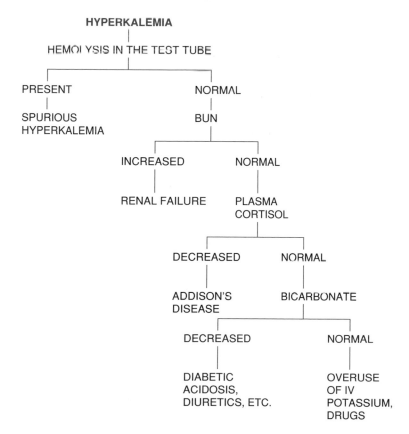

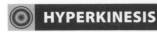

ASK THE FOLLOWING QUESTIONS:

1. **Is there a positive drug history?** Phenothiazines, amphetamines, tricyclic drugs, lithium, and other substances may cause hyperkinesis.
2. **Is there a tremor, a goiter, or tachycardia?** The findings would suggest hyperthyroidism.
3. **Are there other neurologic signs and symptoms?** The presence of other neurologic signs and symptoms would suggest Wilson's disease, Huntington's chorea, Sydenham's chorea, and Parkinson's disease. If there are no other neurologic signs and symptoms, one should look for an attention deficit disorder or Gilles de la Tourette's syndrome.

DIAGNOSTIC WORKUP

Routine studies include a CBC, sedimentation rate, ASO titer, chemistry panel, urine drug screen, and a thyroid panel. A serum copper and ceruloplasmin will usually diagnose Wilson's disease. If all of the above studies are negative, MRI of the brain may be done to rule out tumors or degenerative disease of the nervous system, but why not consult a neurologist first? An EEG may identify epilepsy and brain damage. Referral to a psychiatrist or psychologist is made if all of the above studies are normal.

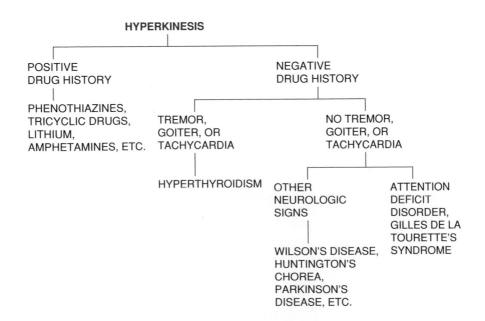

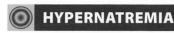

ASK THE FOLLOWING QUESTIONS:

1. **What is the chloride level?** Hypernatremia with an elevated chloride is almost certainly due to dehydration, but renal and hypothalamic diabetes insipidus, heat exhaustion, and hypertonic fluid administration may also be responsible. A low chloride level with hypernatremia may be seen in aldosteronism or Cushing's syndrome.
2. **What is the serum antidiuretic hormone (ADH) assay?** If this is low or absent, hypothalamic diabetes insipidus must be considered. If this is normal, one should consider dehydration, heat exhaustion, prolonged vomiting, renal diabetes insipidus, and hypertonic saline administration as likely causes.

DIAGNOSTIC WORKUP

The workup should include a CBC, urinalysis, chemistry panel, serum and urine osmolality, plasma cortisol, serum ADH, plasma volume studies, serial electrolytes, and consultation with an endocrinologist or nephrologist.

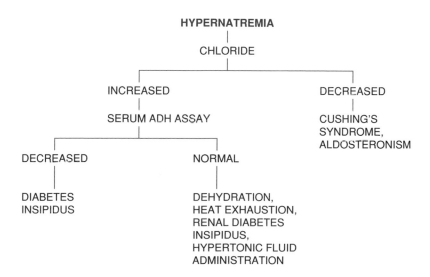

ASK THE FOLLOWING QUESTIONS:

1. **Is there a history of drug ingestion?** Argyria, arsenic poisoning, and methemoglobinemia are among the considerations in taking a drug history.
2. **Is there hepatomegaly?** The presence of hepatomegaly would make one think of hemochromatosis.
3. **Is there significant weight loss?** The presence of significant weight loss would suggest Addison's disease, pellagra, hyperthyroidism, or an ectopic hormone-secreting tumor.
4. **Is there a history of seizures or neuropathy?** The history of seizures or neuropathy should make one consider porphyria.
5. **Is the hyperpigmentation focal?** In addition to melanotic cancer, this should bring to mind acanthosis nigricans and the café au lait spots of neurofibromatosis.

DIAGNOSTIC WORKUP

The serum iron and iron-binding capacity should be measured to rule out hemochromatosis. A thyroid profile will exclude hyperthyroidism. A serum cortisol and ACTH stimulation test will identify Addison's disease. A urine for porphyrins and porphobilinogen will diagnose porphyria. A urine N-methylniacinamide will help diagnose pellagra.

If there is still doubt after these studies are done, a skin or liver biopsy may be done to rule out hemochromatosis, and a CT scan of the abdomen will help identify Addison's disease.

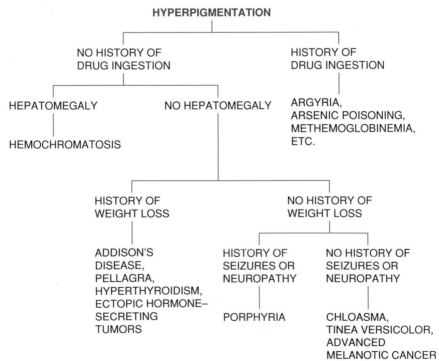

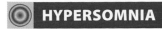

ASK THE FOLLOWING QUESTIONS:

1. **Is there a history of drug or alcohol use?** Alcoholism and barbiturate intoxication are just two of the causes of hypersomnia.
2. **Are there hallucinations, sleep paralysis, and cataplexy?** These findings suggest narcolepsy.
3. **Is there associated loss of appetite and/or libido?** These findings suggest endogenous depression.
4. **Are there abnormalities on the neurologic examination?** Abnormal neurologic findings suggest multiple sclerosis, encephalitis, neurosyphilis, and other disorders.

DIAGNOSTIC WORKUP

The routine workup includes a CBC, sedimentation rate, chemistry panel, VDRL test, and urine drug screen. If there are abnormal neurologic signs, MRI of the brain and spinal tap can be done, but it is advisable to consult a neurologist first. An EEG and sleep study complete the workup.

If all of the above studies are normal, referral to a psychiatrist would be in order.

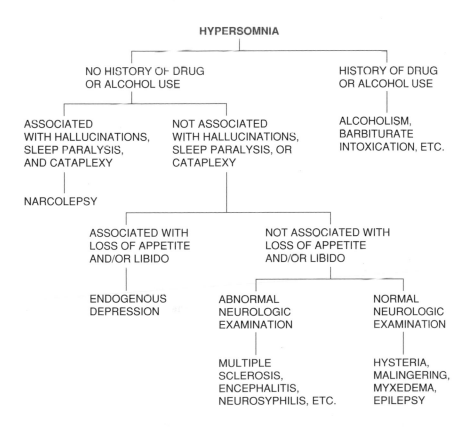

CASE HISTORY

A 34-year-old obese white female presents with a 2-year history of uncontrolled hypertension. Following the algorithm, you find there is elevation of both her systolic and diastolic blood pressure to 180/115. The blood pressure is slightly above that in the lower extremities. There is no flank mass palpable. Examination of the urinary sediment is unremarkable. However, you notice purple abdominal striae. A plasma cortisol level confirms your suspicion of Cushing's syndrome.

ASK THE FOLLOWING QUESTIONS:

1. **Is there systolic hypertension only?** The presence of an elevated systolic pressure only would suggest hyperthyroidism, aortic insufficiency, and atherosclerotic aortitis. Systolic hypertension in the elderly must always be taken seriously.
2. **Is the hypertension paroxysmal?** The presence of paroxysmal hypertension should suggest a pheochromocytoma.
3. **Is there a normal or low blood pressure in the lower extremities?** These findings would suggest a coarctation of the aorta.
4. **Is there a flank mass?** The presence of a flank mass should suggest hypernephroma, hydronephrosis, and polycystic kidneys.
5. **Are there abnormalities of the urinary sediment?** These findings suggest glomerulonephritis, collagen disease, Henoch–Schönlein purpura, and chronic nephritis. All primary care physicians should have this capability in their office. Is the patient ingesting large amounts of cocaine, caffeine, or other stimulating drugs? This is an increasing concern of most physicians.

DIAGNOSTIC WORKUP

Routine diagnostic tests include a CBC, sedimentation rate, chemistry panel, total and high-density lipoprotein (HDL) cholesterol, a VDRL test, urinalysis including microscopic, a urine culture with colony count and sensitivity, a urine drug screen, and an EKG, chest x-ray, and flat plate of the abdomen for kidney size. Remember overuse of diuretics is a cause of resistant hypertension.

If these are normal, a nephrologist should be consulted before undertaking expensive diagnostic tests. It may be wise to observe the results of treatment before further testing also.

Additional tests that may be ordered are an intravenous pyelogram or CT scan of the abdomen, a 24-hr urine catecholamine, a serum cortisol, a plasma renin level, a 24-hr urine aldosterone determination, a cystoscopy, and retrograde pyelography. A 24-hr urine-free cortisol may be more useful in diagnosing Cushing's syndrome than serum-free cortisol. Ultrasonography may pick up a renal artery stenosis. Renal angiography used to be done more frequently, but should be considered in sudden onset of hypertension in the elderly and in hypertension that is resistant to treatment.

Twenty-four-hr blood pressure monitoring can be useful both in diagnosis and in evaluating the results of therapy. Magnetic resonance angiography is a good noninvasive alternative to renal angiography.

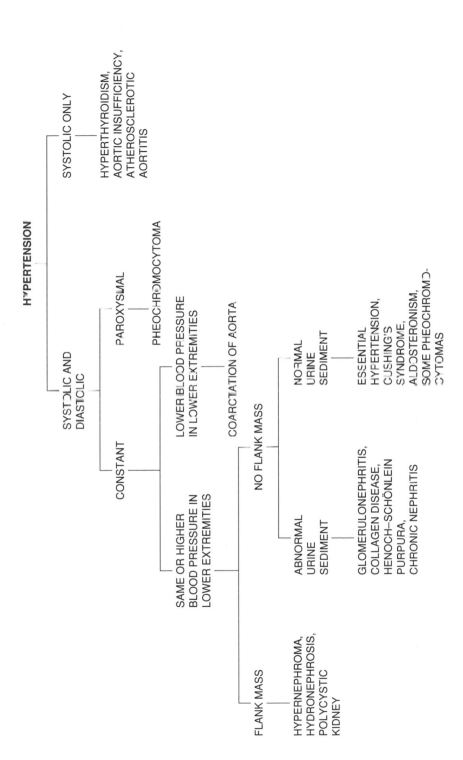

HYPERTENSION

SYSTOLIC AND DIASTOLIC

SYSTOLIC ONLY
HYPERTHYROIDISM,
AORTIC INSUFFICIENCY,
ATHEROSCLEROTIC
AORTITIS

PAROXYSMAL
PHEOCHROMOCYTOMA

CONSTANT

LOWER BLOOD PRESSURE
IN LOWER EXTREMITIES
COARCTATION OF AORTA

SAME OR HIGHER
BLOOD PRESSURE IN
LOWER EXTREMITIES

NO FLANK MASS

NORMAL
URINE
SEDIMENT
ESSENTIAL
HYPERTENSION,
CUSHING'S
SYNDROME,
ALDOSTERONISM,
SOME PHEOCHROMO-
CYTOMAS

ABNORMAL
URINE
SEDIMENT
GLOMERULONEPHRITIS,
COLLAGEN DISEASE,
HENOCH–SCHÖNLEIN
PURPURA,
CHRONIC NEPHRITIS

FLANK MASS
HYPERNEPHROMA,
HYDRONEPHROSIS,
POLYCYSTIC
KIDNEY

HYPERTRIGLYCERIDEMIA

ASK THE FOLLOWING QUESTIONS:

Algorithm A

1. **What is the free T_4?** If this is decreased, hypothyroidism should come to mind.
2. **What is a serum albumin and urine protein?** If the serum albumin is low and there is proteinuria, one should consider nephrotic syndrome.
3. **What is the fasting blood sugar (FBS)?** Hyperglycemia coupled with an elevated triglyceride makes diabetes mellitus the most likely cause. Hypoglycemia should prompt consideration of insulinomas and glycogen storage disease.
4. If all of the above tests are normal, a familial disorder of lipid metabolism (see Algorithm B) should be considered.

Algorithm B

1. **Are the chylomicrons increased?** An increased triglyceride coupled with increased chylomicrons suggest type V and type I lipoproteinemia. Normal chylomicrons suggests the possibility of type III lipoproteinemia.
2. **What is the cholesterol?** An increased triglyceride and chylomicrons should identify type V lipoproteinemia. A normal cholesterol with both increased triglyceride and a marked increase in chylomicrons identifies type I lipoproteinemia. An increased cholesterol with increased triglyceride but normal chylomicrons identifies type III lipoproteinemia. A mild to moderate increased triglyceride with an increased cholesterol but normal chylomicrons should identify type IIB lipoproteinemia without chylomicrons, and a normal or mildly increased cholesterol should point to type IV lipoproteinemia.
3. If neither the chylomicrons nor the triglyceride is elevated, consider type IIA lipoproteinemia or familial hypercholesterolemia. Remember, regular alcohol consumption, estrogen therapy, nicotinic acid treatment, and phenytoin treatment can also produce triglyceridemia.

DIAGNOSTIC WORKUP

The workup of triglyceridemia includes a CBC, urinalysis, chemistry panel, free T_4, glucose tolerance test, 24-hr urine protein, lipoprotein electrophoresis, ultracentrifugation, renal biopsy, liver biopsy, and consultation with a metabolic disease specialist.

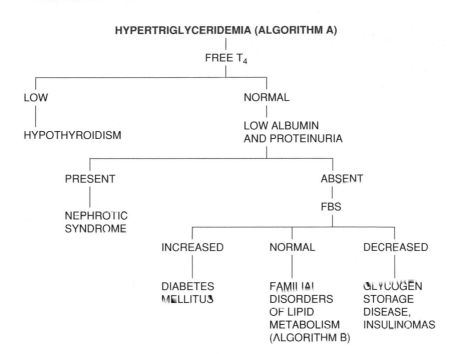

HYPERTRIGLYCERIDEMIA (ALGORITHM A)

FREE T$_4$

LOW — HYPOTHYROIDISM

NORMAL — LOW ALBUMIN AND PROTEINURIA

PRESENT — NEPHROTIC SYNDROME

ABSENT — FBS

INCREASED — DIABETES MELLITUS

NORMAL — FAMILIAL DISORDERS OF LIPID METABOLISM (ALGORITHM B)

DECREASED — GLYCOGEN STORAGE DISEASE, INSULINOMAS

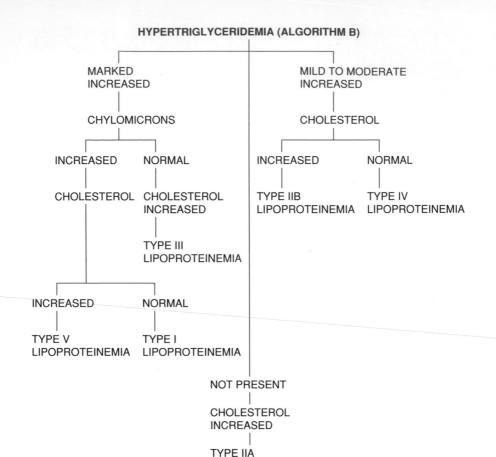

HYPERTRIGLYCERIDEMIA (ALGORITHM B)

MARKED INCREASED

CHYLOMICRONS

INCREASED — CHOLESTEROL

NORMAL — CHOLESTEROL INCREASED — TYPE III LIPOPROTEINEMIA

INCREASED — TYPE V LIPOPROTEINEMIA

NORMAL — TYPE I LIPOPROTEINEMIA

MILD TO MODERATE INCREASED

CHOLESTEROL

INCREASED — TYPE IIB LIPOPROTEINEMIA

NORMAL — TYPE IV LIPOPROTEINEMIA

NOT PRESENT

CHOLESTEROL INCREASED

TYPE IIA LIPOPROTEINEMIA

ASK THE FOLLOWING QUESTIONS:

1. **Is it focal?** Hypoactive reflexes limited to one extremity suggest a herniated disk, plexopathy, or early cauda equina or spinal cord tumor.
2. **If focal, are the hypoactive reflexes involving both the upper and lower extremity?** If the hypoactive reflexes are in both the upper and lower extremity on one side, this may be a normal phenomenon suggesting that the opposite side is pathologic. It may also be a finding in early cerebral vascular accident.
3. **If the hypoactive reflexes are diffuse, was there a sudden onset?** Sudden onset of hypoactive reflexes would suggest acute spinal cord conditions, such as spinal fractures, transverse myelitis, Guillain–Barré syndrome, or poliomyelitis, or acute central nervous system disorders, such as toxic metabolic disease of the central nervous system, concussion, subdural hematoma, or acute increased intercranial pressure. Early basilar artery thrombosis may be associated with hypoactive reflexes also.
4. **Are there other neurologic signs?** The presence of other neurologic signs, particularly cranial nerve involvement, would suggest an early basilar artery thrombosis, cerebral vascular accident, or subdural hematoma. If there are no other neurologic findings or there is simply a disordered state of consciousness, then a head injury or toxic metabolic disease of the central nervous system, increased intercranial pressure, or poliomyelitis might be suspected.

DIAGNOSTIC WORKUP

Focal hypoactive reflexes of the lower extremity require plane x-rays of the lumbosacral spine, a CT scan or MRI of the lumbosacral spine, and nerve conduction velocity and EMG studies. Dermatomal SSEP studies will occasionally show radiculopathy when EMGs are negative.

Hypoactive reflexes of one upper extremity can be worked up with x-rays of the cervical spine, MRI of the cervical spine, nerve conduction velocity studies, EMGs, and dermatomal SSEP studies. X-rays of the chest may be useful to rule out a Pancoast's tumor.

Diffuse hypoactive reflexes associated with other neurologic signs or symptoms require a neuropathy workup (see page 356). A serum B_{12} and folic acid and possibly a Schilling test may need to be done to rule out pernicious anemia. An EMG and muscle biopsy may be done to rule out muscular dystrophy. A spinal tap will be helpful in cases of poliomyelitis and Guillain–Barré syndrome. If the hypoactive reflexes are part of a toxic metabolic or inflammatory disease of the nervous system, the workup will be similar to that of coma (page 88).

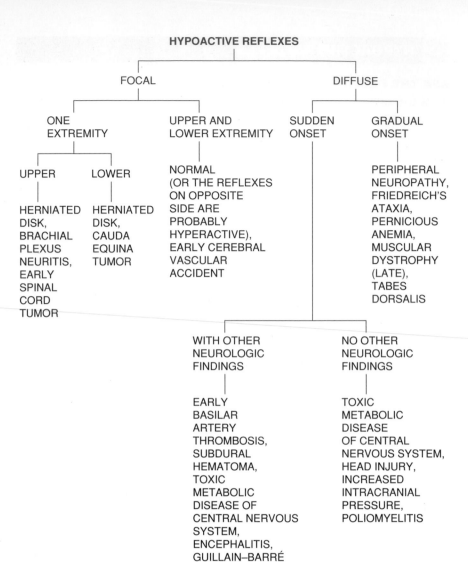

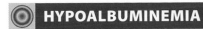

ASK THE FOLLOWING QUESTIONS:

1. **What is the urine protein?** Significant protein in the urine should suggest nephrotic syndrome and other chronic renal disorders as the likely cause.
2. **Are there abnormalities of the liver function tests?** This would point to cirrhosis, viral hepatitis, and other liver diseases as possible causes.
3. **What does the D-xylose absorption test show?** Decreased D-xylose absorption points to malabsorption syndrome.
4. If all of the above tests are normal, look for starvation, protein losing enteropathy, acute burns, hemodilution states such as congestive heart failure, and hypermetabolic states such as hyperthyroidism and metastatic neoplasm. Chronic infectious disease can also lower the albumin.

DIAGNOSTIC WORKUP

Routine tests include a CBC, urinalysis, 24-hr urine protein, chemistry panel, protein electrophoresis, sedimentation rate, a chest x-ray, and EKG. Further considerations include renal function tests, liver and renal biopsy, a CT scan of the abdomen, and consultation with a nephrologist and a hepatologist.

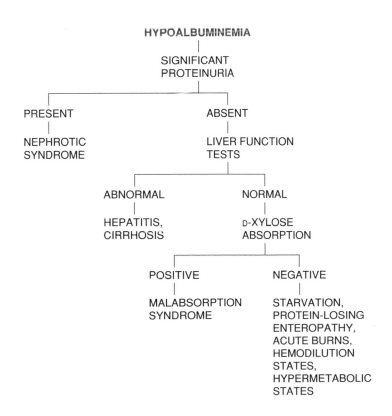

HYPOCALCEMIA

ASK THE FOLLOWING QUESTIONS:

1. **What is the PTH assay?** If this is low, hypoparathyroidism ought to be considered the most likely diagnosis. If it is normal or increased, other causes of hypocalcemia should be investigated.
2. **What is the phosphorus level?** A decreased phosphorus level should prompt a search for malabsorption syndrome, rickets, osteomalacia, renal tubular acidosis, cirrhosis, and nephrotic syndrome. An elevated phosphorus level would be most suggestive of renal disease, but pseudohypoparathyroidism must also be considered.
3. **What is the alkaline phosphatase level?** This would be elevated in hypocalcemia due to malabsorption syndrome, rickets, osteomalacia, renal tubular acidosis, and other chronic renal disease. It would be normal in cirrhosis, nephrosis, alkalosis, and pseudohypoparathyroidism.

DIAGNOSTIC WORKUP

CBC, urinalysis, chemistry panel, 24-hr urine calcium, PTH assay, serum protein electrophoresis, serum 25-OH vitamin D_3, skeletal survey, bone scan, D-xylose absorption test, serum 1,25-$(OH)_2$ vitamin D, and an endocrinology consult should be considered in the workup. Pseudohypoparathyroidism can be further differentiated from primary hypoparathyroidism by the Ellsworth–Howard test, which involves injecting parathyroid hormone intravenously. The blood values of calcium and phosphorus will improve in primary hypoparathyroidism but remain the same in pseudohypoparathyroidism. There is a phosphate diuresis in primary hypoparathyroidism.

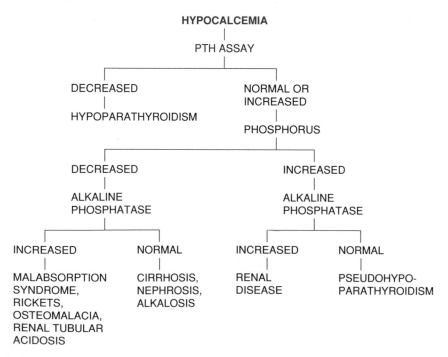

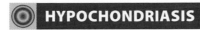

ASK THE FOLLOWING QUESTIONS:

1. **Is there loss of libido and/or appetite?** The findings of loss of libido and appetite would suggest endogenous depression. There may also be insomnia.
2. **Is there loss of memory or concentration?** These findings suggest the possibility of an organic brain syndrome or cerebral arteriosclerosis. Epilepsy may also be involved.
3. **Does extensive testing fail to convince the patient he or she is well?** If extensive testing fails to convince the patient he or she is well, the diagnoses of delusional hypochondriasis and schizophrenia must be considered.

DIAGNOSTIC WORKUP

The diagnostic workup need not be extensive, but certain routine tests should be done. These include a CBC, sedimentation rate, chemistry panel, thyroid profile, EKG, chest x-ray, and flat plate of the abdomen. If there are complaints of memory loss and/or poor concentration, an EEG and CT scan of the brain may be done. A neurologist should be consulted. If the above tests fail to disclose an organic cause for the complaints and the patient is still not convinced he/she is well, referral to a psychiatrist is indicated.

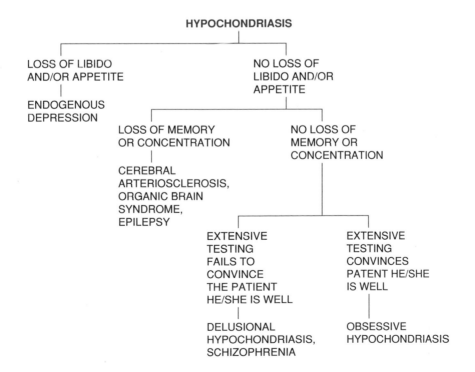

CASE HISTORY

A 36-year-old white male presents to the emergency room with generalized weakness and fatigue which has suddenly gotten worse over the past 24 hours. A stat blood sugar is 48 mg %.

Following the algorithm, you find he is not diabetic and consequently, does not take insulin or oral hypoglycemic agents. There is no history of weight gain and in fact he has lost weight over the past 3 months. He denies any episodes of loss of consciousness. He has a nice tan with hyperpigmentation of the palmar creases. A decreased plasma cortisol confirms your suspicion of Addison's disease.

ASK THE FOLLOWING QUESTIONS:

1. **Is the patient taking oral hypoglycemic drugs or insulin?** If so, the dosage may be too high.
2. **Is there a history of weight gain and/or episodes of loss of consciousness?** This would strongly suggest an insulinoma is the cause.
3. **What is the plasma cortisol?** If this is decreased, look for Addison's disease!
4. **What is the plasma growth hormone?** If this is decreased, look for Simmonds' disease.
5. **What does a D-xylose absorption test show?** If this is abnormal, look for malabsorption syndrome. If the diagnosis is still in doubt, the patient may have cirrhosis, glycogen storage disease, hypothyroidism, or functional hypoglycemia.

DIAGNOSTIC WORKUP

The finding of hypoglycemia on routine blood analysis requires nothing in an asymptomatic patient. If there is doubt, a repeat analysis should be done. If the patient is symptomatic, a 5-hr glucose tolerance test or hospitalization for repeated blood sugar during a 72-hr fast should be done. If these are negative, the patient most likely has functional hypoglycemia. Additional tests to order include a T_4, plasma cortisol, plasma growth hormone assay, plasma proinsulin, C-peptide, plasma insulin, CT scan of the abdomen, and a tolbutamide tolerance test. Obtain an endocrinology consult.

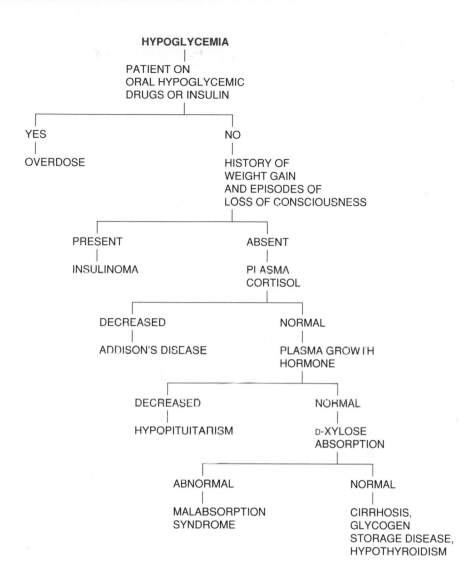

HYPOGLYCEMIA
|
PATIENT ON
ORAL HYPOGLYCEMIC
DRUGS OR INSULIN

- **YES** → OVERDOSE
- **NO** → HISTORY OF WEIGHT GAIN AND EPISODES OF LOSS OF CONSCIOUSNESS
  - **PRESENT** → INSULINOMA
  - **ABSENT** → PLASMA CORTISOL
    - **DECREASED** → ADDISON'S DISEASE
    - **NORMAL** → PLASMA GROWTH HORMONE
      - **DECREASED** → HYPOPITUITARISM
      - **NORMAL** → D-XYLOSE ABSORPTION
        - **ABNORMAL** → MALABSORPTION SYNDROME
        - **NORMAL** → CIRRHOSIS, GLYCOGEN STORAGE DISEASE, HYPOTHYROIDISM

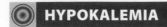

ASK THE FOLLOWING QUESTIONS:

1. **What is the sodium level?** If the sodium is normal or increased, consider aldosteronism, Cushing's syndrome, periodic paralysis, or IV fluid administration without supplemental potassium. If the sodium level is decreased, consider pyloric obstruction, diuretics, severe vomiting, diabetic acidosis, diarrhea, renal tubular acidosis, starvation, and malabsorption syndrome as possibilities.
2. **What is the plasma cortisol?** If it is elevated, look for Cushing's syndrome.
3. **What is the bicarbonate level?** If this is increased with both a low sodium and potassium, look for pyloric obstruction, persistent vomiting, and diuretic administration. If this is low with both a low sodium and potassium, look for diabetic acidosis, renal tubular acidosis, diarrhea, starvation, diuretic effects, and malabsorption syndrome.

DIAGNOSTIC WORKUP

The diagnosis can be pursued by ordering a CBC, urinalysis, 24-hr urine potassium, serial electrolytes, a chemistry panel, plasma renin, 24-hr urine aldosterone, D-xylose absorption test, and plasma cortisol, and obtaining an endocrinology or nephrology consult.

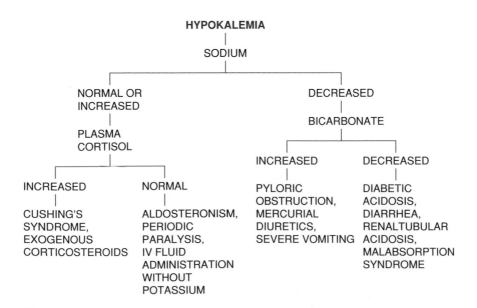

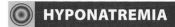

ASK THE FOLLOWING QUESTIONS:

1. **What is the chloride level?** An increased chloride points to diabetic acidosis, Addison's disease, renal tubular acidosis, nephritis, and use of certain diuretics as the cause. A decreased chloride suggests congestive heart failure, syndrome of inappropriate secretion of antidiuretic hormone (SIADH), pyloric obstruction, vomiting, malabsorption syndrome, and diuretic use as the possible cause. SIADH is found in carcinoma of the lung, porphyria, and numerous pulmonary and neurologic conditions.

2. **What is the blood sugar?** An elevated blood sugar level suggests diabetic acidosis or hyperosmolar coma.

3. **What is the plasma cortisol?** A low plasma cortisol coupled with a low sodium and elevated chloride suggests Addison's disease. A low sodium and elevated chloride but normal plasma cortisol should suggest renal tubular acidosis, nephritis, and use of certain diuretics.

4. **What is the blood volume?** Hyponatremia with an increased blood volume is associated with congestive heart failure and SIADH.

DIAGNOSTIC WORKUP

The diagnostic workup should include a CBC, chemistry panel, serial electrolytes, plasma cortisol, serum ADH assay, plasma renin, arterial blood gases, and consultation with an endocrinologist and a nephrologist.

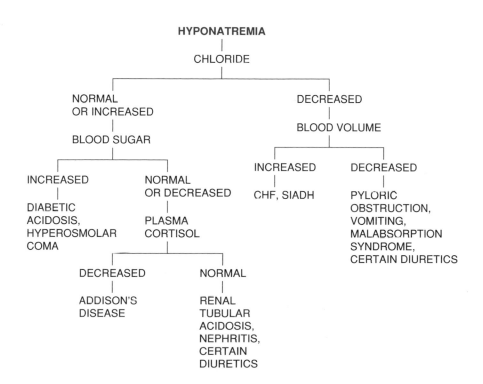

ASK THE FOLLOWING QUESTIONS:

1. **Is the hypotension found only on standing?** The finding of hypotension on standing suggests orthostatic hypotension, which may be due to several causes, including hypopituitarism, diabetic neuropathy, anemia, and various cardiovascular disorders.
2. **Is there a history of drug ingestion?** Many drugs induce hypotension, including nitroglycerin and its analogs, vasodilators, quinidine, and tricyclic drugs.
3. **Is there cardiomegaly or a heart murmur?** These findings suggest mitral valvular disease, aortic stenosis, and congestive heart failure.
4. **Is there pallor?** The finding of pallor suggests anemia.
5. **Is there hyperpigmentation?** The presence of hyperpigmentation suggests Addison's disease.

DIAGNOSTIC WORKUP

Routine studies include a CBC, sedimentation rate, chemistry panel, urinalysis, thyroid panel, EKG, and chest x-ray. A tilt table test is the best way to establish the diagnosis of orthostatic hypotension. Blood volume and arterial blood gas studies may be useful. A urine drug screen should be done. If there is cardiomegaly or a murmur, echocardiography and venous pressure and circulation time should be done. A cardiologist should also be consulted.

If there is hyperpigmentation, a serum cortisol and ACTH stimulation test should be done. A skull x-ray can be done to rule out pituitary tumors. A visual field examination by a qualified ophthalmologist may be helpful in this regard also. Twenty-four-hr blood pressure monitoring may also be useful in the workup.

HYPOTENSION, CHRONIC

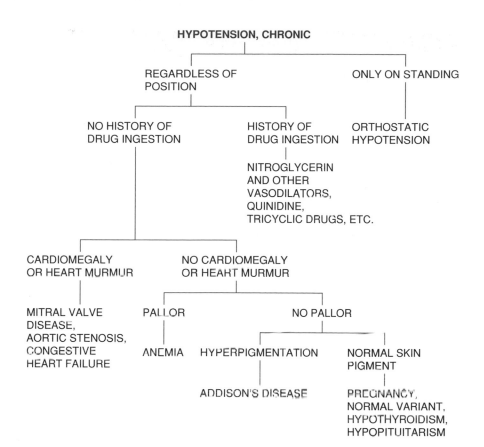

HYPOTHERMIA

ASK THE FOLLOWING QUESTIONS:

1. **Is there a history of drug or alcohol ingestion?** Alcoholic intoxication, opium poisoning, tricyclic antidepressants, and phenothiazine may cause hypothermia.
2. **Is there a history of severe vomiting or diarrhea?** Severe vomiting or diarrhea may induce dehydration and electrolyte disturbances, which will induce hypothermia. Intestinal obstruction, cholera, and peritonitis are among the many disorders that may lead to severe vomiting or diarrhea.
3. **Are there endocrine abnormalities?** Signs of hypothyroidism and Addison's disease may be obvious, but hypopituitarism, hypoglycemia, and diabetes mellitus may also be the cause of hypothermia.
4. **Are there abnormalities on the neurologic examination?** Focal neurologic findings may be seen in a cerebral vascular accident or epidural or subdural hematoma. However, thiamine deficiency may also result in hypothermia.

DIAGNOSTIC WORKUP

Routine laboratory tests include a CBC and differential count, a sedimentation rate and chemistry panel, electrolytes, thyroid profile, blood cultures, urinalysis, and a urine drug screen. An EKG and chest x-ray should also be done. A CT scan of the brain is done if there are focal neurologic abnormalities or disorders of consciousness.

An infusion of dextrose intravenously and thiamine are given as soon as blood studies are drawn in case there is hypoglycemia or thiamine deficiency.

If the above studies are normal, a thorough endocrine workup is indicated, including tests for serum cortisol, FSH, lutein-stimulating hormone (LSH), and growth hormone. A cardiologist, neurologist, or endocrinologist may need to be consulted to help solve the diagnostic dilemma.

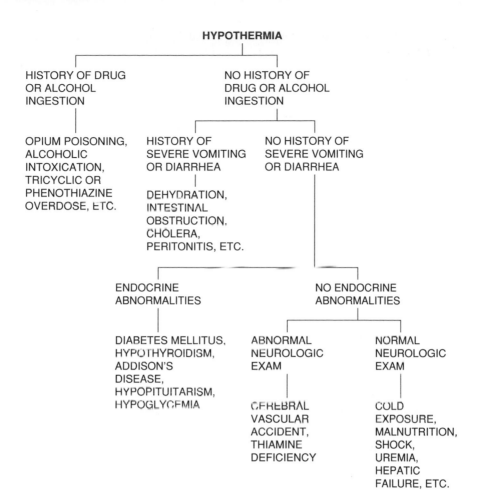

HYPOTHERMIA

HISTORY OF DRUG OR ALCOHOL INGESTION

NO HISTORY OF DRUG OR ALCOHOL INGESTION

OPIUM POISONING, ALCOHOLIC INTOXICATION, TRICYCLIC OR PHENOTHIAZINE OVERDOSE, ETC.

HISTORY OF SEVERE VOMITING OR DIARRHEA

DEHYDRATION, INTESTINAL OBSTRUCTION, CHOLERA, PERITONITIS, ETC.

NO HISTORY OF SEVERE VOMITING OR DIARRHEA

ENDOCRINE ABNORMALITIES

DIABETES MELLITUS, HYPOTHYROIDISM, ADDISON'S DISEASE, HYPOPITUITARISM, HYPOGLYCEMIA

NO ENDOCRINE ABNORMALITIES

ABNORMAL NEUROLOGIC EXAM

CEREBRAL VASCULAR ACCIDENT, THIAMINE DEFICIENCY

NORMAL NEUROLOGIC EXAM

COLD EXPOSURE, MALNUTRITION, SHOCK, UREMIA, HEPATIC FAILURE, ETC.

ASK THE FOLLOWING QUESTIONS:

1. **What is the carbon dioxide level?** An increased carbon dioxide level suggests pulmonary emphysema, asthma, pickwickian syndrome, respiratory paralysis, central nervous system disease, kyphoscoliosis, drug effects, and disorders of the chest wall and spine.

2. **What does spirometry show?** If spirometry shows a decreased 1-second timed vital capacity with an increased carbon dioxide level, consider emphysema and asthma likely. If the timed vital capacity is normal, a diagnosis of pickwickian syndrome, respiratory paralysis, central nervous system disease, drug effects, and chest wall and spine disorders should be considered.

3. **If the carbon dioxide level is normal or decreased, what does the chest radiograph show?** A focal infiltrate suggests pulmonary infarct, congestive heart failure, or pneumonia. A diffuse infiltrate or negative chest x-ray suggests congestive heart failure, pulmonary fibrosis, shock, pulmonary or intracardiac shunt, sarcoidosis, pneumoconiosis, or alveolar proteinosis.

4. **What does a perfusion scan show?** If this is positive, consider pulmonary infarction.

5. **What does the pulmonary capillary wedge pressure show?** If this is increased, consider congestive heart failure. If this is decreased, the patient may have hypovolemic shock. If it is normal, consider a right-to-left shunt, pulmonary fibrosis, pneumoconiosis, or sarcoidosis.

DIAGNOSTIC WORKUP

Repeated arterial blood gases should be done. A CBC, urinalysis, chemistry panel, methemoglobin, sulfhemoglobin, carboxyhemoglobin, venous pressure and circulation time, blood volume, serial ECGs, CT scan of the chest, lung biopsy, additional pulmonary function tests, and consultation with a pulmonologist or cardiologist will be necessary in many cases.

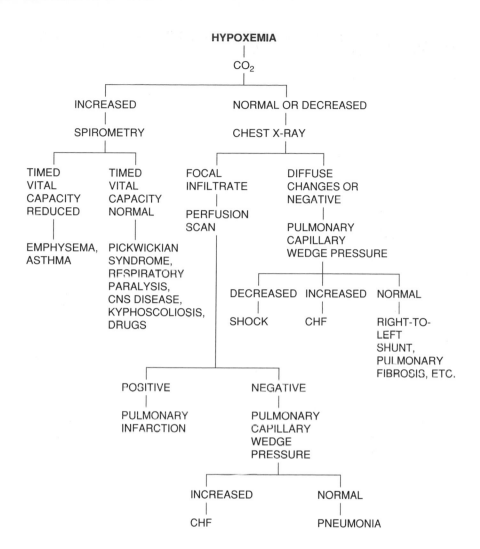

ASK THE FOLLOWING QUESTIONS:

1. **Is there a history of alcohol or drug ingestion?** A host of antihypertensive drugs, including the beta-blockers, may cause impotence. In addition, tricyclic drugs, nicotine, and alcohol intoxication may cause impotence.
2. **Is there loss of secondary sex characteristics?** These findings suggest Fröhlich's syndrome, Klinefelter's syndrome, and other congenital disorders.
3. **Are there abnormalities on urologic examination?** Various conditions such as Peyronie's disease, atrophied testes, prostatitis, and Leriche's syndrome may be found on urologic examination.
4. **Are there abnormalities on the neurologic examination?** Neurologic examination may reveal diabetic neuropathy, spinal cord tumor, multiple sclerosis, and other neurologic disorders.

DIAGNOSTIC WORKUP

A thorough psychiatric and sexual history is necessary before undertaking expensive laboratory tests. However, recent studies suggest that emotional problems are the cause in less than 10% of the cases. It is wise to interview the spouse or sexual partner also because the symptom may be exaggerated by the patient. Do not hesitate to order a drug screen. Routine tests include a CBC and differential count, a urinalysis, a urine culture and colony count, a chemistry panel, VDRL test, thyroid profile, serum testosterone, and gonadotropin assay. A referral to a urologist is probably wise at this point. He will work up the patient further with a nocturnal tumescent study, Doppler ultrasonography, and penile blood pressure studies. In addition, he may want to do a cystoscopy. It may be wise to perform a postage stamp test before referral for a formal tumescence study. A therapeutic trial of sildenafil may be diagnostic!

Nerve conduction velocity studies and EMGs may be needed to rule out diabetic neuropathy. MRI of the spine, cystometric studies, and SSEP studies will help rule out multiple sclerosis and other spinal cord lesions. A sacral reflex latency time may be very helpful in diagnosing sacral nerve injury. A spinal tap may help rule out central nervous system lues. Angiography may be needed to exclude a Leriche's syndrome.

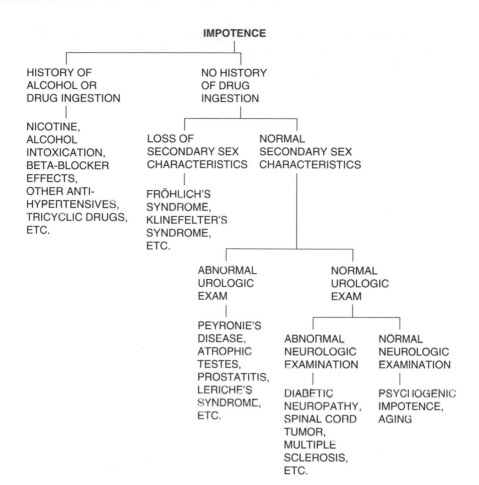

IMPOTENCE

HISTORY OF ALCOHOL OR DRUG INGESTION
|
NICOTINE, ALCOHOL INTOXICATION, BETA-BLOCKER EFFECTS, OTHER ANTI-HYPERTENSIVES, TRICYCLIC DRUGS, ETC.

NO HISTORY OF DRUG INGESTION

LOSS OF SECONDARY SEX CHARACTERISTICS
|
FRÖHLICH'S SYNDROME, KLINEFELTER'S SYNDROME, ETC.

NORMAL SECONDARY SEX CHARACTERISTICS

ABNORMAL UROLOGIC EXAM
|
PEYRONIE'S DISEASE, ATROPHIC TESTES, PROSTATITIS, LERICHE'S SYNDROME, ETC.

NORMAL UROLOGIC EXAM

ABNORMAL NEUROLOGIC EXAMINATION
|
DIABETIC NEUROPATHY, SPINAL CORD TUMOR, MULTIPLE SCLEROSIS, ETC.

NORMAL NEUROLOGIC EXAMINATION
|
PSYCHOGENIC IMPOTENCE, AGING

● INCONTINENCE OF FECES

ASK THE FOLLOWING QUESTIONS:

1. **Is the stool volume small or large?** A small volume of stool should suggest anal fissure; hemorrhoids, diarrhea, or postoperative incontinence from a fistulectomy; or other types of surgery in the perirectal area.
2. **Is the incontinence intermittent?** Intermittent incontinence suggests epilepsy or organic brain syndrome.
3. **Are there hyperactive reflexes in the lower extremities?** Presence of hyperactive reflexes in the lower extremities should suggest a spinal cord tumor or trauma to the spinal cord, multiple sclerosis, a parasagittal meningioma, transverse myelitis, and syringomyelia.
4. **Are there hypoactive reflexes in the lower extremities?** The presence of hypoactive reflexes in the lower extremities should suggest tabes dorsalis, a cauda equina tumor, spinal stenosis, and other conditions of the lumbar spine and lumbosacral area.

DIAGNOSTIC WORKUP

Routine studies include a CBC, sedimentation rate, chemistry panel, and VDRL test. Sigmoidoscopy and barium enema are needed to exclude malignancy. The anorectal area should be carefully inspected for lesions and the sphincter competence determined by a digital examination. If these findings are normal, it would be wise to consult a neurologist. If one is not available, further workup may be done.

If there are hyperactive reflexes with cranial nerve signs, a CT scan or MRI of the brain should be done. If there are hyperactive reflexes of all four extremities with no cranial nerve signs, MRI of the cervical spine should be done. With hyperactive reflexes of the lower extremities only, MRI of the thoracic cord should be done. If there are hypoactive reflexes in the lower extremities, MRI or CT scan of the lumbar spine should be done. If increased intracranial pressure has been excluded, a spinal tap may be done to help diagnose multiple sclerosis or tabes dorsalis. Anorectal manometry and defecography may be used to detect anal and rectal muscle dysfunction.

If the general physical examination and neurologic examination are negative, psychogenic causes should be considered, and cystometric studies might be helpful. The patient should be referred to a psychiatrist.

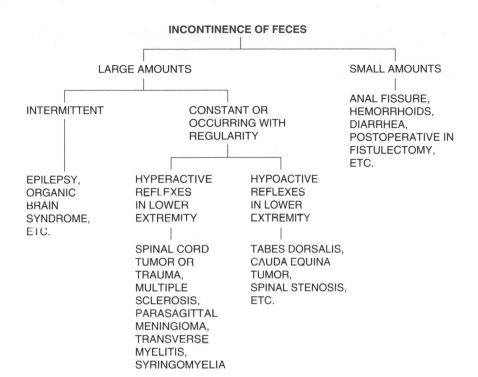

INCONTINENCE OF FECES

LARGE AMOUNTS

SMALL AMOUNTS

INTERMITTENT

CONSTANT OR
OCCURRING WITH
REGULARITY

ANAL FISSURE,
HEMORRHOIDS,
DIARRHEA,
POSTOPERATIVE IN
FISTULECTOMY,
ETC.

EPILEPSY,
ORGANIC
BRAIN
SYNDROME,
ETC.

HYPERACTIVE
REFLEXES
IN LOWER
EXTREMITY

HYPOACTIVE
REFLEXES
IN LOWER
EXTREMITY

SPINAL CORD
TUMOR OR
TRAUMA,
MULTIPLE
SCLEROSIS,
PARASAGITTAL
MENINGIOMA,
TRANSVERSE
MYELITIS,
SYRINGOMYELIA

TABES DORSALIS,
CAUDA EQUINA
TUMOR,
SPINAL STENOSIS,
ETC.

ASK THE FOLLOWING QUESTIONS:

1. **Is the volume of urine large or small?** If the volume of urine released is small, stress incontinence and vesicovaginal fistula should be considered. If the amounts released are large, one should consider a neurologic condition or an enlarged prostate with bladder neck obstruction as the cause.

2. **Are there abnormalities on the neurologic examination?** Neurologic disorders to be considered are spastic neurogenic bladder due to multiple sclerosis, spinal cord tumor, and spinal cord trauma, as well as incompetent sphincter due to cauda equina syndrome, spinal stenosis, poliomyelitis, diabetic neuropathy, and tabes dorsalis. Dementia and Parkinson's disease are significant causes of an overactive bladder.

3. **Are there hyperactive reflexes?** This helps distinguish the disorders of the spinal cord and parasagittal area, such as spastic neurogenic bladder due to multiple sclerosis, spinal cord tumor, spinal cord trauma, and parasagittal meningioma.

4. **Are the reflexes hypoactive?** Hypoactive reflexes suggest poliomyelitis, cauda equina syndrome, spinal stenosis, diabetic neuropathy, and tabes dorsalis.

5. **Is there an enlarged bladder or prostate?** If an enlarged bladder or prostate is palpated, one should consider overflow incontinence from bladder neck obstruction, prostatic hypertrophy, and tuberculosis of the bladder.

DIAGNOSTIC WORKUP

Routine laboratory tests include a CBC, a urinalysis, a urine culture and sensitivity, a chemistry panel, and a VDRL test. An intravenous pyelogram and a voiding cystogram may be helpful. A Q-tip test or stress test may be helpful in diagnosing stress incontinence. The bladder may be catheterized for residual urine, or abdominal ultrasonography may be employed to evaluate residual urine. Fifty milliliters or more is considered abnormal. Cystoscopy may also be necessary to determine if there is chronic bladder inflammation or bladder neck obstruction. Office cystometrography can be considered, but it is usually best to refer the patient to a urologist for cystometric studies. Prostatic size can be determined by transrectal prostatic ultrasonography.

The simplest and most cost-effective approach is to refer the patient to a neurologist if there are abnormalities on the neurologic examination, or refer the patient to a urologist if there are not. If there is stress incontinence and a cystocele is found on vaginal examination, the patient should be referred to a gynecologist. It is not cost-effective to begin ordering MRIs or CT scans of the brain and spinal cord without the assistance of these specialists.

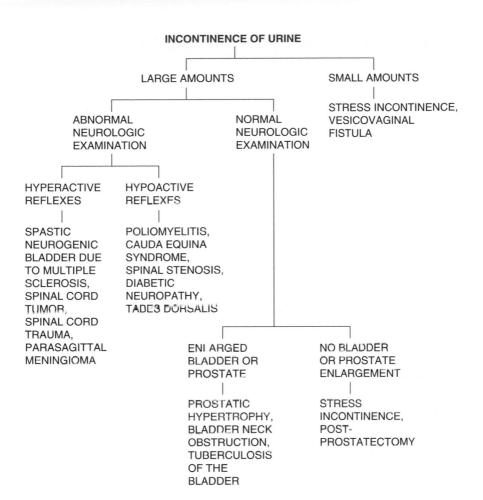

INCONTINENCE OF URINE

LARGE AMOUNTS

SMALL AMOUNTS

ABNORMAL NEUROLOGIC EXAMINATION

NORMAL NEUROLOGIC EXAMINATION

STRESS INCONTINENCE, VESICOVAGINAL FISTULA

HYPERACTIVE REFLEXES

HYPOACTIVE REFLEXES

SPASTIC NEUROGENIC BLADDER DUE TO MULTIPLE SCLEROSIS, SPINAL CORD TUMOR, SPINAL CORD TRAUMA, PARASAGITTAL MENINGIOMA

POLIOMYELITIS, CAUDA EQUINA SYNDROME, SPINAL STENOSIS, DIABETIC NEUROPATHY, TABES DORSALIS

ENLARGED BLADDER OR PROSTATE

NO BLADDER OR PROSTATE ENLARGEMENT

PROSTATIC HYPERTROPHY, BLADDER NECK OBSTRUCTION, TUBERCULOSIS OF THE BLADDER

STRESS INCONTINENCE, POST-PROSTATECTOMY

ASK THE FOLLOWING QUESTIONS:

1. **Is the alkaline phosphatase increased?** An increased alkaline phosphatase along with an increased bilirubin would point to liver disease or obstructive jaundice. An elevated bilirubin without alkaline phosphatase increase is more likely to be associated with hemolytic anemias, Gilbert's disease, or Dubin–Johnson syndrome.

2. **Are the liver enzymes elevated?** If so, the patient likely has hepatitis or cirrhosis of the liver, although occasionally elevation of the liver enzymes is seen in obstructive jaundice.

3. **What is the serum haptoglobin?** An elevated serum haptoglobin indicates hemolytic anemia. If the serum haptoglobin is normal, look for Gilbert's disease or Dubin–Johnson syndrome.

DIAGNOSTIC WORKUP

Hepatitis can be further evaluated by ordering a Hepatitis profile, Monospot test, and serologic tests for leptospirosis and various other liver disorders. Cirrhosis of the liver can be diagnosed by a liver biopsy. Cholestatic hepatitis can be diagnosed by the lowering of serum bilirubin by a course of corticosteroids. Obstructive jaundice is best diagnosed by ultrasound, ERCP or a CT scan of the abdomen, although transhepatic cholangiography is occasionally necessary. Hemolytic anemia can be further evaluated by a CBC, reticulocyte count, direct and indirect Coombs test, and hemoglobin electrophoresis.

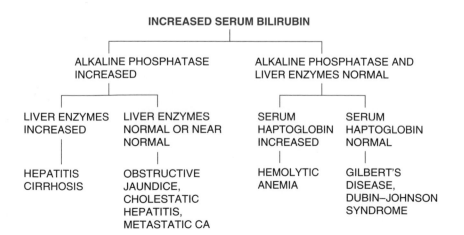

ASK THE FOLLOWING QUESTIONS:

1. **Is there a history of drug or alcohol ingestion?** Alcohol, tobacco, aspirin, other nonsteroidal anti-inflammatory drugs, steroids, caffeine, and antibiotics are just a few of the drugs that may irritate the stomach.

2. **Is the indigestion brought on by exertion?** A history of indigestion brought on by exertion should suggest angina pectoris.

3. **Is there a loss of appetite and weight?** These findings would suggest not only a GI neoplasm but also pernicious anemia, chronic pancreatitis and pyloric obstruction, and chronic gastritis. Chronic organ failure should also be entertained, such as uremia, cirrhosis, or congestive heart failure.

4. **Is the indigestion or pain relieved by food or antacids?** These findings would suggest a duodenal ulcer, hiatal hernia, and esophagitis.

5. **Is the indigestion or pain brought on by food?** These findings would suggest cholecystitis, gastric ulcer, or toxins in food such as monosodium glutamate (MSG) or sulfites.

6. **Is the indigestion or pain unrelated to meals?** These findings would suggest a chronic appendicitis, chronic intestinal obstruction, or tabes dorsalis. It may also suggest air swallowing from chronic anxiety or excessive talking.

7. **Is there no pain associated with the indigestion?** This finding would suggest functional dyspepsia.

DIAGNOSTIC WORKUP

Routine tests include a CBC, urinalysis, chemistry panel, VDRL test, thyroid profile, serum B_{12} and folic acid, an upper GI series, esophagogram, and stools for occult blood and ovum and parasites. A lactose tolerance test can be helpful. The next step is a cholecystogram or gallbladder ultrasound.

If these studies are negative, a gastroenterologist should be consulted. He will do esophagoscopy, gastroscopy, and duodenoscopy. He may also perform esophageal motility studies or esophageal pH monitoring. A Bernstein test may be of value in solving the diagnostic dilemma. He may also want to order a CT scan of the abdomen or a small bowel series.

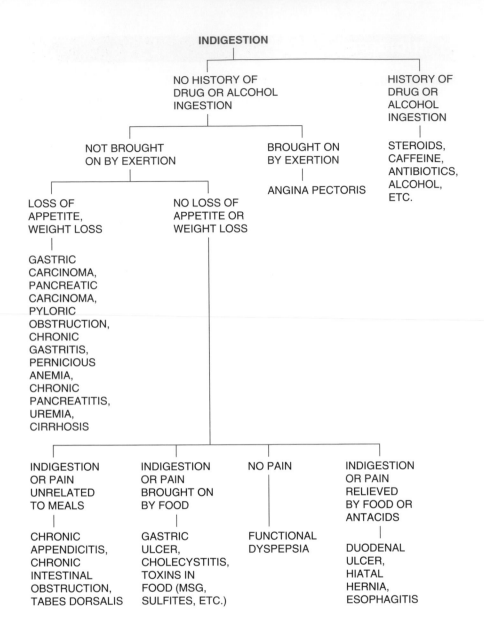

INFERTILITY, FEMALE

ASK THE FOLLOWING QUESTIONS:

1. **Are there abnormalities on pelvic examination?** Abnormalities found on the pelvic examination are cervicitis, stenosis of the cervix, fibroids, retroverted uterus, tubo-ovarian abscesses, and polycystic ovaries.
2. **Are there abnormal secondary sex characteristics?** Patients with Turner's syndrome, Simmonds' disease, Fröhlich's syndrome, and virilism may exhibit abnormal secondary sex characteristics.
3. **Are there other abnormalities in endocrine examination?** The physical examination may disclose hypothyroidism, hyperthyroidism, Simmonds' disease, or acromegaly.

DIAGNOSTIC WORKUP

Routine studies include a CBC, urinalysis, urine culture and colony count, chemistry panel, thyroid profile, VDRL test, and a vaginal smear and culture. Cervicitis should be biopsied and treated. The next logical step is to obtain a specimen of semen from the husband for sperm count.

If the above tests are negative, referral to a gynecologist is in order. If one is not available, further workup can be done, including a serum FSH and LH, serum estradiol, and serum progesterone to determine the presence of pituitary or ovarian causes of ovulatory dysfunction. A hysterosalpingogram can be done. The patient can keep a temperature chart to determine if ovulation occurs. Cervical mucus studies can be done for spinnbarkeit testing and ferning, and the presence of significant white cells should be noted. Pelvic ultrasound may be done, and laparoscopy may be necessary to rule out other conditions that may affect fertility. A trial of clomiphene citrate may be given. Endometrial biopsy may also contribute to solving the diagnostic dilemma.

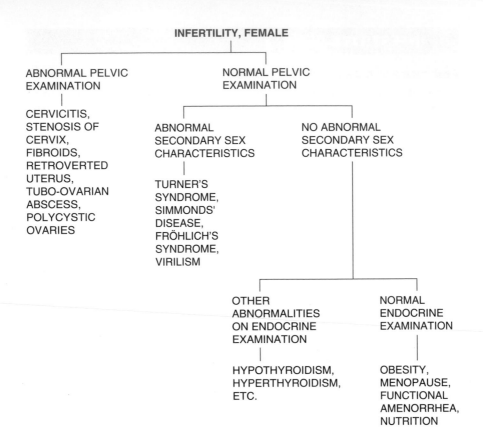

INFERTILITY, FEMALE

ABNORMAL PELVIC EXAMINATION

CERVICITIS, STENOSIS OF CERVIX, FIBROIDS, RETROVERTED UTERUS, TUBO-OVARIAN ABSCESS, POLYCYSTIC OVARIES

NORMAL PELVIC EXAMINATION

ABNORMAL SECONDARY SEX CHARACTERISTICS

TURNER'S SYNDROME, SIMMONDS' DISEASE, FRÖHLICH'S SYNDROME, VIRILISM

NO ABNORMAL SECONDARY SEX CHARACTERISTICS

OTHER ABNORMALITIES ON ENDOCRINE EXAMINATION

HYPOTHYROIDISM, HYPERTHYROIDISM, ETC.

NORMAL ENDOCRINE EXAMINATION

OBESITY, MENOPAUSE, FUNCTIONAL AMENORRHEA, NUTRITION

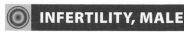

ASK THE FOLLOWING QUESTIONS:

1. **Are there abnormalities on examination of the external genitalia and prostate?** The abnormalities that need to be looked for are Klinefelter's syndrome, epididymitis, testicular atrophy, urethritis, and prostatitis.
2. **Are there abnormalities on the endocrine examination?** The general endocrine examination may reveal hypothyroidism, hyperthyroidism, or hypopituitarism.
3. **Are there stress factors that need to be considered such as marital difficulties or overwork?** Overwork and marital difficulties may lead to drug addiction and alcoholism, among other problems. All these affect fertility.

DIAGNOSTIC WORKUP

Routine laboratory tests include a CBC, urinalysis, chemistry panel, thyroid profile, VDRL test, and sperm count. If there is a urethral discharge, a smear and culture should be done. If the sperm count reveals oligospermia on two separate specimens, referral should be made to a urologist or endocrinologist for further evaluation.

Additional tests that can be ordered include blood tests for LH, FSH, and testosterone. Additional tests of pituitary function may be indicated. Karyotype testing and sperm function tests may be needed. If these are normal, a testicular biopsy may need to be done. Ultrasonography of the testicles may be helpful.

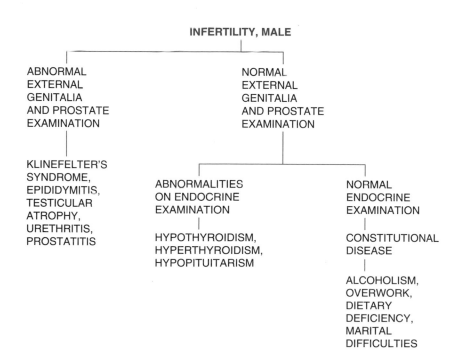

ASK THE FOLLOWING QUESTIONS:

1. **Is it reducible?** If the inguinal swelling is reducible, a femoral hernia or inguinal hernia should be suspected.
2. **Does it transilluminate?** If the mass transilluminates, it is probably a hydrocele and may be a hydrocele of the cord or a hydrocele of Nuck's canal.
3. **Is it tender?** Tenderness in the groin may signify an abscess, hematoma, lymphadenitis, a strangulated hernia, or an obturated hernia.

DIAGNOSTIC WORKUP

The routine workup includes a CBC, sedimentation rate, chemistry panel, VDRL test, and an x-ray of the hips and pelvis. A bone scan may be helpful in ruling out a psoas abscess. Arteriography may be helpful for diagnosing aneurysm. Venography or Doppler ultrasonography will help diagnose saphenous varix. Needle aspiration may be necessary to diagnose an abscess. Exploratory surgery will be necessary in most cases for both diagnosis and treatment.

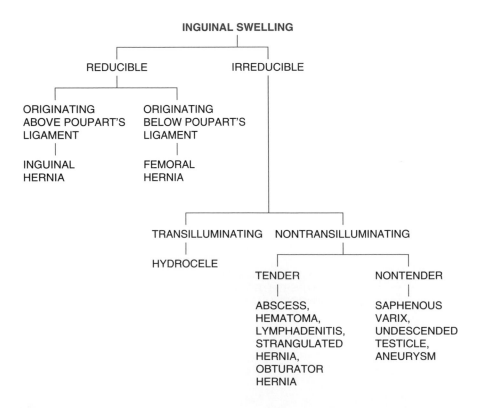

ASK THE FOLLOWING QUESTIONS:

1. **Is there dyspnea?** If there is a history of dyspnea, heart disease or lung disease should be suspected.
2. **Is there a history of drug or alcohol ingestion?** There are many drugs that may cause insomnia, including the amphetamines, theophylline, caffeine, anticonvulsants, nicotine, thyroid hormones, and the sympathomimetics. Alcohol may induce sleep, but patients complain of early morning wakening.
3. **Is there a history of a painful condition?** Abscessed teeth, arthritis, sciatica, bone metastasis, hiatal hernia, and esophagitis are just a few of the conditions that may keep a patient awake because of pain.
4. **Are there other psychiatric symptoms?** Anxiety, loss of libido, loss of appetite, and depression may be associated with hyperthyroidism, general paresis, organic brain syndrome, chronic anxiety, and endogenous depression. In the elderly, look for restless leg syndrome and periodic limb movement disorder.

DIAGNOSTIC WORKUP

The first thing to do is to eliminate caffeinated beverages and chocolate. Routine studies include a CBC, sedimentation rate, urinalysis and drug screen, chemistry panel, thyroid profile, VDRL test, EKG, and chest x-ray. Arterial blood gases and pulmonary function testing should be done to rule out pulmonary disease. A venous pressure and circulation time will help rule out early congestive heart failure. Blood pressure monitoring can be used to rule out paroxysmal hypertension. If an organic brain syndrome is suspected, a CT scan or MRI of the brain should be done. If psychiatric symptoms are present, the patient should be referred to a psychiatrist. Alternatively, a therapeutic trial of psychotherapeutic agents may be initiated if the patient is not suicidal. When all of the above diagnostic tests are negative, a sleep study must be done. However, home monitors for apnea and oxygen desaturation are available and may be an inexpensive alternative to rule out obstructive sleep apnea.

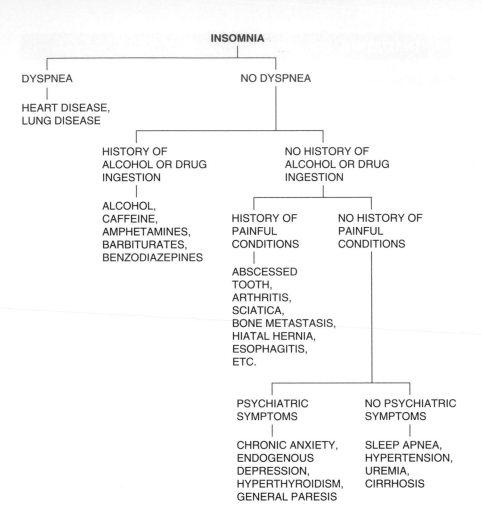

Intracranial bruit may be due to a carotid cavernous sinus fistula or a cerebral angioma. It may also be due to a congenital arteriovenous anomaly. A cerebral aneurysm is rarely big enough to cause a bruit. Severe anemia may cause intracranial bruits without localized pathology being responsible. All intracranial bruits should be investigated with MRI and angiography unless some systemic disease is found (e.g., anemia) that would explain the sign.

Cervical bruits may be due to carotid stenosis, hyperthyroidism, a venous hum, or aortic stenosis with transmission of the bruit to the vessels in the neck. If hyperthyroidism and aortic stenosis can be excluded, a carotid duplex scan and possibly carotid angiography should be done to look for significant carotid stenosis. There is considerable controversy over whether asymptomatic carotid stenosis should be operated on. Nevertheless, a thorough workup should be done so the clinician knows what he is dealing with.

CASE HISTORY

A 42-year-old white male presents to your office because his family noted a yellowish tinge to his skin and eyeballs. You ask about fever and chills or abdominal pain, and he has none.

On examination, he shows icteric sclera, mild hepatomegaly, but no enlargement of the gallbladder or spleen. There is no ascites or pedal edema. Looking at the algorithm, you see that there are three possibilities left: Primary or metastatic carcinoma, toxic hepatitis, and biliary cirrhosis. On further questioning, you find out he has been on ranitidine for reflux esophagitis. Withdrawal of the medication results in the clearing of his jaundice.

ASK THE FOLLOWING QUESTIONS:

1. **Is the jaundice associated with hepatomegaly?** There is little or no hepatomegaly associated with hemolytic anemias, pernicious anemia, Gilbert's disease, and Dubin–Johnson syndrome.
2. **Is the hepatomegaly massive?** Massive hepatomegaly is associated with Gaucher's disease.
3. **Is there associated fever, right upper quadrant pain, or a tender liver?** These findings would suggest viral hepatitis, cholecystitis, infectious mononucleosis, leptospirosis, ascending cholangitis, hepatic vein thrombosis, and toxic hepatitis.
4. **Is the gallbladder enlarged?** The finding of an enlarged gallbladder with the jaundice suggests obstructive jaundice, carcinoma of the pancreas, carcinoma of the bowel ducts, or ampulla of Vater.
5. **Is there skin pigmentation?** The presence of skin pigmentation that is not bilirubin suggests hemochromatosis.
6. **Is there splenomegaly?** The presence of significant splenomegaly suggests infectious mononucleosis, cirrhosis of the liver, hemolytic anemia, Gaucher's disease, kala azar, or agnogenic myeloid metaplasia.
7. **Is there edema and ascites?** The presence of edema and ascites suggests alcoholic cirrhosis.

DIAGNOSTIC WORKUP

The basic workup includes a CBC, sedimentation rate, reticulocyte count, red cell fragility test, urinalysis, chemistry panel, VDRL test, EKG, a chest x-ray, and flat plate of the abdomen.

If infectious hepatitis is suspected, a hepatitis profile, febrile agglutinins, Monospot test, cytomegalic virus antibody titer, and leptospirosis antibody titer should be done. If lupoid hepatitis is suspected, a test for antinuclear antibodies and a smooth muscle antibody should be done. Toxic hepatitis, as in the case above, may be confirmed by a steroid white-wash.

If hemochromatosis is suspected, a serum iron, iron-binding capacity, and ferritin should be done.

If hemolytic anemia is suspected, serum haptoglobins, hemoglobin electrophoresis, and sickle cell preparations may be done.

If obstructive jaundice is suspected, then gallbladder ultrasound should be done to rule out gallstones, and a CT scan of the abdomen may be done to look for GI neoplasm. An upper GI series may assist in finding a primary neoplasm in the GI tract.

ERCP or percutaneous transhepatic cholangiography will assist in determining whether there is definitely obstructive jaundice and whether it is due to a surgically resectable lesion. Peritoneoscopy can also be helpful. An exploratory laparotomy will probably be necessary regardless of whether one performs the above tests. Cholangiopancreatography and endoscopic ultrasonography are two newer methods that may be used to evaluate the biliary tree and pancreatic ducts, especially when a neoplasm is suspected.

Hepatocellular jaundice will often require a needle biopsy of the liver to pin down the diagnosis. Antimitochondrial antibodies will need to be ordered to screen for biliary cirrhosis. An alpha-1-fetoprotein will help diagnose hepatocellular carcinoma. By the time you have reached this point, you have gone to considerable expense in the diagnostic workup. It would be much more prudent to ask for a gastroenterology consultation before ordering all these expensive diagnostic tests.

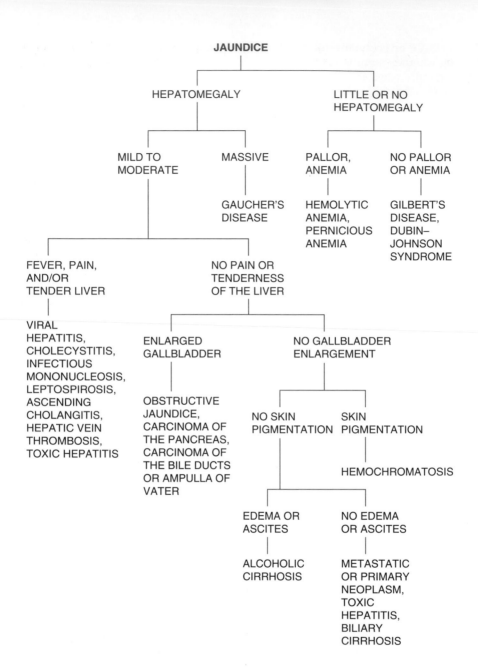

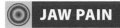

ASK THE FOLLOWING QUESTIONS:

1. **Are there abnormalities on examination of the teeth or gums?** A thorough examination of the teeth and gums may disclose dental caries, gingivitis, oral tumors, or alveolar abscess.
2. **Is the pain intermittent?** Intermittent pain should suggest a trigeminal neuralgia or glossopharyngeal neuralgia.
3. **Is there a rash?** The presence of a rash would suggest herpes zoster. Be sure to examine the eardrum for Ramsay Hunt's syndrome.

DIAGNOSTIC WORKUP

Routine diagnostic studies include a CBC, sedimentation rate, chemistry panel, arthritis panel, and an x-ray of the teeth and jaw. X-ray of the sinuses may be helpful. At this point, referral to a dentist or oral surgeon should be made if there is still diagnostic difficulty. He may order an MRI of the temporomandibular joint, which is the procedure of choice in evaluating this joint. If all tests are negative or equivocal, perhaps a psychiatric referral is in order.

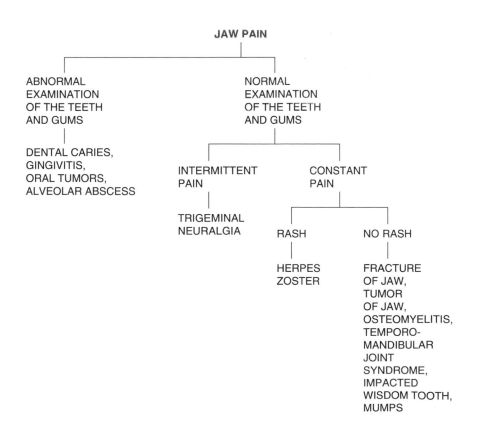

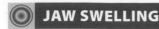

ASK THE FOLLOWING QUESTIONS:

1. **Is the swelling focal or diffuse?** Focal jaw swelling should suggest alveolar abscess, gingivitis, adamantinoma, actinomycosis, epithelioma, a cyst, osteoma, odontoma, or epulis.
2. **Is it painful?** Painful jaw swelling should suggest alveolar abscess, gingivitis, actinomycosis, adamantinoma, cellulitis, fracture, hematoma, necrosis of the jaw, or osteomyelitis.
3. **Is there enlargement of the hands and feet?** Enlargement of the hands and feet should suggest acromegaly.
4. **Is it intermittent?** This would point to a stone in Stensen's duct.

DIAGNOSTIC WORKUP

Routine tests include a CBC, urinalysis, sedimentation rate, chemistry panel, and x-ray of the jaw and teeth. X-rays of the skull and long bones and a serum growth hormone should be done if acromegaly is suspected. PTH assay and x-rays of the skull and long bones should be done if osteitis fibrosa cystica is suspected. Referral to a dentist or oral surgeon should be made if there is still diagnostic confusion at this point.

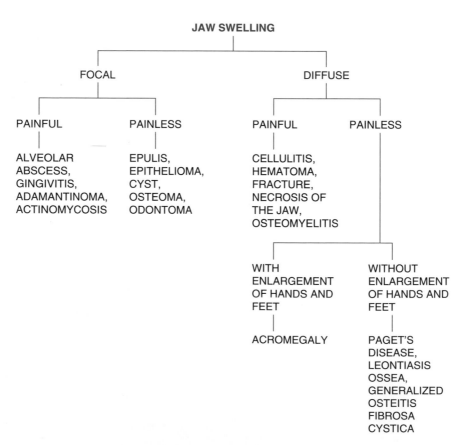

CASE HISTORY

A 23-year-old white male complains of painful wrists and knees of 4 days duration. Following the algorithm, you look for fever and his temperature is 101.3°F.

Your examination shows that his right conjunctiva is red and he has a purulent urethral discharge which on microscopic examination shows Gram-positive diplococci. What is your diagnosis?

ASK THE FOLLOWING QUESTIONS:

1. **Is the joint pain localized to a single joint?** Localization to a single joint should suggest a septic arthritis, gout, tuberculosis, hemophilia, sickle cell disease, trauma, avascular necrosis, and pseudogout. Monoarthritis that is sudden in onset should be considered a septic joint until proven otherwise.
2. **Is there fever?** The presence of fever should make one think of septic arthritis, rheumatic fever, gonococcal arthritis, Reiter's syndrome, lupus erythematosus, Lyme arthritis, polymyalgia rheumatica, Still's disease, and rheumatoid arthritis.
3. **Is there a urethral discharge?** The presence of a urethral discharge should make one think of Reiter's syndrome or gonococcal arthritis.
4. **Is there low back pain?** The presence of low back pain should suggest rheumatoid spondylitis, ochronosis, and gout.
5. **Is the arthritis migratory?** The presence of migratory arthritis should make one think of rheumatic fever and rat-bite fever. Multiple joint involvement with oral or genital ulcers suggests Bechet's disease.
6. **What is the age of the patient?** Younger patients may have sickle cell disease, hemophilia, trauma, rheumatic fever, Still's disease, and gonococcal arthritis. Older patients are more likely to have osteoarthritis, polymyalgia rheumatica, and gout. It should be noted that there is considerable overlap here.

DIAGNOSTIC WORKUP

Routine studies include a CBC, sedimentation rate, ASO titer, ANA, cross-reacting protein (CRP), urinalysis, chemistry panel, arthritis panel, and x-rays of the involved joints. The anticitrullinated protein antibody (ACPA) is more specific for rheumatoid arthritis than the R-A titer. It is also wise at times to order a bone survey. Synovial fluid analysis and culture should be done if there is sufficient joint effusion. A trial of therapy may be initiated at this point and will assist in the diagnosis. For example, a course of colchicine may be given to rule out gout.

If there is still doubt, a rheumatology consultation should be made. Other tests that may be done include a gonococcal antibody titer and a coagulation profile. If there is a urethral discharge, a smear and culture of the material should be made. If there is fever, febrile agglutinins, serologic tests for Lyme disease, brucellin antibody titer, blood cultures, and a Monospot test may be done. If collagen disease is suspected, antinuclear antibodies and anti-DNA antibodies may be sought. If sickle cell anemia is suspected, a sickle cell preparation should be done. A bone scan will help diagnose rheumatoid spondylitis and ochronosis. A urine for homogentisic acid will diagnose ochronosis also. An MRI may diagnose a torn meniscus and other condition.

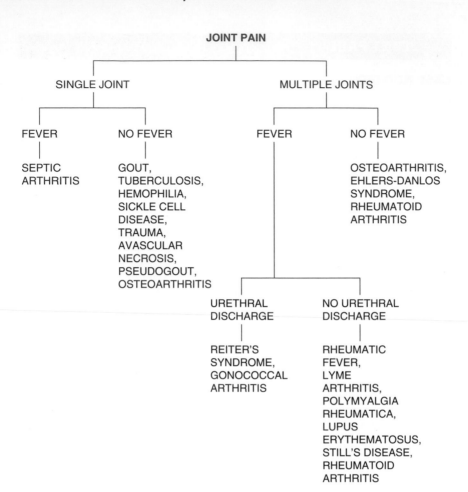

ASK THE FOLLOWING QUESTIONS:

1. **Is it painless?** The presence of joint swelling without pain, especially on motion, would suggest Charcot's disease.

2. **Is the involvement primarily in small or large joints?** Involvement of the small joints is characteristic of rheumatoid arthritis, gonococcal arthritis, and Reiter's syndrome. Involvement of the larger joints is more characteristic of gout and osteoarthritis. However, osteoarthritis and rheumatoid arthritis may involve both.

3. **Is the involvement symmetrical or asymmetrical?** Asymmetrical involvement is more typical of gout, rheumatic fever, hemophilia, neoplasm, septic arthritis, and trauma. Symmetrical involvement is more characteristic of rheumatoid arthritis and osteoarthritis.

4. **Is there fever?** The presence of fever should make one think of rheumatic fever, gonococcal arthritis or other types of septic arthritis, Reiter's syndrome, rheumatoid arthritis, and lupus erythematosus.

5. **What is the age of the patient?** The younger patients with joint swelling most likely have gonococcal arthritis, lupus erythematosus, rheumatoid arthritis, and hemophilia. Gout, osteoarthritis, and neoplasm are more common in older patients. However, there is considerable overlap here.

DIAGNOSTIC WORKUP

Routine tests include a CBC, sedimentation rate, ASO titer, C-reactive protein (CRP), ANA, urinalysis, chemistry panel, arthritis panel, and x-rays of the involved joints. It is also wise to do a bone survey when there is multiple joint involvement. A synovial fluid analysis and culture may be done if there is sufficient joint fluid. A trial of therapy can be initiated and may be diagnostic particularly in gonococcal arthritis. At this point, it is wise to refer the patient to a rheumatologist for further evaluation. Additional tests that may be ordered are found on page 289. Polarized microscopy may reveal positive birefringent crystals of pseudogout.

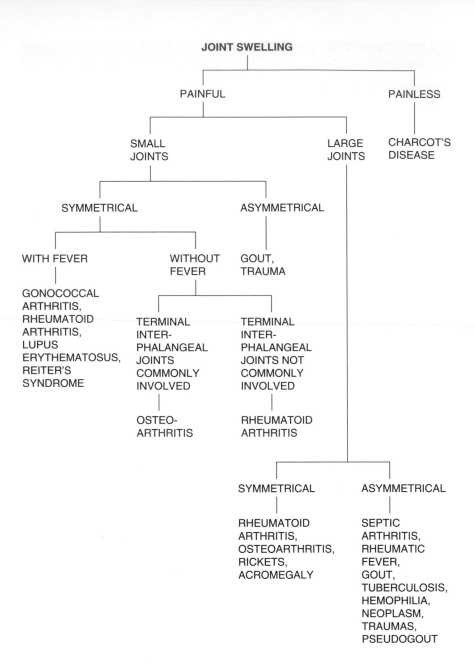

JOINT SWELLING

PAINFUL

PAINLESS

SMALL JOINTS

LARGE JOINTS

CHARCOT'S DISEASE

SYMMETRICAL

ASYMMETRICAL

WITH FEVER

WITHOUT FEVER

GOUT, TRAUMA

GONOCOCCAL ARTHRITIS, RHEUMATOID ARTHRITIS, LUPUS ERYTHEMATOSUS, REITER'S SYNDROME

TERMINAL INTER-PHALANGEAL JOINTS COMMONLY INVOLVED

TERMINAL INTER-PHALANGEAL JOINTS NOT COMMONLY INVOLVED

OSTEO-ARTHRITIS

RHEUMATOID ARTHRITIS

SYMMETRICAL

ASYMMETRICAL

RHEUMATOID ARTHRITIS, OSTEOARTHRITIS, RICKETS, ACROMEGALY

SEPTIC ARTHRITIS, RHEUMATIC FEVER, GOUT, TUBERCULOSIS, HEMOPHILIA, NEOPLASM, TRAUMAS, PSEUDOGOUT

ASK THE FOLLOWING QUESTIONS:

1. **Is it transient?** Transient knee pain may be due to rheumatic fever, sarcoidosis, palindromic rheumatism, or trauma.
2. **Is it unilateral or bilateral?** Unilateral knee pain would suggest gout, septic arthritis, bursitis, hemophilia, pseudogout, osteogenic sarcoma, and traumatic conditions such as torn meniscus, hemarthrosis, sprain of collateral ligaments, and fracture.
3. **Is there a history of trauma?** History of trauma would suggest a sprain, torn meniscus, bruise, or fracture. Perform a McMurray test. Iliotibial band syndrome, compartment syndrome, and patella-femoral syndrome are important to consider in athletes, especially gymnasts and ballet artists.
4. **Are there prominent systemic symptoms?** If there are prominent systemic symptoms, one should consider lupus erythematosus, Reiter's disease, rheumatoid arthritis, other collagen disease, scurvy, and rheumatic fever.
5. **What is the age of the patient?** Younger patients are more likely to have traumatic conditions such as fracture, sprains, bruises, or a torn meniscus. Osgood–Schlatter disease would be more typical of patients in their early teens. Patients in their twenties are more likely to have rheumatoid arthritis, Reiter's disease, and lupus erythematosus, whereas patients in the fourth or fifth decade and older would be more likely to have osteoarthritis, gout, and pseudogout.

DIAGNOSTIC WORKUP

Routine studies include a CBC, sedimentation rate, ASO titer, ANA, CRP, urinalysis, chemistry panel, arthritis panel, and x-rays of the involved joint. X-rays may show a fracture, osteoarthritic changes, and punched-out lesion of gout or chondrocalcinosis (suggesting pseudogout). Stress fractures usually will not be evident on plain films. It is also wise to do a bone survey. Synovial fluid analysis and culture may be done if there is sufficient joint fluid. The anti-citrullinated protein antibody (ACPA) is a new test that is more sensitive than the R-A test. A trial of therapy can be initiated and may be diagnostic.

If further diagnostic workup needs to be done at this point, it is most cost-effective to refer the patient to a rheumatologist or an orthopedic surgeon before ordering MRI or other studies. He may want to do an arthroscopic examination before proceeding with other tests for arthritic conditions. For further workup of knee pain, see page 289.

KNEE PAIN

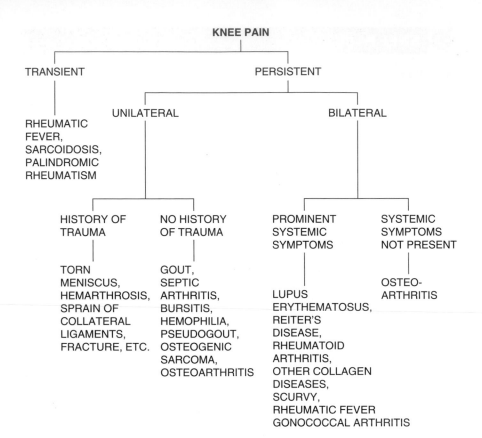

TRANSIENT

PERSISTENT

RHEUMATIC
FEVER,
SARCOIDOSIS,
PALINDROMIC
RHEUMATISM

UNILATERAL

BILATERAL

HISTORY OF
TRAUMA

NO HISTORY
OF TRAUMA

PROMINENT
SYSTEMIC
SYMPTOMS

SYSTEMIC
SYMPTOMS
NOT PRESENT

TORN
MENISCUS,
HEMARTHROSIS,
SPRAIN OF
COLLATERAL
LIGAMENTS,
FRACTURE, ETC.

GOUT,
SEPTIC
ARTHRITIS,
BURSITIS,
HEMOPHILIA,
PSEUDOGOUT,
OSTEOGENIC
SARCOMA,
OSTEOARTHRITIS

LUPUS
ERYTHEMATOSUS,
REITER'S
DISEASE,
RHEUMATOID
ARTHRITIS,
OTHER COLLAGEN
DISEASES,
SCURVY,
RHEUMATIC FEVER
GONOCOCCAL ARTHRITIS

OSTEO-
ARTHRITIS

ASK THE FOLLOWING QUESTIONS:

1. **Is it painless?** Painless swelling of the knee is probably a Charcot's joint.
2. **Is it unilateral or bilateral?** Unilateral knee swelling is most likely due to trauma, gout, pseudogout, hemophilia, septic arthritis, tuberculosis, osteogenic sarcoma, torn meniscus, or osteomyelitis. Bilateral swelling of the knee is more commonly seen in osteoarthritis, lupus erythematosus, Reiter's disease, and rheumatoid arthritis.
3. **Is there fever?** The presence of fever suggests septic arthritis, rheumatic fever, rheumatoid arthritis, osteomyelitis, lupus erythematosus, and Reiter's disease.
4. **Are there systemic symptoms?** Systemic symptoms suggest lupus erythematosus, rheumatoid arthritis, and Reiter's disease, as well as rheumatic fever.
5. **What is the age of the patient?** Knee swelling in younger patients is more likely to be due to rheumatic fever, septic arthritis, lupus erythematosus, Reiter's disease, and rheumatoid arthritis. Older patients are more likely to be affected with gout, pseudogout, and osteoarthritis. Osteogenic sarcoma seems to occur between the ages of 5 and 25 years in most cases.

DIAGNOSTIC WORKUP

Routine diagnostic tests include CBC, sedimentation rate, urinalysis, chemistry panel, arthritis panel, VDRL test, and x-rays of the involved joint or joints. A bone survey should probably also be done. If there is significant swelling, an arthrocentesis for synovial fluid should be done and the fluid analyzed and cultured. A therapeutic trial may be initiated at this point and can assist in the diagnosis.

If there is still doubt about the diagnosis, referral to a rheumatologist or an orthopedic surgeon should be made before ordering MRI or expensive diagnostic tests. An orthopedic surgeon may perform fiberoptic arthroscopy to diagnose the problem. Additional diagnostic tests to order in cases of knee swelling may be found on page 289.

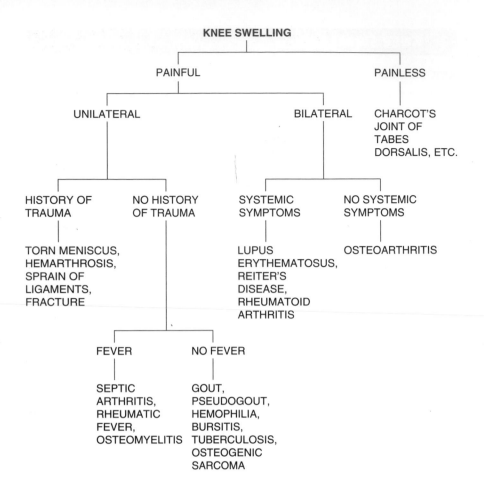

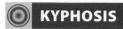

ASK THE FOLLOWING QUESTIONS:

1. **Is there a history of chronic cough?** A history of cough would suggest tuberculosis of the spine, emphysema, and metastatic carcinoma.
2. **What is the sex of the patient?** If the patient is a woman in her forties, menopausal osteoporosis should be suspected.
3. **What is the age of the patient?** Children are more likely to have kyphosis due to rickets, leukopolysaccharidosis, Hurler's disease, Scheuermann's disease, Pott's disease, or Morquio's disease. Adults are more likely to suffer from osteoarthritis, Paget's disease, Parkinson's disease, osteomalacia, osteoporosis, and ankylosing spondylitis.

DIAGNOSTIC WORKUP

Routine diagnostic studies include a CBC, sedimentation rate, urinalysis, chemistry panel, arthritis panel, tuberculin test, and x-rays of the chest, thoracic spine, lumbar spine, and the hips. If there is a productive cough, a sputum for AFB smear and culture should be made.

If muscular disease is suspected, a muscle biopsy may be done. If menopause is suspected, a serum FSH and LH and serum estradiol can be done. A bone scan may identify pathologic fractures and ankylosing spondylitis. An HLA B27 antigen test should be ordered if ankylosing spondylitis is suspected. A bone biopsy may clear up the diagnostic dilemma.

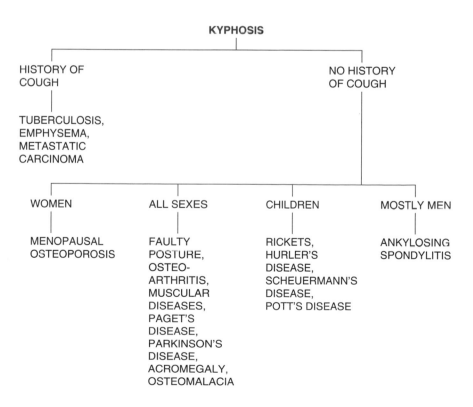

ASK THE FOLLOWING QUESTIONS:

1. **What is the level of creatine phosphokinase isoenzyme containing M and B subunits (MB-CPK)?** An elevated MB-CPK combined with elevated LDH is most likely due to a myocardial infarction, although myocarditis and pericarditis can produce a similar picture.
2. **What is the AST level?** If the MB-CPK or CPK are not also increased, an elevation of both the LDH and AST would point to liver disease.
3. **What are the serum and urine creatine levels?** If these are elevated, muscle disease must be considered likely.
4. **What does the lung scan show?** If positive, a lung scan separates pulmonary infarction from the other conditions in this group.

DIAGNOSTIC WORKUP

The diagnostic workup should include a CBC, urinalysis, chemistry panel, sedimentation rate, ANA, urine and serum creatine, urine myoglobin, serial EKGs, blood gas analysis, LDH isoenzymes, troponin C, chest x-ray, lung scan, EMG, and cardiology and neurology consults. A liver scan, CT scan of the abdomen and liver, and muscle biopsy may be necessary.

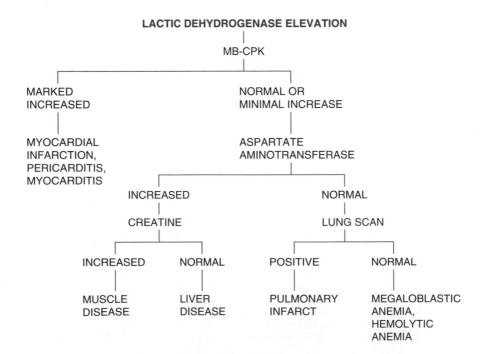

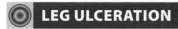

ASK THE FOLLOWING QUESTIONS:

1. **Are the peripheral pulses diminished or absent?** Presence of poor peripheral pulses suggests arteriosclerosis, diabetes mellitus, Buerger's disease, and femoral artery thrombosis.

2. **Are there abnormalities on the neurologic examination?** Neurologic disorders associated with leg ulceration include tabes dorsalis, diabetic neuropathy, hemiplegia, and many other disorders.

3. **Is there a positive smear or culture of the material from the ulcer?** A positive smear or culture of material from the ulcer may be found in osteomyelitis, tuberculosis, syphilis, anthrax, and other fungal diseases.

DIAGNOSTIC WORKUP

Routine studies include a CBC, sedimentation rate, sickle cell preparation, urinalysis, chemistry panel, VDRL test, smear and culture of the material from the ulcer, and x-rays of the involved area. A biopsy may be necessary to establish the diagnosis. Rarely, a dark field examination will be necessary. Arteriography or venography may establish the level of arterial or venous obstruction. A bone scan or MRI will help pin down the diagnosis of osteomyelitis.

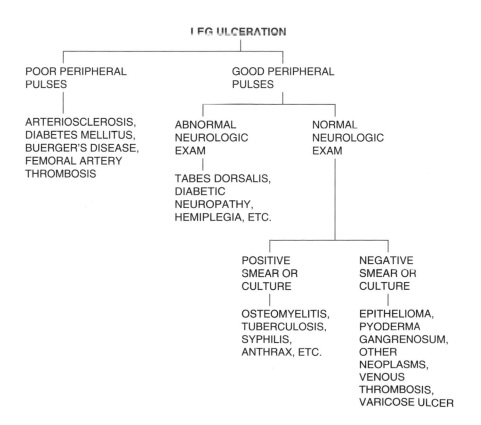

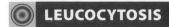 **LEUCOCYTOSIS**

ASK THE FOLLOWING QUESTIONS:

1. **Is the red cell count and platelet elevated?** This would suggest polycythemia vera or hemoconcentration.
2. **Are the neutrophils increased?** This would suggest a bacterial infection, leukemia, or corticosteroid therapy.
3. **Is there an increased percentage of lymphocytes?** This would suggest a viral infection, infectious mononucleosis, or lymphatic leukemia.
4. **Is there an increased percentage of monocytes?** Obviously, in this situation one should consider a monocytic leukemia, but severe infections can also present this picture.
5. **Is the percentage of eosinophils increased?** Allergic disorders (asthma, etc.) and parasitic disease present this picture.
6. **Is the percentage of basophils increased?** This would suggest chronic myelogenous leukemia and other blood dyscrasias.

DIAGNOSTIC WORKUP

On physical examination, one should look for a source of infection. Prostatic abscess and tubo-ovarian abscess are often missed. If there is a massive splenic enlargement, the possibility of myeloid metaplasia must be considered. Cultures should be taken of all body fluids and an unspun drop of urine looked at under the microscope. If there is motile bacteria, it is safe to say that there are more than 100,000 colonies/cc, which is a clear indication of a UTI. A sedimentation rate, chemistry panel, blood and bone marrow smear examination, serial blood cultures, blood smears for malarial parasites, and Monospot test, all have their place in the workup, but a hematology consult is wise before undertaking more expensive tests.

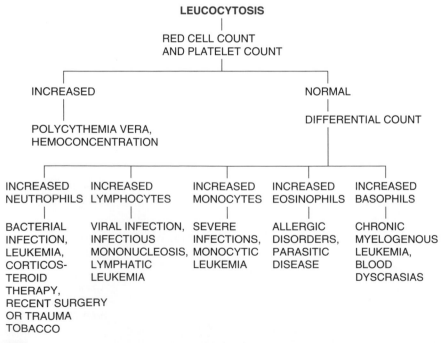

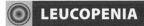

ASK THE FOLLOWING QUESTIONS:

1. **Are the red blood cell (RBC) and platelet counts decreased?** If so, this suggests hypersplenism, aplastic anemia, aleukemic leukemia, myelophthisic anemia, megaloblastic anemia, or paroxysmal nocturnal hemoglobinuria. If not, one should look for a viral infection, agranulocytosis, or idiopathic leucopenia.

2. **Is there an enlarged spleen?** An enlarged spleen should suggest hypersplenism of various causes, even though it may be associated with the other disorders listed above on occasion.

3. **What is the serum B_{12} level?** A decreased serum B_{12} will separate pernicious anemia from the other disorders on the list.

DIAGNOSTIC WORKUP

A CBC, sedimentation rate, chemistry panel, serum protein electrophoresis, urinalysis, platelet count, serum haptoglobins, serum B_{12} and folic acid, and Donath–Landsteiner test may need to be done. A hematologist should be consulted before ordering a bone marrow examination, liver-spleen scan, CT scans, or other expensive tests.

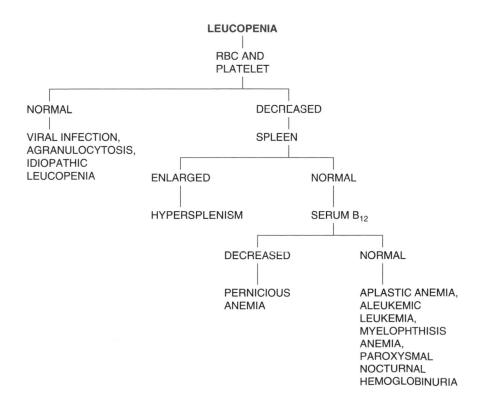

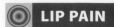

ASK THE FOLLOWING QUESTIONS:

1. **Is there ulceration or swelling?** Presence of ulceration would suggest herpes simplex, syphilis, and carcinoma. Swelling would suggest there was trauma, a carbuncle, insect bites or stings, and angioneurotic edema.
2. **Is there a rash?** The presence of a rash would suggest herpes zoster, particularly if it is unilateral.
3. **Is there a history of trauma, insect bite, or sting?** These historical findings are important in determining if the swelling is due to trauma, insect bites, or stings.

DIAGNOSTIC WORKUP

Routine studies include a CBC, sedimentation rate, urinalysis, chemistry panel, VDRL test, and culture of any material that can be obtained from ulceration if present. A therapeutic trial of antibiotics or antiviral medication can be done at this point. If this is unsuccessful, the patient should be referred to an oral surgeon or a dermatologist.

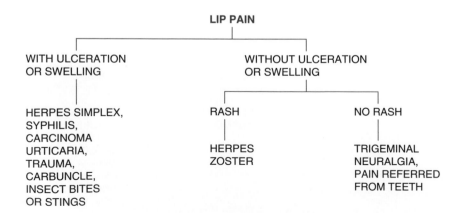

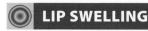

ASK THE FOLLOWING QUESTION:

1. **Is it painful or nonpainful?** Painful swelling of the lip is more likely to be herpes zoster, herpes simplex, pyoderma granulosa, insect bites or stings, alveolar abscess, and trauma. Painless swellings of the lip are more likely to be due to syphilis, allergic urticaria, angioneurotic edema, contact dermatitis, carcinoma, myxedema, and cretinism.

DIAGNOSTIC WORKUP

Routine laboratory tests include a CBC, sedimentation rate, urinalysis, chemistry panel, VDRL test, and culture of any material that can be obtained from an ulcer if present. An x-ray of the teeth and jaw may be necessary also. A therapeutic trial of antibiotics or antiviral therapy can be tried. If this is unsuccessful, a referral to an oral surgeon or a dermatologist should be made.

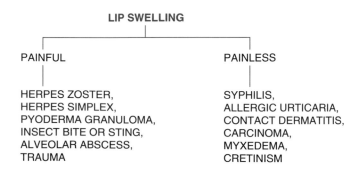

LORDOSIS

This is often a congenital effusion or backward curvature of the spine causing the person to appear "high and mighty." However, it may be seen in untreated bilateral congenital dislocation of the hips, muscular dystrophy, tuberculosis, and spondylolisthesis. Lordosis is also seen in orthostatic albuminuria and chondrodystrophy.

An x-ray of the lumbosacral spine and hips will usually establish the diagnosis in cases of congenital dislocation of the hips and spondylolisthesis. A family history and muscle biopsy will assist in the diagnosis of muscular dystrophy.

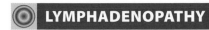
LYMPHADENOPATHY

ASK THE FOLLOWING QUESTIONS:

1. **Is there a history of drug ingestion?** Many drugs can cause lymphaden-opathy; the most notable is Dilantin, but the antibiotics, aspirin, iodides, and certain antihypertensive drugs can also cause lymphadenopathy.
2. **Is the lymphadenopathy focal or diffuse?** If the adenopathy is focal, one should look for an infectious process in the area supplied by the respective lymph nodes. For example, if there is occipital node enlargement, one would look for ringworm, dermatitis of the scalp, furunculosis, pediculosis, and cellu-litis. However, infectious mononucleosis and rubella may begin with enlarge-ment of these nodes.
3. **Is there fever?** The presence of fever should make one think of infectious mononucleosis, brucellosis, dengue fever, toxoplasmosis, and Still's disease, among other diseases. Is the adenopathy primarily cervical? In these cases, consider infectious mononucleosis, strep throat, and Kawasaki disease.

DIAGNOSTIC WORKUP

Routine diagnostic tests include a CBC, sedimentation rate, nose and throat culture, and culture of material from any area supplied by the enlarged lymph nodes. Blood cultures are indicated in generalized lymphadenopathy. In addition, a chemistry panel should be done, as well as a heterophile antibody titer, brucellin antibody titer, febrile agglutinins, and VDRL test. A chest x-ray and flat plate of the abdomen may be helpful in diagnosing generalized lymphadenopathy. HIV testing is done in patients with a history of high-risk sexual behavior.

X-ray of the long bones may identify metastatic carcinoma, and x-ray of the hands may identify sarcoidosis. A bone marrow examination may identify leuke-mia or lymphoma. If an infectious process has been ruled out, biopsy of the local node may turn up metastatic carcinoma, Hodgkin's disease, and sarcoidosis. A tuberculin skin test should be done; a Brucellergen skin test and Kveim test may also need to be done. ANA and rheumatoid arthritis factor testing may need to be done to rule out a collagen disease. A lymphangiogram may turn up a lympho-sarcoma or multiple metastatic lymph nodes. Liver biopsy is also occasionally necessary. Imaging studies of the abdomen and pelvis and the mediastinum are occasionally necessary. Mediastinoscopy may facilitate getting a tissue diagnosis. Before ordering these, consultation with a hematologist or an infectious disease specialist would be prudent.

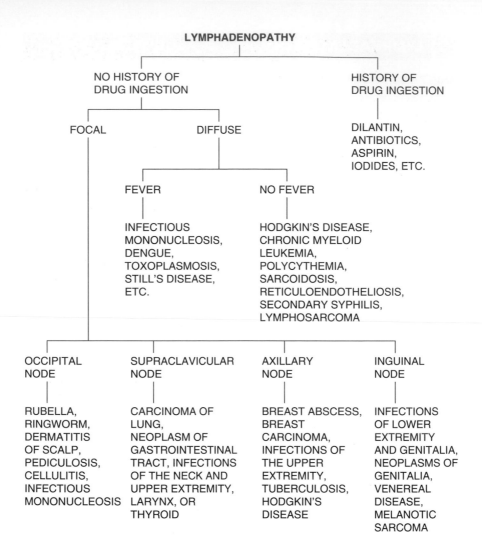

ASK THE FOLLOWING QUESTIONS:

1. **Is it true or false melena?** False melena may be induced by iron ingestion, bismuth ingestion, charcoal ingestion, red wine ingestion, and many other substances.
2. **Is there a history of alcohol or drug ingestion?** It is surprising how often the ingestion of alcohol is overlooked. Aspirin, other NSAIDs, caffeine, anticoagulants, and reserpine are among the other drugs that may cause melena.
3. **Is there associated hematemesis?** The presence of hematemesis should prompt a search for esophageal varices, peptic ulcer, gastritis, and many other conditions. For a more thorough discussion of this topic, one is referred to the section on hematemesis (page 217).
4. **Is there abdominal pain?** The presence of abdominal pain and heartburn should make one think of duodenal ulcer, esophagitis, gastritis, gastric ulcer, mesenteric embolism or thrombosis, and Meckel's diverticulum. On the other hand, the absence of abdominal pain would be more consistent with a blood dyscrasia or hereditary telangiectasia.

DIAGNOSTIC WORKUP

Routine laboratory tests include a CBC, sedimentation rate, urinalysis, chemistry panel, coagulation panel, VDRL test, and stool for occult blood. A stool for ovum and parasites may also need to be done. If these tests are inconclusive, an upper GI series and esophagogram would be the next step. Perhaps a small bowel series should be added to the above studies.

If all of these tests are negative or still inconclusive, referral to a gastroenterologist should be made. The gastroenterologist will probably perform panendoscopy and resolve the diagnostic dilemma. Occasionally, a fluorescein string test may be useful. A radioactive scan following intravenous chromium or technetium-99 may show the site of bleeding in obscure cases. When bleeding continues despite therapy, mesenteric angiography or splenic venography may assist in the diagnosis. Exploratory laparotomy may be necessary in some cases. Needless to say, a gastroenterologist should be consulted before undertaking this.

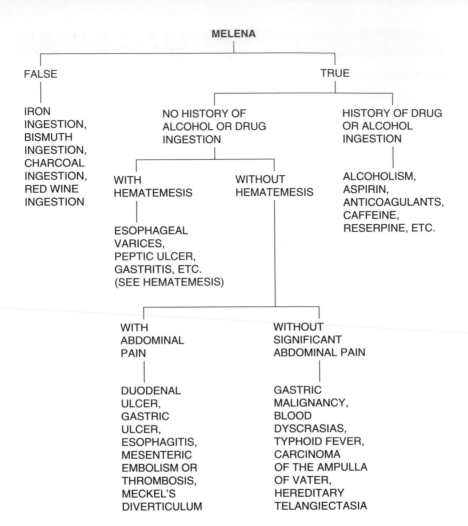

MELENA

FALSE

IRON
INGESTION,
BISMUTH
INGESTION,
CHARCOAL
INGESTION,
RED WINE
INGESTION

TRUE

NO HISTORY OF
ALCOHOL OR DRUG
INGESTION

HISTORY OF DRUG
OR ALCOHOL
INGESTION

WITH
HEMATEMESIS

WITHOUT
HEMATEMESIS

ALCOHOLISM,
ASPIRIN,
ANTICOAGULANTS,
CAFFEINE,
RESERPINE, ETC.

ESOPHAGEAL
VARICES,
PEPTIC ULCER,
GASTRITIS, ETC.
(SEE HEMATEMESIS)

WITH
ABDOMINAL
PAIN

WITHOUT
SIGNIFICANT
ABDOMINAL PAIN

DUODENAL
ULCER,
GASTRIC
ULCER,
ESOPHAGITIS,
MESENTERIC
EMBOLISM OR
THROMBOSIS,
MECKEL'S
DIVERTICULUM

GASTRIC
MALIGNANCY,
BLOOD
DYSCRASIAS,
TYPHOID FEVER,
CARCINOMA
OF THE AMPULLA
OF VATER,
HEREDITARY
TELANGIECTASIA

CASE HISTORY

You are called to the urology ward to evaluate a 52-year-old Hispanic male who developed confusion and disorientation following a radical prostatectomy for prostatic carcinoma 4 weeks ago.

Following the algorithm, you find no history of trauma. His family denies he has ever abused alcohol or drugs. Looking over the list of drugs he is on, you fail to find anything that will likely cause delirium or memory loss. However, he has had frequent loose stools post-operatively and examination of his extremities discloses a maculopapular eruption. You suspect pellagra and begin him on a course of vitamin B Complex which clears his symptoms.

ASK THE FOLLOWING QUESTIONS:

1. **Is there a history of trauma?** A history of trauma would suggest concussion, intracranial hematoma, and posttraumatic epilepsy, among other conditions.
2. **Is there a history of alcohol or drug ingestion?** Chronic alcoholism is associated with Korsakoff's syndrome and Wernicke's encephalopathy. Drugs such as bromides, barbiturates, cocaine, and LSD may induce memory loss. Heavy metals such as lead may cause a chronic encephalopathy with memory loss.
3. **Are there systemic signs and symptoms?** If there is anemia and memory loss, one should consider pernicious anemia. Pellagra, beriberi, myxedema, lupus erythematosus, uremia, and liver failure may be associated with memory loss.
4. **Are there other focal neurologic signs?** Extrapyramidal symptoms may be found in Wilson's disease, Huntington's chorea, and Parkinson's disease. Long tract signs may be found in multiple sclerosis, Creutzfeldt–Jakob disease, general paresis, and normal pressure hydrocephalus. When there is memory loss without focal neurologic signs, Alzheimer's disease and Pick's disease should be considered, as well as malingering.

DIAGNOSTIC WORKUP

It is wise to start with simple tests of mental status such as the Kendrick cognitive tests for the elderly or Mini-Mental Status Examination. Routine laboratory tests include a CBC, sedimentation rate, urinalysis, chemistry panel, ANA, serum B_{12} and folic acid, and VDRL test. In the elderly, a chest x-ray should be done to look for a primary neoplasm. A urine drug screen is essential.

If these studies are negative, the patient may be referred to a neurologist, or a CT scan or MRI may be done. The neurology consultation is much less expensive. Ultimately, a spinal tap may need to be done to look for multiple sclerosis and central nervous system lues. A lumbar isotope cisternography may need to be done to rule out normal pressure hydrocephalus. A referral to a psychologist can be made for psychometric testing.

MEMORY LOSS

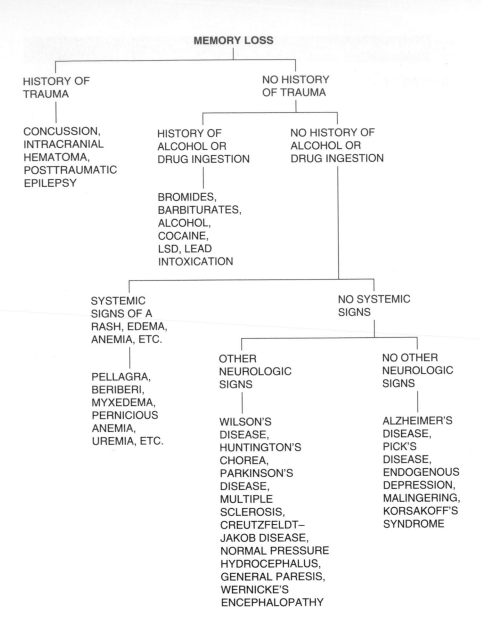

HISTORY OF
TRAUMA

CONCUSSION,
INTRACRANIAL
HEMATOMA,
POSTTRAUMATIC
EPILEPSY

NO HISTORY
OF TRAUMA

HISTORY OF
ALCOHOL OR
DRUG INGESTION

BROMIDES,
BARBITURATES,
ALCOHOL,
COCAINE,
LSD, LEAD
INTOXICATION

NO HISTORY OF
ALCOHOL OR
DRUG INGESTION

SYSTEMIC
SIGNS OF A
RASH, EDEMA,
ANEMIA, ETC.

PELLAGRA,
BERIBERI,
MYXEDEMA,
PERNICIOUS
ANEMIA,
UREMIA, ETC.

NO SYSTEMIC
SIGNS

OTHER
NEUROLOGIC
SIGNS

WILSON'S
DISEASE,
HUNTINGTON'S
CHOREA,
PARKINSON'S
DISEASE,
MULTIPLE
SCLEROSIS,
CREUTZFELDT–
JAKOB DISEASE,
NORMAL PRESSURE
HYDROCEPHALUS,
GENERAL PARESIS,
WERNICKE'S
ENCEPHALOPATHY

NO OTHER
NEUROLOGIC
SIGNS

ALZHEIMER'S
DISEASE,
PICK'S
DISEASE,
ENDOGENOUS
DEPRESSION,
MALINGERING,
KORSAKOFF'S
SYNDROME

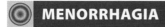

ASK THE FOLLOWING QUESTIONS:

1. **Is there persistent or recurring abdominal or pelvic pain?** The presence of pain with menorrhagia should make one suspect PID, endometriosis, and ectopic pregnancy.
2. **Are there abnormalities on the pelvic examination?** The pelvic examination will usually be positive in cases of uterine fibroid, pregnancy, cervical polyp, pelvic inflammatory disease, and ectopic pregnancy. Endometriosis may not always be detected on pelvic examination.
3. **Is there anemia or other systemic symptoms or signs?** The clinician should remember that iron deficiency anemia, hypothyroidism, lupus erythematosus, and cirrhosis of the liver are just a few of the systemic conditions that may present with menorrhagia.

DIAGNOSTIC WORKUP

Routine studies include a CBC, sedimentation rate, urinalysis, pregnancy test, chemistry panel, ANA titer, VDRL test, coagulation profile, thyroid profile, and flat plate of the abdomen. A Pap smear and vaginal smear and culture should be done.

If these tests are negative, referral to a gynecologist should be made before undertaking expensive tests such as pelvic ultrasound or CT scan of the abdomen and pelvis. Some clinicians will probably ignore this advice. A gynecologist will often be able to resolve the diagnostic dilemma with a good pelvic examination. Laparoscopy, culdocentesis, endometrial biopsy, and dilation and curettage are just a few of the diagnostic tools at his disposal.

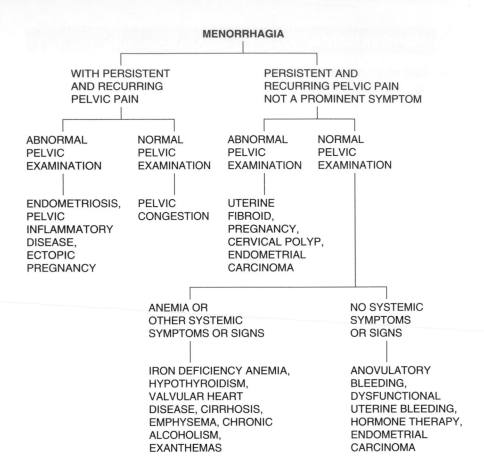

MENORRHAGIA

WITH PERSISTENT AND RECURRING PELVIC PAIN

ABNORMAL PELVIC EXAMINATION

ENDOMETRIOSIS, PELVIC INFLAMMATORY DISEASE, ECTOPIC PREGNANCY

NORMAL PELVIC EXAMINATION

PELVIC CONGESTION

PERSISTENT AND RECURRING PELVIC PAIN NOT A PROMINENT SYMPTOM

ABNORMAL PELVIC EXAMINATION

UTERINE FIBROID, PREGNANCY, CERVICAL POLYP, ENDOMETRIAL CARCINOMA

NORMAL PELVIC EXAMINATION

ANEMIA OR OTHER SYSTEMIC SYMPTOMS OR SIGNS

IRON DEFICIENCY ANEMIA, HYPOTHYROIDISM, VALVULAR HEART DISEASE, CIRRHOSIS, EMPHYSEMA, CHRONIC ALCOHOLISM, EXANTHEMAS

NO SYSTEMIC SYMPTOMS OR SIGNS

ANOVULATORY BLEEDING, DYSFUNCTIONAL UTERINE BLEEDING, HORMONE THERAPY, ENDOMETRIAL CARCINOMA

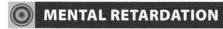

ASK THE FOLLOWING QUESTIONS:

1. **Is there decreased hair and skin pigment?** These findings would suggest phenylketonuria.
2. **Are there abnormal secondary sex characteristics?** These findings would suggest Klinefelter's syndrome, Turner's syndrome, and Laurence–Moon–Bardet–Biedl syndrome.
3. **Are there abnormalities of the skull present?** Findings of deformities or enlargement of the skull should suggest rickets, microcephaly, hypertelorism, oxycephaly, and hydrocephalus, among other things.
4. **Is there hepatosplenomegaly?** The findings of hepatosplenomegaly suggest galactosemia, Hurler's disease, and Gaucher's disease, among other diagnostic possibilities.
5. **Are there skin changes?** Sturge–Weber syndrome, tuberous sclerosis, neurofibromatosis, and cretinism may present with skin changes. Kernicterus is associated with jaundice.
6. **Are there other neurologic signs?** Tay–Sachs disease, congenital syphilis, Arnold–Chiari malformation, and cerebral diplegia are just a few of the causes of mental retardation that may present with other neurologic signs.

DIAGNOSTIC WORKUP

Routine laboratory tests include a CBC, sedimentation rate, chemistry panel, serum galactose level, VDRL test, thyroid profile, and urine screen for carbohydrates, amino acids, and organic acids. Chromosomal analysis may detect Klinefelter's syndrome, Turner's syndrome, mongolism, and other disorders. If there are deformities of the skull present, a skull x-ray should be done.

An EEG, CT scan of the brain, and psychometric testing will often need to be done, but a referral to a neurologist should be made before ordering these expensive tests.

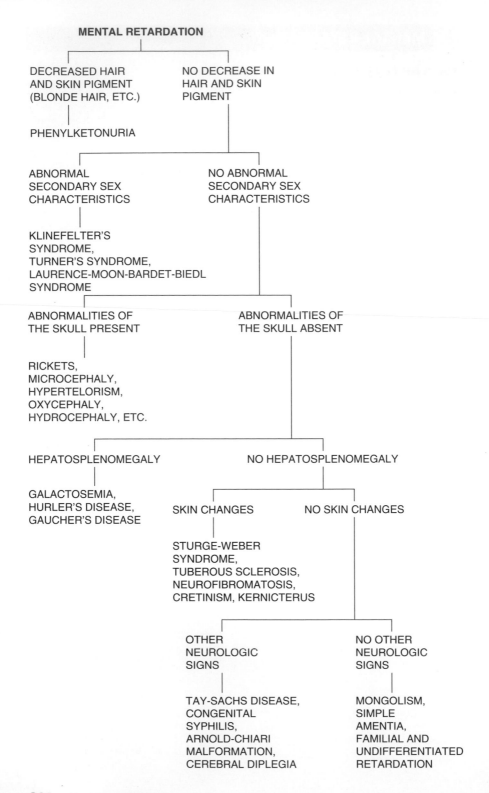

MENTAL RETARDATION

DECREASED HAIR
AND SKIN PIGMENT
(BLONDE HAIR, ETC.)

PHENYLKETONURIA

NO DECREASE IN
HAIR AND SKIN
PIGMENT

ABNORMAL
SECONDARY SEX
CHARACTERISTICS

KLINEFELTER'S
SYNDROME,
TURNER'S SYNDROME,
LAURENCE-MOON-BARDET-BIEDL
SYNDROME

NO ABNORMAL
SECONDARY SEX
CHARACTERISTICS

ABNORMALITIES OF
THE SKULL PRESENT

RICKETS,
MICROCEPHALY,
HYPERTELORISM,
OXYCEPHALY,
HYDROCEPHALY, ETC.

ABNORMALITIES OF
THE SKULL ABSENT

HEPATOSPLENOMEGALY

GALACTOSEMIA,
HURLER'S DISEASE,
GAUCHER'S DISEASE

NO HEPATOSPLENOMEGALY

SKIN CHANGES

STURGE-WEBER
SYNDROME,
TUBEROUS SCLEROSIS,
NEUROFIBROMATOSIS,
CRETINISM, KERNICTERUS

NO SKIN CHANGES

OTHER
NEUROLOGIC
SIGNS

TAY-SACHS DISEASE,
CONGENITAL
SYPHILIS,
ARNOLD-CHIARI
MALFORMATION,
CEREBRAL DIPLEGIA

NO OTHER
NEUROLOGIC
SIGNS

MONGOLISM,
SIMPLE
AMENTIA,
FAMILIAL AND
UNDIFFERENTIATED
RETARDATION

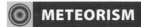

ASK THE FOLLOWING QUESTIONS:

1. **Are there hyperactive bowel sounds?** These findings should suggest intestinal obstruction, and in that case one would look for strangulated hernia, adhesions, volvulus, mesenteric embolism or thrombosis, and other disorders. Perhaps the problem is a fecal impaction.
2. **Is there blood in the stool?** Blood in the stool along with hyperactive bowel sounds would suggest a mesenteric embolism or thrombosis or intussusception.
3. **Are there systemic symptoms?** The clinician should keep in mind that systemic diseases may present with meteorism. These include diabetes mellitus, lobar pneumonia, typhoid fever, acute pancreatitis, and steatorrhea.
4. **Are there neurologic signs?** Spinal cord trauma and transverse myelitis are among the many disorders that may present with meteorism.

DIAGNOSTIC WORKUP

Routine laboratory tests include a stat CBC, sedimentation rate, serum amylase and lipase, urinalysis, chemistry panel, stool for occult blood, culture, ovum and parasites, and quantitative fat. A chest x-ray and flat plate of the abdomen should also be done. If these tests are negative, referral to a gastroenterologist or general surgeon is in order before ordering CT scans, ultrasonography, or contrast radiography.

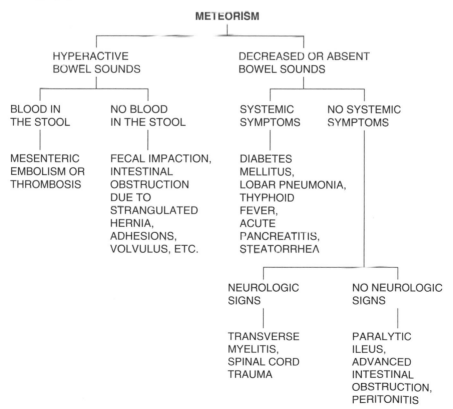

CASE HISTORY

A 26-year-old white female, gravid 3 para 3 comes to your office for a routine annual physical examination. On examination, you note a slight amount of vaginal bleeding but no other abnormalities. When you bring this to her attention, she admits she's had irregular periods and spotting between periods for sometime now. She is not on birth control pills.

Following the algorithm, you look for pallor and find none. However, she has a slight tension tremor and her pulse is 110 per minute. You examine her neck and palpate a diffusely enlarged thyroid. A TSH and Free T_4 confirm your suspicion of hyperthyroidism.

ASK THE FOLLOWING QUESTIONS:

1. **Are there abnormalities found on the vaginal examination?** An enlarged uterus suggests pregnancy, fibroids, retained secundina, hydatiform mole, choriocarcinoma, endometrial carcinoma, or endometrial polyp. An adnexal mass suggests a granulosa cell tumor, salpingitis, or ectopic pregnancy. Cervical lesions that cause metrorrhagia are cervicitis, carcinoma of the cervix, and cervical polyp. Vaginal lesions include vaginal carcinoma and senile vaginitis.

2. **Is there a history of hormone therapy?** If the patient has been taking estrogen or progesterone, withdrawal or breakthrough bleeding should be considered.

3. **Is there pallor or other signs of anemia?** Most types of anemia, but particularly iron deficiency anemia, are associated with metrorrhagia.

4. **Is there a history of tremor, tachycardia, or edema?** Both hyperthyroidism and hypothyroidism may be associated with metrorrhagia.

5. **Is there hirsutism or virilism?** Look for an adrenal or ovarian neoplasm and polycystic ovary syndrome in these cases.

   If all of these questions fail to turn up any positive answers, then dysfunctional uterine bleeding, collagen disease, or a coagulation disorder should be strongly considered.

6. **Is the patient past menopause?** If so, then endometrial carcinoma should be strongly considered.

DIAGNOSTIC WORKUP

Routine studies include a CBC, sedimentation rate, urinalysis, pregnancy test, chemistry panel, ANA test, coagulation profile, thyroid profile, and flat plate of the abdomen. A pap smear and vaginal smear and culture for gonorrhea and chlamydia should also be done.

If these are negative, referral to a gynecologist should be made before undertaking expensive diagnostic tests such as pelvic or transvaginal ultrasound or CT scans of the abdomen and pelvis. Alternatively, a trial of cyclical estrogen and progesterone hormones may be done if dysfunctional bleeding is suspected before referral is made. A gynecologist may be able to resolve the diagnostic dilemma with a good pelvic examination or, if that is unsuccessful, may perform laparoscopy or culdocentesis. A dilation and curettage or office endometrial biopsy are among the additional procedures at the gynecologist's disposal. An endocrinologist may be of help in deciding whether pituitary or ovarian dysfunction is responsible. An FSH of greater than 40 mIU/ml suggests ovarian failure. The endocrinologist may note hirsutism and order a free testosterone and 17-hydroxy progesterone to rule out adrenal or ovarian neoplasm.

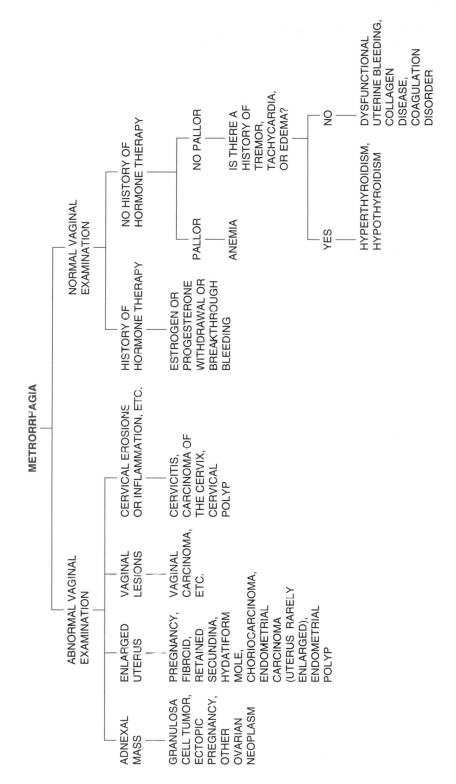

METRORRHAGIA

ABNORMAL VAGINAL EXAMINATION

- ADNEXAL MASS
  - GRANULOSA CELL TUMOR, ECTOPIC PREGNANCY, OTHER OVARIAN NEOPLASM

- ENLARGED UTERUS
  - PREGNANCY, FIBROID, RETAINED SECUNDINA, HYDATIFORM MOLE, CHORIOCARCINOMA, ENDOMETRIAL CARCINOMA (UTERUS RARELY ENLARGED), ENDOMETRIAL POLYP

- VAGINAL LESIONS
  - VAGINAL CARCINOMA, ETC.

- CERVICAL EROSIONS OR INFLAMMATION, ETC.
  - CERVICITIS, CARCINOMA OF THE CERVIX, CERVICAL POLYP

NORMAL VAGINAL EXAMINATION

- HISTORY OF HORMONE THERAPY
  - ESTROGEN OR PROGESTERONE WITHDRAWAL OR BREAKTHROUGH BLEEDING

- NO HISTORY OF HORMONE THERAPY
  - PALLOR
    - ANEMIA
  - NO PALLOR
    - IS THERE A HISTORY OF TREMOR, TACHYCARDIA, OR EDEMA?
      - YES
        - HYPERTHYROIDISM, HYPOTHYROIDISM
      - NO
        - DYSFUNCTIONAL UTERINE BLEEDING, COLLAGEN DISEASE, COAGULATION DISORDER

● MONOPLEGIA

ASK THE FOLLOWING QUESTIONS:

1. **Are there hyperactive or pathologic reflexes of the involved extremity?** These findings suggest spinal cord tumor, parasagittal tumor, amyotrophic lateral sclerosis, anterior cerebral artery occlusion, spinal cord injury, transverse myelitis, and multiple sclerosis.

2. **Are there decreased or absent reflexes of the involved extremity?** These findings suggest a herniated disk, a cauda equina tumor or early cervical cord tumor, progressive muscular atrophy, brachial plexus neuropathy, sciatic neuritis, or peripheral neuropathy.

3. **Is the onset acute or gradual?** An acute onset would suggest a vascular lesion such as anterior cerebral artery occlusion, a spinal cord injury, transverse myelitis, and multiple sclerosis. A gradual onset suggests a space-occupying lesion such as spinal cord tumor, parasagittal tumor, and degenerative diseases such as amyotrophic lateral sclerosis.

4. **Are there exacerbations or remissions?** The presence of exacerbations or remissions should suggest multiple sclerosis, transient ischemic attack, and migraine.

DIAGNOSTIC WORKUP

Monoplegia of the upper extremities with hyperactive reflexes should suggest the need to order a CT scan or MRI of the brain and/or MRI of the cervical spine.

Monoplegia of the lower extremities with hyperactive reflexes or pathologic reflexes would suggest the need to order MRI of the thoracic spine. However, because an anterior cerebral artery occlusion or parasagittal tumor may cause similar findings, a CT scan of the brain may be necessary. Rather than make this difficult choice yourself, a neurologist should be consulted. He may want to do a spinal fluid analysis or evoked potential studies as well. If he believes a vascular lesion is possible, then he may want to do a four-vessel angiography, MRA or simply a carotid scan.

The findings of monoplegia with hypoactive reflexes, especially of gradual onset, would suggest a radiculopathy, peripheral neuropathy, or plexopathy. In the lower extremities, these findings would indicate the need for a CT scan or MRI of the lumbosacral spine. In the upper extremities, these findings would suggest the need for MRI of the cervical spine.

A neuropathy workup is also indicated in monoplegia of the upper or lower extremity (page 356). Nerve conduction velocity studies and EMG studies of the involved extremities are also extremely valuable. The most cost-effective approach is to refer the patient to a neurologist at the outset.

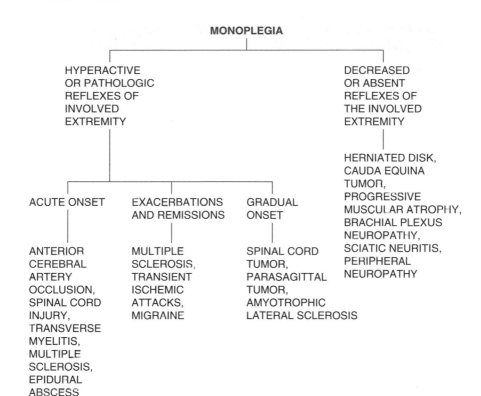

MONOPLEGIA

HYPERACTIVE OR PATHOLOGIC REFLEXES OF INVOLVED EXTREMITY

DECREASED OR ABSENT REFLEXES OF THE INVOLVED EXTREMITY

HERNIATED DISK, CAUDA EQUINA TUMOR, PROGRESSIVE MUSCULAR ATROPHY, BRACHIAL PLEXUS NEUROPATHY, SCIATIC NEURITIS, PERIPHERAL NEUROPATHY

ACUTE ONSET

EXACERBATIONS AND REMISSIONS

GRADUAL ONSET

ANTERIOR CEREBRAL ARTERY OCCLUSION, SPINAL CORD INJURY, TRANSVERSE MYELITIS, MULTIPLE SCLEROSIS, EPIDURAL ABSCESS

MULTIPLE SCLEROSIS, TRANSIENT ISCHEMIC ATTACKS, MIGRAINE

SPINAL CORD TUMOR, PARASAGITTAL TUMOR, AMYOTROPHIC LATERAL SCLEROSIS

MOUTH PIGMENTATION

ASK THE FOLLOWING QUESTIONS:

1. **Is there generalized pigmentation?** The findings of generalized pigmentation would suggest Addison's disease, arsenic poisoning, and occasionally hemochromatosis. When there is no generalized pigmentation, one should suspect Peutz–Jeghers syndrome, chronic cachectic conditions, and acanthosis nigricans.
2. **Is there hypotension or weight loss?** These findings suggest Addison's disease and arsenic poisoning. If there is no hypotension or weight loss, then the mouth pigmentation and generalized pigmentation may be associated with African ancestry or Fabry's disease.

DIAGNOSTIC WORKUP

Routine laboratory workup includes a CBC, sedimentation rate, urinalysis, chemistry panel, and VDRL test. If arsenic poisoning is suspected, hair analysis for arsenic should be done. If Addison's disease is suspected, a 24-hr urine collection for 17-hydroxysteroids and 17-ketosteroids should be done. The rapid ACTH test is a suitable alternative but usually more expensive. If Peutz–Jeghers syndrome or acanthosis nigricans is suspected, a GI series with a small bowel follow-through and a barium enema may be necessary. Endoscopy procedures may also be useful in certain cases.

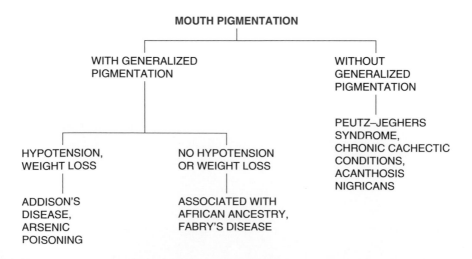

MUSCULAR ATROPHY

ASK THE FOLLOWING QUESTIONS:

1. **Is it focal or diffuse?** Focal muscular atrophy would suggest poliomyelitis, early spinal muscular atrophy, peripheral vascular disease, and sympathetic dystrophy. However, occasionally it is an indication of an early spinal cord tumor, herniated disk, or peroneal muscular atrophy. It can also be a sign of an entrapment syndrome of one of the peripheral nerves. Focal muscular atrophy with hyperactive reflexes suggests amyotrophic lateral sclerosis, multiple sclerosis, spinal cord tumors, or syringomyelia.

2. **Are the reflexes hypoactive or hyperactive?** Muscular atrophy with hypoactive reflexes suggests peripheral neuropathy, poliomyelitis, spinal muscular atrophy, myasthenia gravis, peripheral vascular disease, sympathetic dystrophy, herniated disk, early spinal cord tumor, and peroneal muscular atrophy. Muscular atrophy with hyperactive reflexes suggests multiple sclerosis, spinal cord tumors, syringomyelia, and amyotrophic lateral sclerosis.

3. **Are there associated sensory changes?** The finding of muscular atrophy with sensory changes suggests a peripheral neuropathy, Guillain–Barré syndrome, Friedreich's ataxia, multiple sclerosis, transverse myelitis, a herniated disk, spinal cord tumor, and peroneal muscular atrophy. It may also suggest syringomyelia.

4. **Are the reflexes normal?** The presence of normal reflexes suggests anorexia nervosa, tuberculosis, metastatic malignancy, and hyperthyroidism.

DIAGNOSTIC WORKUP

The basic workup includes a CBC, sedimentation rate, urinalysis, chemistry panel, ANA titer, serum protein electrophoresis, and VDRL test. Additional muscle enzymes may be ordered such as serum aldolase and CPK. A 24-hr urine collection for creatinine and creatine may be done.

At this point, it is best to consult a neurologist. He will probably order nerve conduction velocity studies and EMGs of the involved extremities. He also will be best qualified to determine the need for CT scans or MRIs of the brain or spine, as well as the particular study to order in each individual case. At times, spinal fluid analysis and muscle biopsies may be necessary to solve the problem. Also, a Tensilon test or acetylcholine receptor antibody titer may be ordered in suspected myasthenia gravis.

MUSCULAR ATROPHY

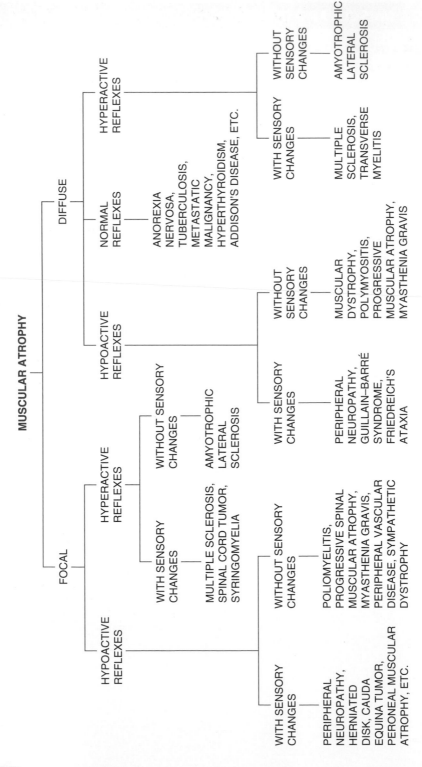

MUSCULOSKELETAL PAIN, GENERALIZED

ASK THE FOLLOWING QUESTIONS:

1. **Is there fever?** Musculoskeletal pain with fever suggests dengue fever, which is also called break-bone fever, poliomyelitis, Bornholm disease, acute trichinosis, epidemic myalgia, viral influenza, and meningitis, as well as almost any other febrile illness.

2. **Is there paralysis?** The presence of paralysis, especially if it is focal, would suggest poliomyelitis, but porphyria, polyneuritis, Guillain–Barré syndrome, dermatomyositis, and other collagen diseases may present with generalized musculoskeletal pain and paralysis. If there is diffuse pain without paralysis, one should consider trichinosis and chronic fibromyositis. Polymyalgia rheumatica may also present in this fashion.

3. **Is it transient?** Transient musculoskeletal pain may occur with fever, but it may also occur after injury, fatigue, and anxiety, and especially extensive physical workouts.

4. **Are there electrolyte abnormalities?** One should always remember that electrolyte abnormalities, such as hypokalemia, hyponatremia, and hypocalcemia, will cause generalized musculoskeletal pain.

5. **What drugs is the patient on?** The statins and other drugs can cause myalgia and frank muscle necrosis.

DIAGNOSTIC WORKUP

Routine studies include a CBC, sedimentation rate, urinalysis, chemistry panel including electrolytes, ANA test, serum protein electrophoresis, febrile agglutinins, chest x-ray, and EKG.

If muscular disease is strongly suspected, then a 24-hr collection for urine creatine and creatinine should be done, as well as serial muscle enzymes. A urine myoglobin should be done to exclude muscle injury. Perhaps a *Trichinella* skin test or antibody titer will be helpful. An EMG and a nerve conduction velocity study may be helpful in both muscular disease and peripheral neuropathies.

A muscle biopsy may be necessary to diagnose dermatomyositis, trichinosis, cysticercosis, and various collagen diseases. Urine for porphyrins and porphobilinogen should be done in difficult diagnostic cases also.

Twenty-four-hour urine quantitative potassium, sodium, or calcium will be helpful in the electrolyte disorders, as the serum electrolytes do not always reflect the decrease in intracellular electrolytes.

A spinal tap will help diagnose poliomyelitis, meningitis, and Guillain–Barré syndrome. It may be necessary to seek the help of a rheumatologist, a neurologist, or an infectious disease specialist. If chronic fibromyositis is suspected, a psychiatrist should be consulted. There is no convincing proof that this is an organic disease.

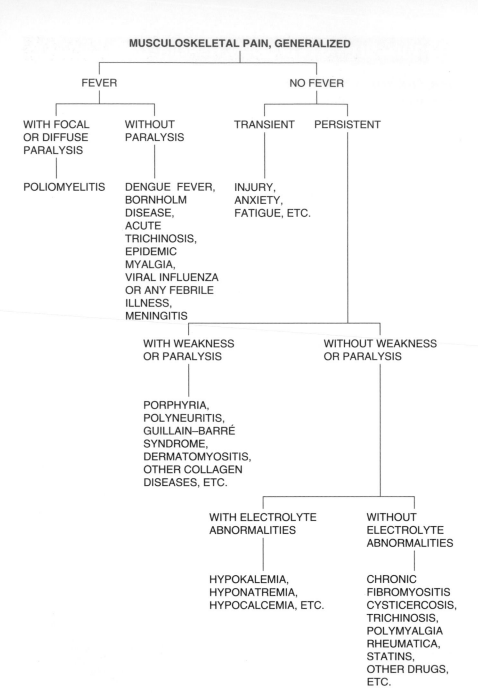

MUSCULOSKELETAL PAIN, GENERALIZED

FEVER

NO FEVER

WITH FOCAL OR DIFFUSE PARALYSIS

POLIOMYELITIS

WITHOUT PARALYSIS

DENGUE FEVER, BORNHOLM DISEASE, ACUTE TRICHINOSIS, EPIDEMIC MYALGIA, VIRAL INFLUENZA OR ANY FEBRILE ILLNESS, MENINGITIS

TRANSIENT

PERSISTENT

INJURY, ANXIETY, FATIGUE, ETC.

WITH WEAKNESS OR PARALYSIS

PORPHYRIA, POLYNEURITIS, GUILLAIN–BARRÉ SYNDROME, DERMATOMYOSITIS, OTHER COLLAGEN DISEASES, ETC.

WITHOUT WEAKNESS OR PARALYSIS

WITH ELECTROLYTE ABNORMALITIES

HYPOKALEMIA, HYPONATREMIA, HYPOCALCEMIA, ETC.

WITHOUT ELECTROLYTE ABNORMALITIES

CHRONIC FIBROMYOSITIS CYSTICERCOSIS, TRICHINOSIS, POLYMYALGIA RHEUMATICA, STATINS, OTHER DRUGS, ETC.

ASK THE FOLLOWING QUESTION:

1. **Are the abnormalities focal or diffuse?** Focal abnormalities include thickening, which is often due to fungus infections; inflammation, which is usually due to a paronychia, onychia, fungal infection, or syphilis; hemorrhages under the nail, which may be due to trauma, subacute bacterial endocarditis, or trichinosis; pitting of the nail, which may be due to psoriasis; and atrophy or dystrophy of the nail, which may be due to peripheral vascular diseases, epidermolysis bullosa, nail biting, peripheral neuropathy, and various other dermatoses. Diffuse abnormalities of the nail may include thickening due to syphilis, hyperthyroidism or hypothyroidism, clubbing, cyanotic heart disease, bronchiectasis, carcinoma of the lungs, and other disorders; yellow nails due to lymphedema or chest conditions; and spoon nails due to iron-deficiency anemia.

Diffuse spoon nails may be caused by iron-deficiency anemia. Yellow nails may be due to lymphedema or chest conditions. Clubbing may be due to cyanotic heart disease, bronchiectasis, or carcinoma of the lung (see page 86). Thickening may result from syphilis, hyperthyroidism, or hypothyroidism. Hemorrhages may be due to trauma, subacute bacterial endocarditis, or trichinosis. Pitting may be due to psoriasis. Focal thickening may be due to fungus infections. Focal inflammation may be due to paronychia, onychia, or syphilis. Focal atrophy or dystrophy may be due to peripheral vascular disease, peripheral neuropathy, epidermolysis bullosa, nail biting, or other dermatoses.

DIAGNOSTIC WORKUP

Focal abnormalities of one nail warrant a culture and sensitivity of any scrapings or exudates from the area, as well as an x-ray of the digit or extremity. A CBC and sedimentation rate will help identify an infectious process. A glucose tolerance test will help identify diabetes mellitus. Careful assessment of the area for vascular insufficiency includes Doppler studies and possibly arteriography. A nerve conduction velocity study and EMG may be necessary if peripheral neuropathy is suspected. A skin or nail biopsy may be helpful.

Routine tests for diffuse nail changes include a CBC, sedimentation rate, chemistry panel, VDRL test, ANA, thyroid profile, chest x-ray, and EKG. Arterial blood gases and pulmonary function studies should be done if clubbing is suspected. Other tests for clubbing will be found on page 86. Serial blood cultures should be done if subacute bacterial endocarditis is suspected. *Trichinella* skin test or antibody titer should be done in cases in which there are splintered nails with negative cultures for subacute bacterial endocarditis. Muscle or skin biopsy will be useful not only for trichinosis but also for collagen disease. Nerve conduction velocity studies and EMGs will be helpful in diagnosing peripheral neuropathy.

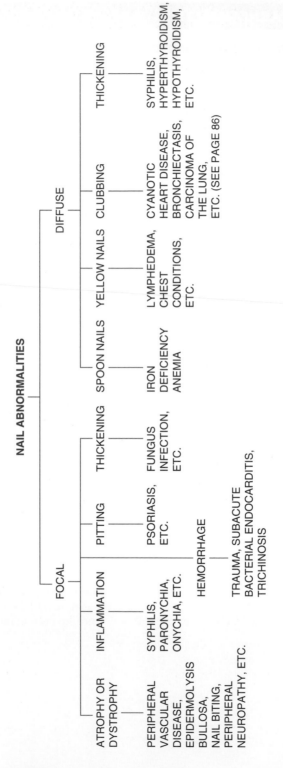

NAIL ABNORMALITIES

FOCAL

- ATROPHY OR DYSTROPHY
  - PERIPHERAL VASCULAR DISEASE, EPIDERMOLYSIS BULLOSA, NAIL BITING, PERIPHERAL NEUROPATHY, ETC.
- INFLAMMATION
  - SYPHILIS, PARONYCHIA, ONYCHIA, ETC.
- HEMORRHAGE
  - TRAUMA, SUBACUTE BACTERIAL ENDOCARDITIS, TRICHINOSIS
- PITTING
  - PSORIASIS, ETC.
- THICKENING
  - FUNGUS INFECTION, ETC.

DIFFUSE

- SPOON NAILS
  - IRON DEFICIENCY ANEMIA
- YELLOW NAILS
  - LYMPHEDEMA, CHEST CONDITIONS, ETC.
- CLUBBING
  - CYANOTIC HEART DISEASE, BRONCHIECTASIS, CARCINOMA OF THE LUNG, ETC. (SEE PAGE 86)
- THICKENING
  - SYPHILIS, HYPERTHYROIDISM, HYPOTHYROIDISM, ETC.

NASAL DISCHARGE

ASK THE FOLLOWING QUESTIONS:

1. **Is it unilateral or bilateral?** Unilateral nasal discharge, especially if it is purulent, suggests acute sinusitis, Wegener's granulomatosis, neoplasm, foreign body, and syphilis. If the discharge is clear or mucoid, it could be just simply chronic sinusitis. Bilateral nasal discharge suggests a URI, especially if it is an acute onset. If it is a chronic condition and is mucoid or clear, allergic rhinitis, chronic sinusitis, or vasomotor rhinitis should be suspected. Rarely, cerebral spinal fluid rhinorrhea is the problem.

2. **Is there fever?** The presence of fever makes acute sinusitis most likely if the discharge is unilateral, but if it is bilateral, one should suspect an acute viral URI. However, if there is significant pain associated with the fever, one should consider the possibility that there is an acute sinusitis.

3. **Is it purulent, mucoid, or clear?** The presence of a purulent discharge suggests acute sinusitis, chronic bacterial sinusitis, mucormycosis, Wegener's granulomatosis, neoplasm, foreign body, and syphilis. The presence of a mucoid discharge suggests allergic rhinitis or a chronic sinusitis. The presence of a clear discharge suggests cerebral spinal fluid rhinorrhea and senile rhinorrhea, especially if the patient is older. If there is unilateral face pain, one should consider cluster headache or migraine.

4. **Is there pain?** The presence of pain with fever or purulent discharge certainly suggests acute sinusitis. However, when there is pain with a clear discharge, one should think of cluster headache or migraine.

5. **Is there sneezing or an allergy history?** The presence of sneezing or an allergic history should suggest allergic rhinitis and sinusitis. However, allergic rhinitis and sinusitis may also occur without sneezing or an allergic history.

6. **Is the patient abusing cocaine or nasal sprays?** These are common causes of a chronic nasal discharge.

DIAGNOSTIC WORKUP

Routine orders for the workup of a nasal discharge include a CBC, sedimentation rate, chemistry panel, VDRL test, smear and culture of the nasal discharge, and x-rays of the sinuses. CT scans of the sinuses are the preferred imaging study to diagnose sinusitis. If the discharge is chronic and mucoid or clear, one should do a nasal smear for eosinophils and serum IgE level to look for allergic rhinitis. A trial of therapy may be indicated in these cases also. If Wegener's granulomatosis is suspected, serum for ANCA should be done. A RISA study can be done to rule out cerebrospinal rhinorrhea.

If there is still diagnostic confusion after the above tests have been done, referral to an ear, nose, and throat specialist or an allergist is indicated. The specialist will perform nasopharyngoscopy and is in a better position to evaluate whether CT scans or bone scans are needed. Also, the specialist can better evaluate when the patient should undergo allergy skin testing, inhalation testing, or radioallergosorbent tests (RASTs). Idiopathic vasomotor rhinitis can be diagnosed by a trial of Atrovent.

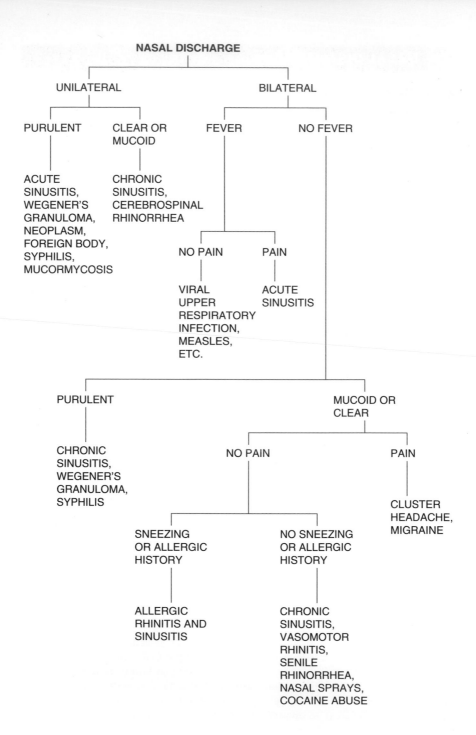

NASAL DISCHARGE

UNILATERAL

PURULENT

ACUTE
SINUSITIS,
WEGENER'S
GRANULOMA,
NEOPLASM,
FOREIGN BODY,
SYPHILIS,
MUCORMYCOSIS

CLEAR OR
MUCOID

CHRONIC
SINUSITIS,
CEREBROSPINAL
RHINORRHEA

BILATERAL

FEVER

NO FEVER

NO PAIN

VIRAL
UPPER
RESPIRATORY
INFECTION,
MEASLES,
ETC.

PAIN

ACUTE
SINUSITIS

PURULENT

CHRONIC
SINUSITIS,
WEGENER'S
GRANULOMA,
SYPHILIS

MUCOID OR
CLEAR

NO PAIN

SNEEZING
OR ALLERGIC
HISTORY

ALLERGIC
RHINITIS AND
SINUSITIS

NO SNEEZING
OR ALLERGIC
HISTORY

CHRONIC
SINUSITIS,
VASOMOTOR
RHINITIS,
SENILE
RHINORRHEA,
NASAL SPRAYS,
COCAINE ABUSE

PAIN

CLUSTER
HEADACHE,
MIGRAINE

NASAL OBSTRUCTION

ASK THE FOLLOWING QUESTIONS:

1. **Is it acute or chronic?** The presence of acute nasal obstruction should suggest acute sinusitis, acute rhinitis, a viral URI, allergic rhinitis, nasal diphtheria, cluster headache, migraine, foreign body, and trauma. The presence of chronic nasal obstruction, particularly if it is unilateral, would suggest sinusitis, foreign bodies, neoplasm, deviated septum, polyps, Wegener's granulomatosis, mucormycosis, and nasal gumma. If it is bilateral, it would suggest allergic rhinitis, vasomotor rhinitis, adenoid enlargement, rhinitis medicamentosa, and ingestion of drugs such as reserpine.

2. **Is it unilateral or bilateral?** The presence of unilateral nasal obstruction suggests acute purulent sinusitis, foreign body, neoplasm, mucormycosis, Wegener's granulomatosis, polyps, and neoplasms. It also suggests a deviated septum. The presence of bilateral nasal obstruction suggests allergic rhinitis, acute viral URI, nasal diphtheria, rhinitis medicamentosa, adenoids, and vasomotor rhinitis.

3. **Is there fever?** The presence of fever with unilateral nasal obstruction would suggest acute sinusitis. The presence of fever with bilateral nasal obstruction would suggest acute rhinitis and acute viral URI. Nasal diphtheria may occasionally present with this picture, even in modern times.

DIAGNOSTIC WORKUP

Routine diagnostic studies include a CBC, sedimentation rate, chemistry panel, VDRL test, ANA, a nasal smear and culture for bacteria and fungi, and x-rays of the sinuses. A nasal smear for eosinophils and serum IgE antibodies should be done if allergy is suspected. A trial of antibiotics or antihistamines may assist in the diagnosis. If Wegener's granulomatosis is suspected, serum for ANCA should be done.

If there is still confusion regarding the diagnosis at this point, a referral to an ear, nose, and throat specialist or allergist would be indicated. The ear, nose, and throat specialist may do a nasopharyngoscopy and is in a better position to determine when CT scans or bone scans are indicated. The allergist can best determine whether allergy skin testing, inhalation testing, or RAST studies would be indicated.

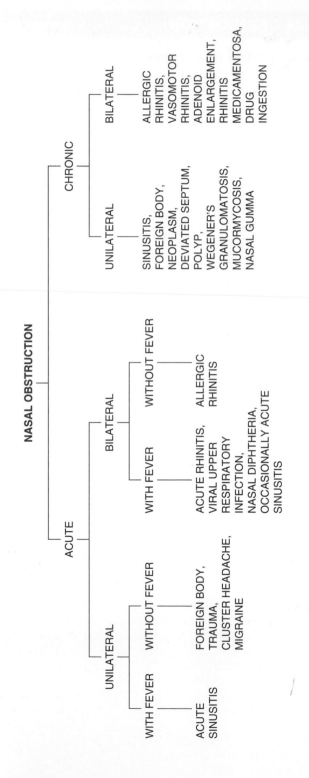

NASAL OBSTRUCTION

ACUTE

UNILATERAL

WITH FEVER
ACUTE SINUSITIS

WITHOUT FEVER
FOREIGN BODY, TRAUMA, CLUSTER HEADACHE, MIGRAINE

BILATERAL

WITH FEVER
ACUTE RHINITIS, VIRAL UPPER RESPIRATORY INFECTION, NASAL DIPHTHERIA, OCCASIONALLY ACUTE SINUSITIS

WITHOUT FEVER
ALLERGIC RHINITIS

CHRONIC

UNILATERAL
SINUSITIS, FOREIGN BODY, NEOPLASM, DEVIATED SEPTUM, POLYP, WEGENER'S GRANULOMATOSIS, MUCORMYCOSIS, NASAL GUMMA

BILATERAL
ALLERGIC RHINITIS, VASOMOTOR RHINITIS, ADENOID ENLARGEMENT, RHINITIS MEDICAMENTOSA, DRUG INGESTION

ASK THE FOLLOWING QUESTIONS:

1. **Is there a history of alcohol or drug ingestion?** Alcohol and many drugs such as digitalis, aspirin, nonsteroidal anti-inflammatory agents, antihypertensives, and antibiotics may cause gastric irritation or gastritis.
2. **Is there fever?** Fever may point to a localized abdominal condition such as acute cholecystitis or acute appendicitis, as well as a systemic condition such as tuberculosis, brucellosis, yellow fever, and other febrile illnesses.
3. **Is there abdominal pain?** Abdominal pain suggests the possibility of acute cholecystitis, acute appendicitis, pyelonephritis, pancreatitis, renal calculus, and peritonitis.
4. **Is there an abdominal mass?** The presence of an abdominal mass suggests pyloric or intestinal obstruction, a pancreatic neoplasm, acute cholecystitis, Crohn's disease, perinephric abscess, diverticulitis, and other abscesses and neoplasms.
5. **Is there vertigo?** The clinician should remember that inner ear diseases such as Ménière's disease and labyrinthitis may be associated with vomiting, and sometimes the patient does not mention vertigo.
6. **Is there headache?** Migraine, concussion, cerebral tumors or other space-occupying lesions, meningitis, and subarachnoid hemorrhage are associated with headaches, nausea, and vomiting. Migraine has been known to cause vomiting without headache.

DIAGNOSTIC WORKUP

A patient presenting with nausea, vomiting and diarrhea almost always has a viral or bacterial gastroenteritis. However, appendicitis, pancreatitis and cholecystitis must always be kept in mind as does botulism. The basic workup includes a CBC, sedimentation rate, urinalysis, urine drug screen, chemistry panel and electrolytes, serum amylase, arterial blood gases, stools for occult blood, chest x-ray, EKG, and flat plate of the abdomen. Acute onset of nausea and vomiting with ataxia requires an immediate CT scan of the brain to rule out a cerebellar hemorrhage. A pregnancy test should be routine in women of child-bearing age. If there is fever, febrile agglutinins and a heterophile antibody titer should be done. If there is an abdominal mass, a gallbladder ultrasound and intravenous pyelogram may need to be done. Isotope scanning with iminodiacetic acid derivatives is extremely useful to detect acute cholecystitis. If there is chronic vomiting and abdominal pain, the diagnosis can often be made with an upper GI series, small bowel series, or barium enema.

When there is persistent vomiting with abdominal pain, an exploratory laparotomy may need to be considered. The presence of an abdominal mass or suspected pancreatic or biliary disease merits consideration of a CT scan. However, before ordering expensive diagnostic tests, a general surgeon or gastroenterologist ought to be consulted. Laparoscopy, gastroscopy, esophagoscopy, duodenoscopy, and colonoscopy all need to be considered in the workup. Gastroparesis and intestinal pseudo-obstruction can be ruled out by radioisotope studies and manometry of the stomach and small intestine. Angiography is useful to diagnose mesenteric artery ischemia.

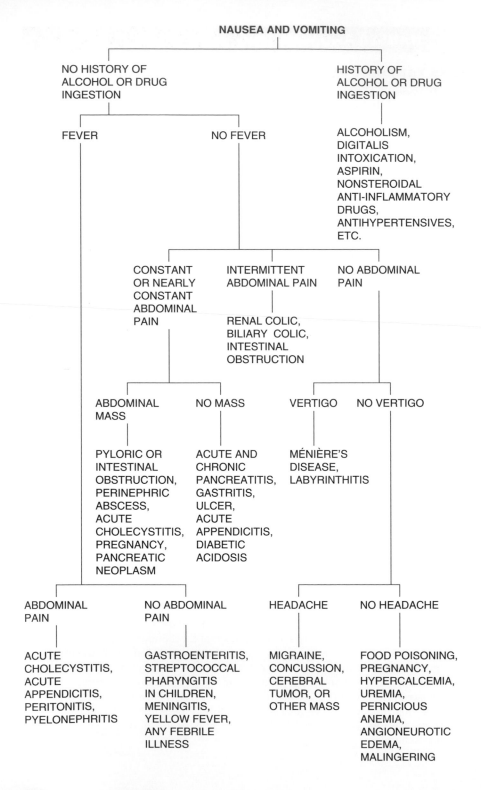

NAUSEA AND VOMITING

NO HISTORY OF ALCOHOL OR DRUG INGESTION

HISTORY OF ALCOHOL OR DRUG INGESTION

FEVER

NO FEVER

ALCOHOLISM, DIGITALIS INTOXICATION, ASPIRIN, NONSTEROIDAL ANTI-INFLAMMATORY DRUGS, ANTIHYPERTENSIVES, ETC.

CONSTANT OR NEARLY CONSTANT ABDOMINAL PAIN

INTERMITTENT ABDOMINAL PAIN

NO ABDOMINAL PAIN

RENAL COLIC, BILIARY COLIC, INTESTINAL OBSTRUCTION

ABDOMINAL MASS

NO MASS

VERTIGO

NO VERTIGO

PYLORIC OR INTESTINAL OBSTRUCTION, PERINEPHRIC ABSCESS, ACUTE CHOLECYSTITIS, PREGNANCY, PANCREATIC NEOPLASM

ACUTE AND CHRONIC PANCREATITIS, GASTRITIS, ULCER, ACUTE APPENDICITIS, DIABETIC ACIDOSIS

MÉNIÈRE'S DISEASE, LABYRINTHITIS

ABDOMINAL PAIN

NO ABDOMINAL PAIN

HEADACHE

NO HEADACHE

ACUTE CHOLECYSTITIS, ACUTE APPENDICITIS, PERITONITIS, PYELONEPHRITIS

GASTROENTERITIS, STREPTOCOCCAL PHARYNGITIS IN CHILDREN, MENINGITIS, YELLOW FEVER, ANY FEBRILE ILLNESS

MIGRAINE, CONCUSSION, CEREBRAL TUMOR, OR OTHER MASS

FOOD POISONING, PREGNANCY, HYPERCALCEMIA, UREMIA, PERNICIOUS ANEMIA, ANGIONEUROTIC EDEMA, MALINGERING

ASK THE FOLLOWING QUESTIONS:

1. **Is there radiation of the pain to one or both upper extremities?** The finding of radiation of the pain to one or both upper extremities would suggest a space-occupying lesion such as a herniated disk, spinal cord tumor, fracture, or cervical spondylosis.
2. **Are there focal neurologic findings?** The presence of focal neurologic findings make a space-occupying lesion even more likely, and the conditions that should be considered are fracture, herniated disk, spinal cord tumor, and cervical spondylosis. One should not forget a Pancoast's tumor.
3. **Is there nuchal rigidity?** The finding of nuchal rigidity suggests meningitis or subarachnoid hemorrhage.

DIAGNOSTIC WORKUP

Routine tests include a CBC, sedimentation rate, urinalysis, chemistry panel, arthritis panel, and plain films of the cervical spine. At this point, it is best to observe the results of conservative treatment before an expensive workup is begun. If there are focal neurologic findings, MRI of the cervical spine, as well as EMG examinations, nerve conduction velocity studies, and dermatomal SSEP studies may need to be done.

It is wise to consult a neurologist or neurosurgeon before ordering these expensive tests. If there is nuchal rigidity, a CT scan of the brain should be done before performing a spinal tap unless there are clear-cut clinical findings of meningitis. If possible, a neurologist should be consulted first in these circumstances.

NECK PAIN

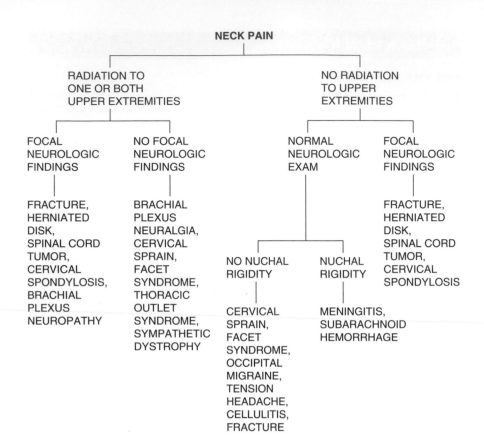

RADIATION TO ONE OR BOTH UPPER EXTREMITIES

FOCAL NEUROLOGIC FINDINGS

FRACTURE, HERNIATED DISK, SPINAL CORD TUMOR, CERVICAL SPONDYLOSIS, BRACHIAL PLEXUS NEUROPATHY

NO FOCAL NEUROLOGIC FINDINGS

BRACHIAL PLEXUS NEURALGIA, CERVICAL SPRAIN, FACET SYNDROME, THORACIC OUTLET SYNDROME, SYMPATHETIC DYSTROPHY

NO RADIATION TO UPPER EXTREMITIES

NORMAL NEUROLOGIC EXAM

NO NUCHAL RIGIDITY

CERVICAL SPRAIN, FACET SYNDROME, OCCIPITAL MIGRAINE, TENSION HEADACHE, CELLULITIS, FRACTURE

NUCHAL RIGIDITY

MENINGITIS, SUBARACHNOID HEMORRHAGE

FOCAL NEUROLOGIC FINDINGS

FRACTURE, HERNIATED DISK, SPINAL CORD TUMOR, CERVICAL SPONDYLOSIS

ASK THE FOLLOWING QUESTIONS:

1. **Is it acute or chronic?** Acute stiffness of the neck should make one look for nuchal rigidity. If there is nuchal rigidity, meningitis or subarachnoid hemorrhage would be high on the list of possibilities. If there is chronic neck stiffness, one should consider rheumatoid arthritis, cervical spondylosis, and idiopathic torticollis. With a history of trauma, the possibility of flexion–extension injury and fracture is more likely.

2. **Is there nuchal rigidity or fever?** The presence of nuchal rigidity or fever should make one think of meningitis, subarachnoid hemorrhage, or meningismus due to some systemic infectious disease. Retropharyngeal abscess must also be considered.

3. **Is it congenital or acquired?** The presence of congenital stiffness of the neck should make one think of congenital torticollis or Klippel–Feil syndrome. Chronic acquired neck stiffness should make one think of cervical spondylosis, Parkinson's disease, idiopathic torticollis, rheumatoid arthritis, tuberculosis, fractures of the spine, flexion–extension injuries, and inflammation of the lymph nodes.

4. **Are there x-ray changes?** Plain films of the cervical spine will often reveal cervical spondylosis, fractures, and tuberculosis. However, one should not jump to the conclusion that this is the cause of the condition.

DIAGNOSTIC WORKUP

If there is nuchal rigidity and fever, a CT scan of the brain should be done to rule out a space-occupying lesion, and, following that, a spinal tap for analysis, smear, and culture should be done.

If there is no nuchal rigidity or fever, plain films of the cervical spine are a good place to start the diagnostic workup. A CBC, sedimentation rate, urinalysis, chemistry panel, and arthritis profile may also be helpful. If the stiffness is associated with pain radiating into the upper extremities, EMG and nerve conduction velocity studies may be useful. If the stiffness persists, MRI of the cervical spine may be necessary. A bone scan may identify a subtle fracture or osteomyelitis. A neurologic specialist should be consulted before ordering expensive diagnostic tests.

NECK STIFFNESS

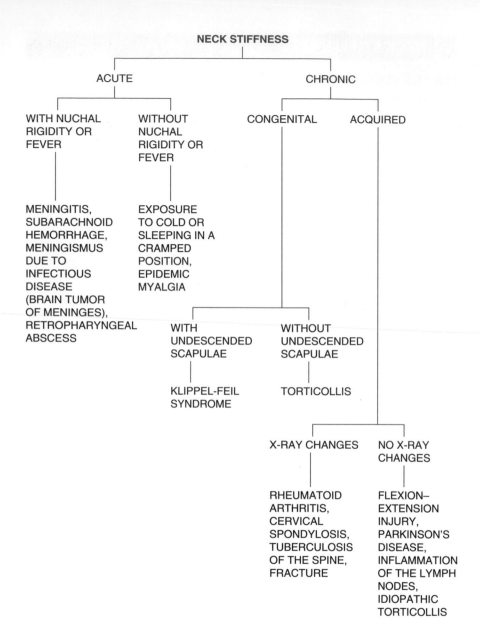

NECK STIFFNESS

ACUTE
- WITH NUCHAL RIGIDITY OR FEVER
  - MENINGITIS, SUBARACHNOID HEMORRHAGE, MENINGISMUS DUE TO INFECTIOUS DISEASE (BRAIN TUMOR OF MENINGES), RETROPHARYNGEAL ABSCESS
- WITHOUT NUCHAL RIGIDITY OR FEVER
  - EXPOSURE TO COLD OR SLEEPING IN A CRAMPED POSITION, EPIDEMIC MYALGIA

CHRONIC
- CONGENITAL
  - WITH UNDESCENDED SCAPULAE
    - KLIPPEL-FEIL SYNDROME
  - WITHOUT UNDESCENDED SCAPULAE
    - TORTICOLLIS
- ACQUIRED
  - X-RAY CHANGES
    - RHEUMATOID ARTHRITIS, CERVICAL SPONDYLOSIS, TUBERCULOSIS OF THE SPINE, FRACTURE
  - NO X-RAY CHANGES
    - FLEXION–EXTENSION INJURY, PARKINSON'S DISEASE, INFLAMMATION OF THE LYMPH NODES, IDIOPATHIC TORTICOLLIS

ASK THE FOLLOWING QUESTIONS:

1. **Is it focal or diffuse?** Focal masses or swellings may be thyroglossal cyst, branchial cleft cyst, aneurysm, an enlarged lymph node due to Hodgkin's disease, metastatic carcinoma, sarcoidosis, a cystic hygroma, carotid body tumor, Riedel's struma, and thyroid adenomas and carcinomas. Diffuse masses would be Graves' disease, subacute thyroiditis, nontoxic goiter, venous distention of congestive heart failure or superior vena cava syndrome, and subcutaneous emphysema. An acute diffuse neck swelling must be considered Ludwig's angina (neck extension of an abscessed tooth) until proven otherwise.

2. **If the lesion is focal, is it in the midline or lateral to the midline?** Midline masses are thyroglossal cysts, adenoma of the thyroid, Riedel's struma, and thyroid cyst. Lateral masses include a pharyngeal pouch, bronchial cyst, pulsion diverticulum, stone of Wharton's duct, Virchow's node, cervical rib, metastatic lymph nodes or Hodgkin's lymphoma, metastatic carcinoma, cystic hygroma, carotid body tumor, and some thyroid masses.

3. **Is the swelling intermittent?** The presence of an intermittent swelling suggests a pulsion diverticulum, venous distention of congestive heart failure, a bronchial cyst, a stone of Wharton's duct, and aneurysms.

4. **Is there crepitus?** Subcutaneous crepitus is present in subcutaneous emphysema.

5. **Is the swelling associated with a tremor or tachycardia?** The presence of tremor or tachycardia would make one think of Graves' disease and subacute thyroiditis.

DIAGNOSTIC WORKUP

Routine tests include a CBC, sedimentation rate, urinalysis, chemistry panel, thyroid profile, chest x-ray, and EKG. If these are negative, the next best step is a CT scan of the neck.

Measurement of venous pressure and circulation time, BNP and pulmonary function studies will help differentiate congestive heart failure. A radioactive iodine uptake and scan will help differentiate thyroid tumors and enlargements. Ultrasound and needle aspiration will be needed in differentiating cystic adenomas. A lymph node biopsy will be useful in diagnosing sarcoidosis, lymphomas, and metastatic carcinoma. Esophagogram will help detect Zenker's diverticulum. Angiography will be useful in diagnosing aortic aneurysms, innominate aneurysms, and subclavian aneurysms. A CT scan of the mediastinum will help diagnose superior vena cava syndrome.

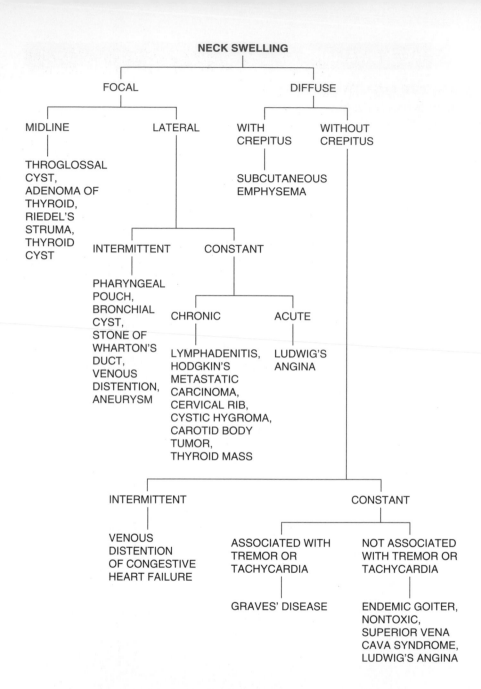

NECK SWELLING

FOCAL

MIDLINE

THROGLOSSAL
CYST,
ADENOMA OF
THYROID,
RIEDEL'S
STRUMA,
THYROID
CYST

LATERAL

INTERMITTENT

PHARYNGEAL
POUCH,
BRONCHIAL
CYST,
STONE OF
WHARTON'S
DUCT,
VENOUS
DISTENTION,
ANEURYSM

CONSTANT

CHRONIC

LYMPHADENITIS,
HODGKIN'S
METASTATIC
CARCINOMA,
CERVICAL RIB,
CYSTIC HYGROMA,
CAROTID BODY
TUMOR,
THYROID MASS

ACUTE

LUDWIG'S
ANGINA

DIFFUSE

WITH
CREPITUS

SUBCUTANEOUS
EMPHYSEMA

WITHOUT
CREPITUS

INTERMITTENT

VENOUS
DISTENTION
OF CONGESTIVE
HEART FAILURE

CONSTANT

ASSOCIATED WITH
TREMOR OR
TACHYCARDIA

GRAVES' DISEASE

NOT ASSOCIATED
WITH TREMOR OR
TACHYCARDIA

ENDEMIC GOITER,
NONTOXIC,
SUPERIOR VENA
CAVA SYNDROME,
LUDWIG'S ANGINA

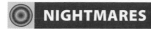

ASK THE FOLLOWING QUESTIONS:

1. **Are they acute or chronic?** The presence of acute nightmares should make one think of the possibility of infectious disease, acute situational maladjustment, or a head injury. Remember, there may be amnesia from the head injury. Chronic nightmares may be associated with drug or alcohol use, epilepsy, and neuroses or psychoses.
2. **Is there a history of trauma?** Nightmares following trauma may be due to the acute anxiety associated with the trauma or actually to a head injury.
3. **Is there a history of drug or alcohol use?** Acute alcoholic intoxication can create hallucinations and nightmares. Chronic alcoholism can lead to delirium tremens. Benzodiazepines and numerous other drugs may cause nightmares.
4. **Is there a history of tongue biting or incontinence?** These findings suggest grand mal epilepsy. Nightmares may result from complex partial seizures without tongue biting or incontinence.

DIAGNOSTIC WORKUP

A CBC, sedimentation rate, and chemistry panel will help rule out infectious diseases. A urine drug screen will help rule out the possibility of drug-induced nightmares. A wake-and-sleep EEG will help diagnose epilepsy. If epilepsy is strongly suspected, a therapeutic trial of anticonvulsants may be necessary. If the workup is negative, referral to a psychiatrist or psychologist is in order.

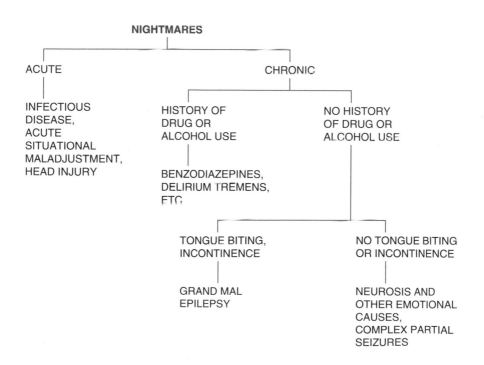

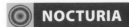
ASK THE FOLLOWING QUESTIONS:

1. **Is there daytime frequency of urination also?** If there is daytime frequency, the differential diagnosis of polyuria should be considered (page 379).
2. **Is there associated pain or difficulty voiding?** These findings would suggest cystitis, prostatitis, and urethritis.
3. **Is there dyspnea, orthopnea, or peripheral edema?** These findings would suggest congestive heart failure. If there is no dyspnea or edema, one should consider chronic nephritis.

DIAGNOSTIC WORKUP

Routine laboratory tests should include a CBC, sedimentation rate, urinalysis, chemistry panel, and urine culture and sensitivity. A quantitative 24-hr urine volume should be determined. If this is above normal, the differential diagnosis of polyuria should be considered and additional workup can be found on page 379.

Catheterization for residual urine will help determine if there is bladder neck obstruction. If congestive heart failure is suspected, a chest x-ray, EKG, and venous pressure and circulation time should be done. For further evaluation, a nephrologist or urologist may be consulted.

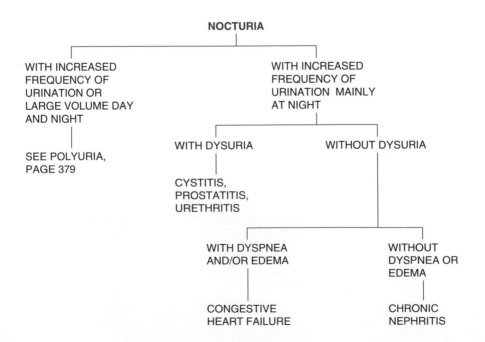

ASK THE FOLLOWING QUESTIONS:

1. **Are there structural abnormalities on examination of the nasopharynx?** Structural abnormalities of the palate indicate cleft palate, congenital short soft palate, trauma, tuberculosis, syphilis, carcinoma, leprosy, and post-tonsillectomy scarring.

2. **Are the abnormalities congenital or acquired?** Congenital abnormalities of the palate include cleft palate and congenital short soft palate. Acquired abnormalities of the palate include trauma, syphilis, tuberculosis, carcinoma, leprosy, and post-tonsillectomy scarring.

3. **Is there paralysis of the soft palate?** The finding of paralysis of the soft palate may suggest myasthenia gravis, poliomyelitis, Guillain–Barré syndrome, pseudobulbar palsy, brain tumor, basilar artery insufficiency, and syphilitic meningitis.

4. **Is the paralysis of the soft palate intermittent or constant?** Intermittent paralysis of the soft palate should suggest myasthenia gravis.

5. **Are there associated hypoactive or hyperactive reflexes?** The presence of hypoactive reflexes would suggest poliomyelitis or Guillain–Barré syndrome. The presence of hyperactive reflexes or sensory findings would suggest pseudobulbar palsy, a brain tumor, basilar artery insufficiency, and syphilitic meningitis, among other conditions.

DIAGNOSTIC WORKUP

Routine laboratory tests include a CBC, sedimentation rate, urinalysis, chemistry panel, VDRL test, smear and culture from the lesions in the nasopharynx, and a tuberculin test. A chest x-ray also should be done if tuberculosis is suspected. A neurologic workup consists of MRI of the brain, EMG and nerve conduction velocity studies, spinal fluid analysis, acetylcholine receptor antibody titers, and Tensilon tests. It is best to consult an ear, nose, and throat specialist or a neurologic specialist before ordering expensive diagnostic tests.

NOSE, REGURGITATION OF FOOD THROUGH

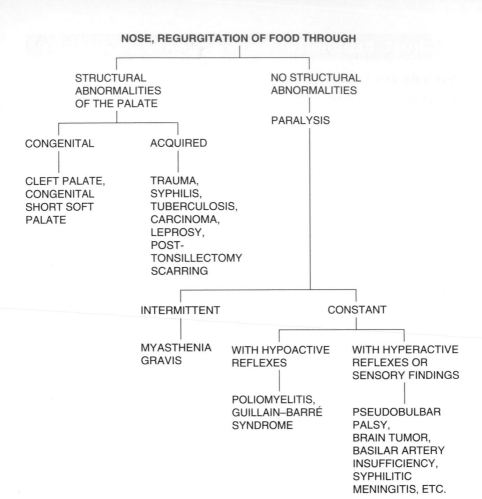

STRUCTURAL
ABNORMALITIES
OF THE PALATE

NO STRUCTURAL
ABNORMALITIES

PARALYSIS

CONGENITAL

ACQUIRED

CLEFT PALATE,
CONGENITAL
SHORT SOFT
PALATE

TRAUMA,
SYPHILIS,
TUBERCULOSIS,
CARCINOMA,
LEPROSY,
POST-
TONSILLECTOMY
SCARRING

INTERMITTENT

CONSTANT

MYASTHENIA
GRAVIS

WITH HYPOACTIVE
REFLEXES

WITH HYPERACTIVE
REFLEXES OR
SENSORY FINDINGS

POLIOMYELITIS,
GUILLAIN–BARRÉ
SYNDROME

PSEUDOBULBAR
PALSY,
BRAIN TUMOR,
BASILAR ARTERY
INSUFFICIENCY,
SYPHILITIC
MENINGITIS, ETC.

ASK THE FOLLOWING QUESTIONS:

1. **Is the nystagmus pendular?** Pendular nystagmus without a fast or slow component suggests ocular nystagmus due to albinism, partial blindness, or other ocular disorders.

2. **Is it intermittent or fatigable?** Intermittent or fatigable nystagmus suggests otologic disorders such as acoustic neuroma, Ménière's disease, vestibular neuronitis, and acute labyrinthitis.

3. **Is there associated tinnitus or deafness?** The presence of nystagmus with tinnitus or deafness also suggests otologic disorders such as acoustic neuroma, Ménière's disease, or cholesteatoma. If there are long tract signs, multiple sclerosis and brain stem tumors must be considered.

4. **Is the nystagmus brought on by change of position?** Nystagmus brought on by certain changes of position suggests benign positional vertigo. However, this also may be found in post-traumatic labyrinthitis and postconcussion syndrome.

5. **Are there associated long tract signs?** The presence of long tract signs suggests multiple sclerosis, basilar artery insufficiency, syringomyelia, and Friedreich's ataxia. Certain brain stem tumors may also be associated with long tract signs.

DIAGNOSTIC WORKUP

The basic diagnostic workup includes visual acuity, visual fields, audiogram, caloric testing, and x-rays of the skull, mastoids, and petrous bones. If these are negative or indefinite, a CT scan or MRI of the brain will be necessary. A spinal fluid analysis will help diagnose central nervous system lues and multiple sclerosis. A BSEP or VEP study may be needed to diagnose multiple sclerosis. The help of a neurologic specialist should be sought before ordering expensive diagnostic tests. Cisternography, tomography, and vertebral–basilar angiography are occasionally necessary to establish the diagnosis. Magnetic resonance angiography is an excellent noninvasive means of visualizing the vertebral–basilar circulation.

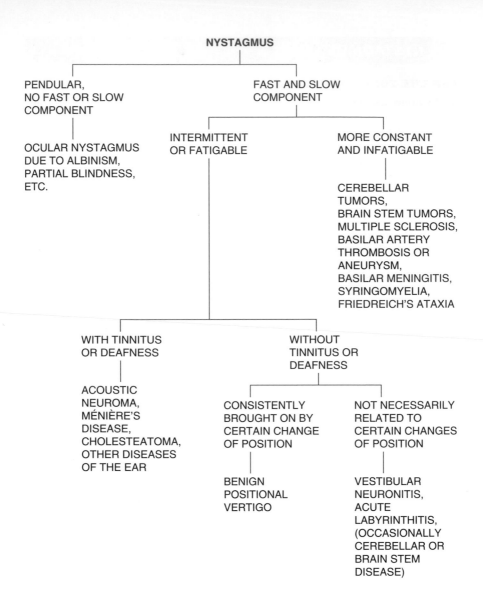

NYSTAGMUS

PENDULAR,
NO FAST OR SLOW
COMPONENT

OCULAR NYSTAGMUS
DUE TO ALBINISM,
PARTIAL BLINDNESS,
ETC.

FAST AND SLOW
COMPONENT

INTERMITTENT
OR FATIGABLE

MORE CONSTANT
AND INFATIGABLE

CEREBELLAR
TUMORS,
BRAIN STEM TUMORS,
MULTIPLE SCLEROSIS,
BASILAR ARTERY
THROMBOSIS OR
ANEURYSM,
BASILAR MENINGITIS,
SYRINGOMYELIA,
FRIEDREICH'S ATAXIA

WITH TINNITUS
OR DEAFNESS

ACOUSTIC
NEUROMA,
MÉNIÈRE'S
DISEASE,
CHOLESTEATOMA,
OTHER DISEASES
OF THE EAR

WITHOUT
TINNITUS OR
DEAFNESS

CONSISTENTLY
BROUGHT ON BY
CERTAIN CHANGE
OF POSITION

BENIGN
POSITIONAL
VERTIGO

NOT NECESSARILY
RELATED TO
CERTAIN CHANGES
OF POSITION

VESTIBULAR
NEURONITIS,
ACUTE
LABYRINTHITIS,
(OCCASIONALLY
CEREBELLAR OR
BRAIN STEM
DISEASE)

OBESITY, PATHOLOGIC

ASK THE FOLLOWING QUESTIONS:

1. **Is there associated hyperphagia?** If the patient recognizes that he or she has a ravenous appetite or eats more than is necessary, the possibility of an insulinoma or Fröhlich's syndrome should be considered.
2. **Is the obesity centripetal?** The presence of centripetal obesity, especially with moon facies, should suggest Cushing's syndrome.
3. **Is the obesity mainly of the lower extremities?** This finding would suggest lipodystrophy.
4. **Is there mental retardation?** The presence of mental retardation should suggest Laurence–Moon–Bardet–Biedl syndrome.
5. **What is the sex of the patient?** In male patients, one should consider Klinefelter's syndrome, and in female patients, one should consider polycystic ovary.
6. **What drugs is the patient on?**

Many drugs may cause obesity, most notably the tricyclic antidepressants and corticosteroids.

DIAGNOSTIC WORKUP

Routine laboratory tests include a CBC, urinalysis, chemistry panel, 2-hr post-prandial blood sugar, and thyroid profile. If an insulinoma is strongly suspected, a 24- to 36-hr fast, a 5-hr glucose tolerance test, and tolbutamide tolerance test may be done. If Cushing's syndrome is suspected, a 24-hr urine free cortisol and cortisol suppression test should be done. Pelvic ultrasound will help diagnose polycystic ovaries. Chromosomal analysis will help diagnose Klinefelter's syndrome. Perhaps a psychiatrist should be consulted.

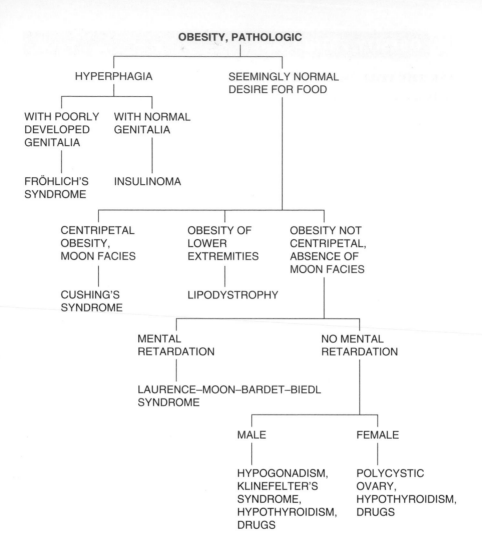

OBESITY, PATHOLOGIC

HYPERPHAGIA

SEEMINGLY NORMAL DESIRE FOR FOOD

WITH POORLY DEVELOPED GENITALIA

WITH NORMAL GENITALIA

FRÖHLICH'S SYNDROME

INSULINOMA

CENTRIPETAL OBESITY, MOON FACIES

OBESITY OF LOWER EXTREMITIES

OBESITY NOT CENTRIPETAL, ABSENCE OF MOON FACIES

CUSHING'S SYNDROME

LIPODYSTROPHY

MENTAL RETARDATION

NO MENTAL RETARDATION

LAURENCE–MOON–BARDET–BIEDL SYNDROME

MALE

FEMALE

HYPOGONADISM, KLINEFELTER'S SYNDROME, HYPOTHYROIDISM, DRUGS

POLYCYSTIC OVARY, HYPOTHYROIDISM, DRUGS

ASK THE FOLLOWING QUESTIONS:

1. **Is there coma or disturbances of consciousness?** The presence of coma or disturbances of consciousness should suggest alcoholism, diabetic acidosis, uremia, and hepatic coma.
2. **Is the odor sweet?** The presence of a sweet odor to the breath should suggest diabetic acidosis, alcoholism, and maple syrup urine disease.
3. **Is the odor unpleasant or foul?** The presence of an unpleasant or foul odor should suggest uremia, hepatic coma, anaerobic infections in the mouth or nasopharynx, and isovaleric aciduria.

DIAGNOSTIC WORKUP

Routine laboratory work includes a CBC, urinalysis, chemistry panel, blood alcohol level, and tests for serum acetone and serum amino acids. Urine for chromatography may help pick up certain keto acids. A culture of the mouth, gums, and nasopharynx may be necessary to diagnose anaerobic infections.

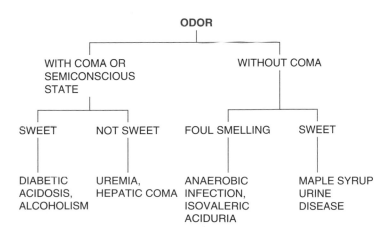

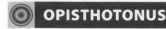
ASK THE FOLLOWING QUESTIONS:

1. **Is it acute?** If it is acute, strychnine poisoning, tetanus, and phenothiazine intoxication should be considered. Also, consider meningitis and uremia.
2. **Is there a history of oral or intravenous drug use or a recent wound infection?** If there is a recent wound infection, one should consider tetanus. If there is no recent wound infection, but a history of oral or intravenous drug use, tetanus and strychnine poisoning are both possibilities. Phenothiazine intoxication must also be considered.
3. **Is the opisthotonus chronic or recurring?** The presence of chronic or recurring opisthotonus should suggest epilepsy, stiff-man syndrome, and hysteria.
4. **If it is chronic and recurring, is there incontinence or tongue biting?** The presence of incontinence or tongue biting in a chronic recurring form of opisthotonus should suggest epilepsy.
5. **Is there fever?** If the opisthotonus is acute and there is a significant fever, one should consider meningitis. However, strychnine poisoning and tetanus may also induce fever in the later stages.

DIAGNOSTIC WORKUP

Routine studies include a CBC, sedimentation rate, urinalysis, chemistry panel including electrolytes, blood cultures, urine drug screen, and VDRL test. A spinal fluid analysis, smear, and culture are indicated if meningitis is suspected. An EEG is indicated in the chronic recurring form.

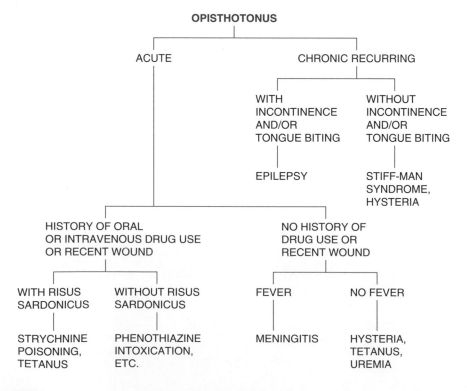

ORTHOPNEA

A patient with orthopnea is able to breathe without significant subjective difficulty in the sitting or upright position but almost invariably develops shortness of breath in the recumbent position. This symptom is the most characteristic of congestive heart failure, especially left ventricular failure. The differential diagnosis and workup are the same as for dyspnea (page 137).

ASK THE FOLLOWING QUESTIONS:

1. **Is the pain mostly during micturition?** If the pain is mostly during micturition, one should consider the possibilities of urethritis, cystitis, bladder calculus, prostatitis, urethral stricture, carcinoma of the bladder, seminal vesiculitis, anal fissure, and hemorrhoids.

2. **If the pain is during micturition, is it mostly at the end of micturition?** If the pain in the penis is at the end of micturition, chronic prostatitis, seminal vesiculitis, anal fissure, hemorrhoids, and bladder calculi should be suspected.

3. **Is the pain mostly during an erection?** If the pain is mostly during an erection, Peyronie's disease should be considered.

4. **Is the pain unrelated to micturition or erection?** If the pain is not related to micturition or erection, renal colic, epithelioma, appendicitis, anxiety, chancroid, and herpes simplex should be considered.

5. **Is there a discharge?** The presence of a urethral discharge should make one think of gonorrhea and nonspecific urethritis.

DIAGNOSTIC WORKUP

The most important diagnostic procedure is a urinalysis, urine culture and sensitivity, and smear and culture of any urethral discharge. It may be necessary to massage the prostate to obtain an adequate specimen! An intravenous pyelogram or CT scan of the abdomen should be done if obstructive uropathy or bladder or renal calculi are suspected. If the above studies are negative, referral to a urologist should be made. He will probably do cystoscopy and retrograde pyelography as well as other diagnostic tests.

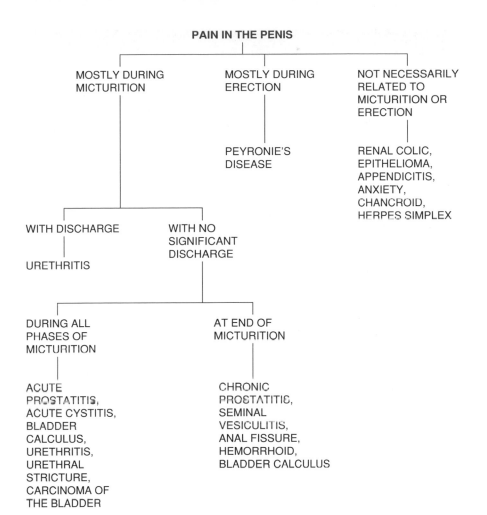

PAIN IN THE PENIS

MOSTLY DURING MICTURITION

MOSTLY DURING ERECTION

NOT NECESSARILY RELATED TO MICTURITION OR ERECTION

PEYRONIE'S DISEASE

RENAL COLIC, EPITHELIOMA, APPENDICITIS, ANXIETY, CHANCROID, HERPES SIMPLEX

WITH DISCHARGE

URETHRITIS

WITH NO SIGNIFICANT DISCHARGE

DURING ALL PHASES OF MICTURITION

ACUTE PROSTATITIS, ACUTE CYSTITIS, BLADDER CALCULUS, URETHRITIS, URETHRAL STRICTURE, CARCINOMA OF THE BLADDER

AT END OF MICTURITION

CHRONIC PROSTATITIS, SEMINAL VESICULITIS, ANAL FISSURE, HEMORRHOID, BLADDER CALCULUS

CASE HISTORY

A 27-year-old stenographer complains of palpitations. Following the algorithm, you examine for murmurs, cardiomegaly, pallor, and fever and find none. Her blood pressure is 135/85 and pulse is 120 per minute. There is no thyromegaly but her hands are sweaty and tremulous. On further questioning, you find she has been drinking a pot of coffee a day and working overtime for several months. Eliminating coffee, tea, and other caffeinated beverages relieved her symptomatology.

ASK THE FOLLOWING QUESTIONS:

1. **Are the palpitations constant or intermittent?** Constant palpitations may signify tachycardia, and that would suggest hyperthyroidism or overuse of caffeine and other drugs. Intermittent palpitations are more likely related to a cardiac arrhythmia, particularly extrasystoles. WPW and other disorders of the conduction system need to be considered here. Also, constant palpitations may indicate a fever of unknown origin.

2. **Are there associated symptoms?** Palpitations with weight loss, increased appetite, and polyuria would suggest hyperthyroidism. Palpitations with shortness of breath and pitting edema would suggest congestive heart failure.

3. **Are there positive physical findings?** If there is cardiomegaly, one must think of the possibility of congestive heart failure or valvular heart disease. If one finds a cardiac murmur, it is more likely that there is valvular heart disease such as acute or chronic rheumatic fever. Mitral valve prolapse is a cause of palpitations. Cardiomegaly, murmur, and/or fever would suggest bacterial endocarditis. Cardiomegaly without a murmur would suggest myocardiopathy, congestive heart failure, and hypothyroidism. Palpitations with no cardiomegaly but with hypertension would suggest pheochromocytoma, particularly if it is systolic hypertension, but it can also be found in hyperthyroidism. Persistent or intermittent palpitations with a totally normal physical examination suggest sensitivity to caffeine or the use of other drugs.

DIAGNOSTIC WORKUP

Before initiating an expensive workup, the patient should eliminate use of all drugs, alcohol, caffeine, and nicotine, if possible, for several days. If this does not eliminate the palpitations, a careful inquiry into the dietary habits should be made, and a CBC should be done to eliminate anemia. In the presence of tachycardia, weight loss, and increased appetite, it is obvious that a thyroid profile should be drawn. If there are palpitations and fever, a workup for an infectious disease, particularly rheumatic fever and bacterial endocarditis, is in order. Blood cultures, ASO titers, sedimentation rate, and echocardiography are useful. If the palpitations are intermittent, a pheochromocytoma should be considered, and 24-hr urine collection for VMA or metanephrines should be ordered. A drug screen may be necessary to ensure patient cooperation in eliminating all drugs. Twenty-four-hour blood-pressure monitoring is also useful. In addition, 24-hr or 48-hr Holter monitoring is very useful in the diagnosis of intermittent palpitations. Newer technology involving a continuous-loop event recorder allows monitoring for 2 weeks at a time. Arm-to-tongue circulation times as well as spirometry may diagnose early congestive heart failure.

PALPITATIONS

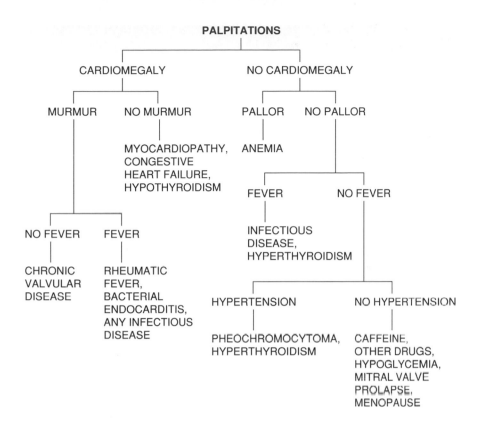

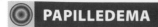

ASK THE FOLLOWING QUESTIONS:

1. **Is the onset acute or gradual?** An acute onset would suggest optic neuritis, hypertensive encephalopathy, cerebral hemorrhage, extradural hematoma, brain abscess, dural sinus thrombosis, meningitis, and subarachnoid hemorrhage. On the other hand, a gradual onset would suggest a space-occupying lesion such as brain tumor, abscess, or subdural hematoma.

2. **If the onset is acute, is there coma or focal neurologic signs?** Findings of coma or focal neurologic signs should suggest cerebral hemorrhage, extradural hematoma, brain abscess, dural sinus thrombosis, meningitis, and subarachnoid hemorrhage. An acute onset without focal neurologic signs or coma would suggest hypertensive encephalopathy and optic neuritis.

3. **If the onset is gradual, are there focal neurologic signs?** A gradual onset of papilledema with focal neurologic signs suggests a brain tumor, abscess, or subdural hematoma.

4. **Is there hypertension?** The presence of hypertension and papilledema suggests hypertensive encephalopathy, acute glomerulonephritis, and certain collagen diseases. If there is no hypertension and no focal neurologic signs, then a diagnosis of pseudotumor cerebri or pseudopapilledema should be suspected.

DIAGNOSTIC WORKUP

Regardless of whether there are focal neurologic signs or hypertension, a CT scan or MRI should be done, and a consultation with a neurologist should be made when papilledema is suspected.

If there is significant hypertension and the CT scan or MRI is negative, a hypertensive workup should be done (see page 248).

With a normal CT scan or MRI and no focal neurologic signs or hypertension, a spinal tap and visual field examination will assist in the diagnosis of pseudotumor cerebri. However, a blood lead level should be done to rule out lead poisoning. Also, the visual field examination may show optic neuritis when the clinical examination is inconclusive.

An ophthalmologist will help diagnose optic neuritis and pseudopapilledema.

PAPILLEDEMA

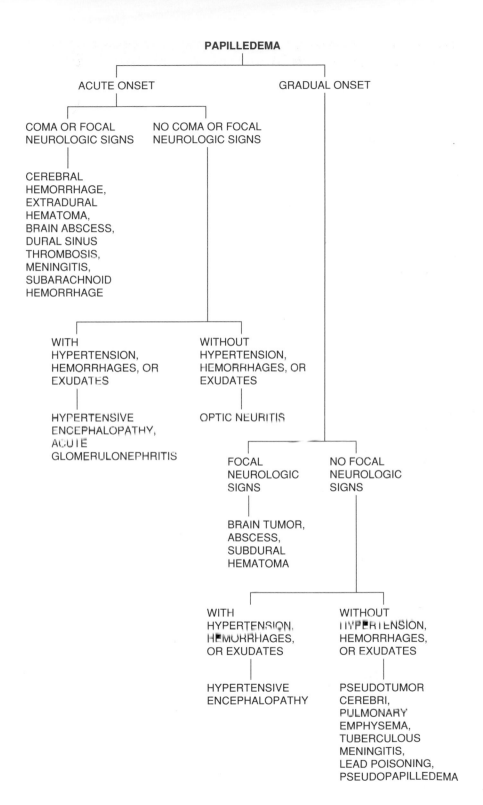

ACUTE ONSET

GRADUAL ONSET

COMA OR FOCAL
NEUROLOGIC SIGNS

NO COMA OR FOCAL
NEUROLOGIC SIGNS

CEREBRAL
HEMORRHAGE,
EXTRADURAL
HEMATOMA,
BRAIN ABSCESS,
DURAL SINUS
THROMBOSIS,
MENINGITIS,
SUBARACHNOID
HEMORRHAGE

WITH
HYPERTENSION,
HEMORRHAGES, OR
EXUDATES

WITHOUT
HYPERTENSION,
HEMORRHAGES, OR
EXUDATES

HYPERTENSIVE
ENCEPHALOPATHY,
ACUTE
GLOMERULONEPHRITIS

OPTIC NEURITIS

FOCAL
NEUROLOGIC
SIGNS

NO FOCAL
NEUROLOGIC
SIGNS

BRAIN TUMOR,
ABSCESS,
SUBDURAL
HEMATOMA

WITH
HYPERTENSION,
HEMORRHAGES,
OR EXUDATES

WITHOUT
HYPERTENSION,
HEMORRHAGES,
OR EXUDATES

HYPERTENSIVE
ENCEPHALOPATHY

PSEUDOTUMOR
CEREBRI,
PULMONARY
EMPHYSEMA,
TUBERCULOUS
MENINGITIS,
LEAD POISONING,
PSEUDOPAPILLEDEMA

ASK THE FOLLOWING QUESTIONS:

1. **Are the pulses diminished?** The presence of diminished pulses should suggest peripheral arteriosclerosis or Leriche's syndrome.
2. **Is there associated pain in the involved extremity?** The presence of pain in the involved extremity should suggest lumbar spondylosis, spinal stenosis, cauda equina tumor, spondylolisthesis, herniated disk, and pelvic tumors.
3. **Is there a positive straight-leg raising test and/or decreased Achilles reflex?** These findings suggest a herniated disk of L4 to 5 or L5 to S1, lumbar spondylosis, spinal stenosis, a cauda equina tumor, or spondylolisthesis.
4. **Is there a positive femoral stretch test or decreased knee jerk?** These findings suggest a herniated disk of L3–4 or L2–3 or lumbar spondylosis.
5. **Are there diffuse hyperactive reflexes?** These findings suggest multiple sclerosis, pernicious anemia, degenerative diseases of the spinal cord such as syringomyelia, spinal cord tumor, or other space-occupying lesions. It may also suggest anterior spinal artery occlusion.
6. **Are there diffuse hypoactive reflexes?** The presence of diffuse hypoactive reflexes would suggest poliomyelitis, Guillain–Barré syndrome, cauda equina tumor, metastatic tumor of the lumbar spine, and, occasionally, pernicious anemia or peroneal neuropathy. Also, peripheral neuropathy will present with diffuse hypoactive reflexes.
7. **Is there incontinence associated with the hypoactive reflexes?** The presence of incontinence with the hypoactive reflexes may indicate poliomyelitis, cauda equina tumor, or metastatic tumors to the lumbar spine.
8. Paresthesias limited to the foot and toes may indicate Morton's neuroma or tarsal tunnel syndrome.

DIAGNOSTIC WORKUP

The basic diagnostic workup includes a CBC, sedimentation rate, urinalysis, chemistry panel, arthritis panel, VDRL test, and x-ray of the lumbosacral spine. Serum B_{12} and folic acid tests should be done if pernicious anemia is suspected. If these tests are negative, an orthopedic or neurologic specialist should be consulted. A CT scan of the lumbosacral spine, a nerve conduction velocity study, and an EMG may all be necessary in the workup. MRI is more expensive and often unnecessary.

Combined myelography and CT scan is often useful in evaluating the need for surgery. A bone scan may be helpful in diagnosing occult fractures, metastases, or osteomyelitis.

If multiple sclerosis, Guillain–Barré syndrome, or central nervous system lues is suspected, a spinal tap may be done. SSEP studies are useful in diagnosing multiple sclerosis.

A neuropathy workup may be necessary. This involves a glucose tolerance test to rule out diabetes; urine tests for porphyrins and porphobilinogen to rule out porphyria; quantitative urine niacin, thiamine, pyridoxine, and other B vitamins after loading, an ANA and anti-dsDNA test to rule out collagen disease; serum protein electrophoresis and immunoelectrophoresis to diagnose various collagen diseases and macroglobulinemia; a lymph node biopsy and Kveim test for sarcoidosis; nerve conduction velocity studies and EMG to establish the presence of a neuropathy; thyroid profile to rule out hypothyroidism or hyperthyroidism;

HIV antibody titers; blood levels for heavy metals such as lead to rule out lead or arsenic neuropathy; and skin and muscle biopsies to rule out various collagen diseases. A trial of therapy is often necessary to rule out the nutritional neuropathies.

Lumbar puncture, as already mentioned, is useful in diagnosing Guillain–Barré syndrome. Nerve biopsy may be necessary when all the above procedures are negative.

RBC transketolase activity is decreased in beriberi and the serum pyruvate and lactate levels are elevated.

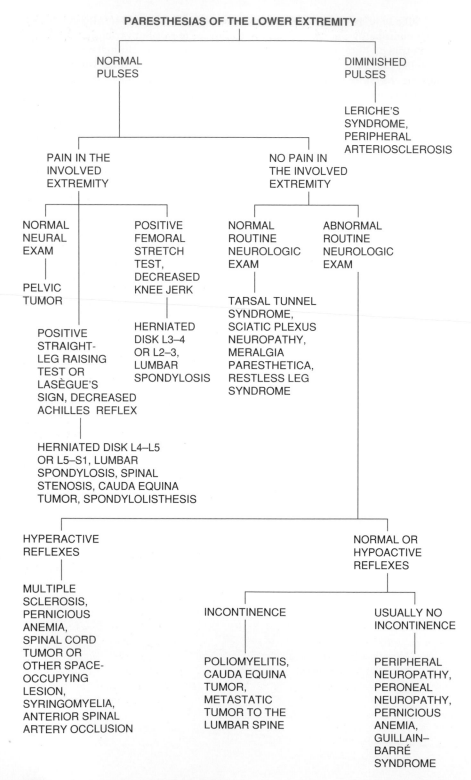

PARESTHESIAS OF THE LOWER EXTREMITY

NORMAL PULSES

DIMINISHED PULSES

LERICHE'S SYNDROME, PERIPHERAL ARTERIOSCLEROSIS

PAIN IN THE INVOLVED EXTREMITY

NO PAIN IN THE INVOLVED EXTREMITY

NORMAL NEURAL EXAM

POSITIVE FEMORAL STRETCH TEST, DECREASED KNEE JERK

NORMAL ROUTINE NEUROLOGIC EXAM

ABNORMAL ROUTINE NEUROLOGIC EXAM

PELVIC TUMOR

POSITIVE STRAIGHT-LEG RAISING TEST OR LASÈGUE'S SIGN, DECREASED ACHILLES REFLEX

HERNIATED DISK L3–4 OR L2–3, LUMBAR SPONDYLOSIS

TARSAL TUNNEL SYNDROME, SCIATIC PLEXUS NEUROPATHY, MERALGIA PARESTHETICA, RESTLESS LEG SYNDROME

HERNIATED DISK L4–L5 OR L5–S1, LUMBAR SPONDYLOSIS, SPINAL STENOSIS, CAUDA EQUINA TUMOR, SPONDYLOLISTHESIS

HYPERACTIVE REFLEXES

NORMAL OR HYPOACTIVE REFLEXES

MULTIPLE SCLEROSIS, PERNICIOUS ANEMIA, SPINAL CORD TUMOR OR OTHER SPACE-OCCUPYING LESION, SYRINGOMYELIA, ANTERIOR SPINAL ARTERY OCCLUSION

INCONTINENCE

USUALLY NO INCONTINENCE

POLIOMYELITIS, CAUDA EQUINA TUMOR, METASTATIC TUMOR TO THE LUMBAR SPINE

PERIPHERAL NEUROPATHY, PERONEAL NEUROPATHY, PERNICIOUS ANEMIA, GUILLAIN–BARRÉ SYNDROME

ASK THE FOLLOWING QUESTIONS:

1. **Are there paresthesias of the face or cranial nerve signs?** These findings would suggest a diagnosis of cerebral vascular disease, a space-occupying lesion of the brain, migraine, or multiple sclerosis.

2. **Is there pain in the involved extremity?** Pain in the involved extremity, particularly radicular pain, should suggest a herniated cervical disk, spinal cord tumor, or cervical spondylosis. However, many other conditions, such as brachial plexus neuropathy, thoracic outlet syndrome, a cervical rib, Pancoast's tumor, Raynaud's disease, and sympathetic dystrophy, should also be considered. Finally, the various entrapment syndromes should be considered, such as carpal tunnel syndrome and ulnar nerve entrapment at the elbow.

3. **Are the Adson's tests positive?** If the radial pulse diminishes in certain positions of the neck and shoulders, a thoracic outlet syndrome or cervical rib should be considered. *(Thoracic outlet x)*

4. **Is the Tinel's sign positive at the wrist or elbow?** A positive Tinel's sign at the wrist would suggest a carpal tunnel syndrome and can be confirmed by a positive Phalen's test. A positive Tinel's sign at the elbow would suggest ulnar entrapment syndrome. The ulnar nerve may also be entrapped in Guyon's canal and the median nerve may be trapped at the elbow in a pronator syndrome.

5. **Is the cervical compression test positive?** The presence of a positive cervical compression test or a positive Spurling's test would suggest cervical spondylosis and herniated cervical disk. *(head to side, downward pressure to top of head)*

6. **Are there hyperactive reflexes?** The presence of hyperactive reflexes in the upper or lower extremity would suggest a spinal cord tumor, multiple sclerosis, degenerative disease of the spinal cord such as syringomyelia or amyotrophic lateral sclerosis, anterior spinal artery occlusion, and cervical spondylosis.

7. **Are there normal or hypoactive reflexes noted?** The presence of normal or hypoactive reflexes in the involved extremity should prompt consideration of peripheral neuropathy, pernicious anemia, and brachial plexus neuropathy.

DIAGNOSTIC WORKUP

A CBC, sedimentation rate, urinalysis, chemistry panel, serum B12 and folic acid, arthritis panel, and plain films of the cervical spine constitute the basic workup of paresthesias of the upper extremities. If these are negative, the next logical step is to consult a neurologist or neurosurgeon.

If there are paresthesias of the face or cranial nerve signs, MRI or CT scan of the brain will probably be the most logical test to order next. If not, MRI of the cervical spine will be useful. Nerve conduction velocity studies, EMG, and dermatomal SSEP studies complete the workup in most cases. However, SSEP studies and a spinal tap may be necessary to diagnose multiple sclerosis. If tabes dorsalis is suspected, a blood or spinal fluid fluorescent *Treponema pallidum* antibody test may be done. Immunoelectrophoresis may diagnose a monoclonal gammopathy A therapeutic trial of vitamin B6 or corticosteroids may diagnose carpal tunnel syndrome if a neurologist is not available.

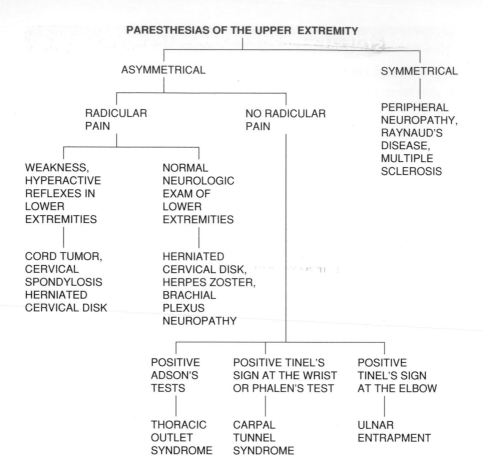

PARESTHESIAS OF THE UPPER EXTREMITY

ASYMMETRICAL

SYMMETRICAL

RADICULAR PAIN

NO RADICULAR PAIN

PERIPHERAL NEUROPATHY, RAYNAUD'S DISEASE, MULTIPLE SCLEROSIS

WEAKNESS, HYPERACTIVE REFLEXES IN LOWER EXTREMITIES

NORMAL NEUROLOGIC EXAM OF LOWER EXTREMITIES

CORD TUMOR, CERVICAL SPONDYLOSIS HERNIATED CERVICAL DISK

HERNIATED CERVICAL DISK, HERPES ZOSTER, BRACHIAL PLEXUS NEUROPATHY

POSITIVE ADSON'S TESTS

POSITIVE TINEL'S SIGN AT THE WRIST OR PHALEN'S TEST

POSITIVE TINEL'S SIGN AT THE ELBOW

THORACIC OUTLET SYNDROME

CARPAL TUNNEL SYNDROME

ULNAR ENTRAPMENT

ASK THE FOLLOWING QUESTIONS:

1. **Are the findings intermittent?** If the pathologic reflexes come and go, transient ischemic attacks, multiple sclerosis, migraine, epilepsy, and hypoglycemia should be considered in the differential diagnosis.
2. **Are they unilateral or bilateral?** Unilateral pathologic reflexes should signify either a brain tumor or vascular lesion. Bilateral pathologic reflexes should suggest an inflammatory or degenerative disease. However, multiple sclerosis may present with either unilateral or bilateral pathologic reflexes. Vascular lesions in the basilar circulation may also present with bilateral pathologic reflexes. It should be pointed out that there is no hard-and-fast rule.
3. **Is there associated facial palsy or other cranial nerve signs?** The presence of facial palsy or other cranial nerve signs should make one look for a lesion in the brain or brain stem.
4. **Is there headache or papilledema?** The presence of headache or papilledema should prompt the investigation for a space-occupying lesion of the brain or brain stem.
5. **Is there hypertension or a possible source for an embolism?** These findings would suggest a cerebral vascular accident such as cerebral hemorrhage or embolism.
6. **Is the sensory examination normal?** The findings of bilateral pathologic reflexes or unilateral pathologic reflexes with a normal sensory exam and no cranial nerve signs would suggest amyotrophic lateral sclerosis or primary lateral sclerosis.

DIAGNOSTIC WORKUP

Routine studies include a CBC, sedimentation rate, urinalysis, chemistry panel, ANA assay, serum B_{12} and folic acid, VDRL test, chest x-ray, and EKG. If there are cranial nerve signs, a CT scan or MRI of the brain will usually be necessary. However, it is wise to get a neurology consultation before undertaking these expensive tests. A spinal tap may be done if the imaging study is negative.

If vascular disease is suspected, carotid scans to rule out carotid stenosis or plaque and a search for an embolic source using echocardiography and blood culture should be done. A cardiologist can assist in this search. Four-vessel cerebral angiography or an MRA may be necessary. In fact, if a cerebral hemorrhage has been ruled out and there is no significant hypertension, a four-vessel cerebral angiographic study should probably be done. Evoked potential studies and HIV antibody titers should also be done. If there are no cranial nerve signs, MRI of the cervical spine or thoracic spine should be done, depending on the level of the lesion. Myelography may also be helpful. Serum protein electrophoresis and immunoelectrophoresis all may be necessary in the workup.

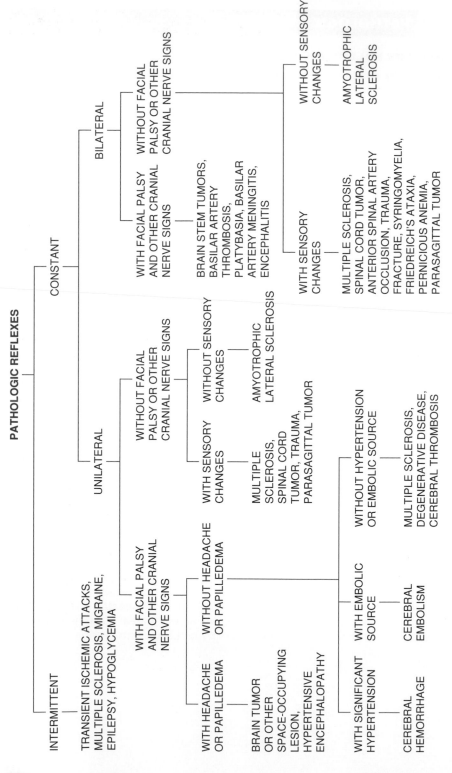

PATHOLOGIC REFLEXES

INTERMITTENT

TRANSIENT ISCHEMIC ATTACKS,
MULTIPLE SCLEROSIS, MIGRAINE,
EPILEPSY, HYPOGLYCEMIA

CONSTANT

UNILATERAL

WITH FACIAL PALSY
AND OTHER CRANIAL
NERVE SIGNS

WITH HEADACHE
OR PAPILLEDEMA

BRAIN TUMOR
OR OTHER
SPACE-OCCUPYING
LESION,
HYPERTENSIVE
ENCEPHALOPATHY

WITHOUT HEADACHE
OR PAPILLEDEMA

WITH SIGNIFICANT
HYPERTENSION

CEREBRAL
HEMORRHAGE

WITH EMBOLIC
SOURCE

CEREBRAL
EMBOLISM

WITHOUT HYPERTENSION
OR EMBOLIC SOURCE

MULTIPLE SCLEROSIS,
DEGENERATIVE DISEASE,
CEREBRAL THROMBOSIS

WITHOUT FACIAL
PALSY OR OTHER
CRANIAL NERVE SIGNS

WITH SENSORY
CHANGES

MULTIPLE
SCLEROSIS,
SPINAL CORD
TUMOR, TRAUMA,
PARASAGITTAL TUMOR

WITHOUT SENSORY
CHANGES

AMYOTROPHIC
LATERAL SCLEROSIS

BILATERAL

WITH FACIAL PALSY
AND OTHER CRANIAL
NERVE SIGNS

BRAIN STEM TUMORS,
BASILAR ARTERY
THROMBOSIS,
PLATYBASIA, BASILAR
ARTERY MENINGITIS,
ENCEPHALITIS

WITHOUT FACIAL
PALSY OR OTHER
CRANIAL NERVE SIGNS

WITH SENSORY
CHANGES

MULTIPLE SCLEROSIS,
SPINAL CORD TUMOR,
ANTERIOR SPINAL ARTERY
OCCLUSION, TRAUMA,
FRACTURE, SYRINGOMYELIA,
FRIEDREICH'S ATAXIA,
PERNICIOUS ANEMIA,
PARASAGITTAL TUMOR

WITHOUT SENSORY
CHANGES

AMYOTROPHIC
LATERAL
SCLEROSIS

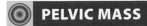

ASK THE FOLLOWING QUESTIONS:

1. **Is there abdominal pain?** The presence of abdominal pain suggests PID, ectopic pregnancy, and endometriosis, among other things. It should also suggest pelvic appendix.

2. **Is there fever or vaginal discharge?** The presence of fever or vaginal discharge would be most suggestive of PID.

3. **Is there a history of menorrhagia or metrorrhagia?** The history of menorrhagia or metrorrhagia should suggest ectopic pregnancy, endometriosis, and threatened abortion, as well as retained secundinae.

4. **Is the pregnancy test positive?** A positive pregnancy test is the key to a diagnosis of ectopic pregnancy when there is abdominal pain along with the abdominal mass. If there is no pain, the pregnancy test will help diagnose a normal pregnancy.

DIAGNOSTIC WORKUP

Routine diagnostic studies include a CBC, sedimentation rate, pregnancy test, urinalysis, urine culture, chemistry panel, VDRL test, and Pap smear. If there is a vaginal discharge, a smear and culture of the material should be made. If a distended bladder is suspected, catheterization for residual urine must be done. Pelvic ultrasound or a CT scan will often be useful, but why not consult a gynecologist before ordering these more expensive tests? The gynecologist may do a laparoscopy, a culdocentesis, and, ultimately, an exploratory laparotomy.

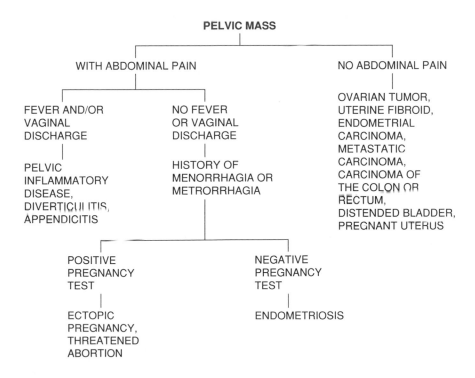

CASE HISTORY

A 39-year-old female, gravid iii, para ii, presents to your office with a history of recurrent hypogastric pain. Following the algorithm, you look for a vaginal discharge and fever. These are absent. There is a history of heavy periods and on examination, she had an enlarged asymmetrical uterus. The pregnancy test is negative so, you suspect either uterine fibroids or endometriosis. Pelvic ultrasound confirms the diagnosis of uterine fibroids.

ASK THE FOLLOWING QUESTIONS:

1. **Is there a pelvic mass?** The presence of a pelvic mass would suggest salpingo-oophoritis, ectopic pregnancy, endometriosis, uterine fibroid, or an ovarian tumor that is twisting on its pedicle. Be sure to do a recto-vaginal examination as there may be a mass or fluid in the cul de sac.
2. **Is there fever or purulent vaginal discharge?** The presence of fever or purulent vaginal discharge would suggest PID, diverticulitis, and appendicitis.
3. **Is there a history of metrorrhagia or menorrhagia?** The history of metrorrhagia or menorrhagia would suggest ectopic pregnancy, threatened abortion, retained secundinae, uterine fibroids, and endometriosis.
4. **Is there a positive pregnancy test?** The presence of a positive pregnancy test would suggest an ectopic pregnancy or threatened abortion.
5. **Is the pain related to the menstrual cycle?** If the pain is related to the menstrual cycle, mittelschmerz should be considered.

DIAGNOSTIC WORKUP

Routine studies include a CBC, sedimentation rate, pregnancy test, urinalysis, urine culture, chemistry panel, VDRL test, and Pap smear. A vaginal smear and culture should also be done routinely.

The next step would logically be a pelvic or transvaginal ultrasound, but it is wise to consult a gynecologist before ordering expensive tests. The gynecologist may proceed with laparoscopy, culdocentesis, and, ultimately, an exploratory laparotomy. A CT scan of the abdomen and pelvis may also be necessary. If there is fever, a trial of antibiotics may be appropriate even if the workup is negative.

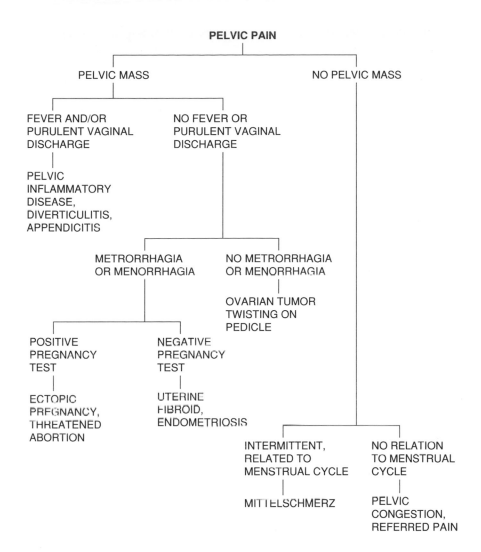

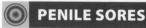
ASK THE FOLLOWING QUESTIONS:

1. **Is it painful?** The presence of a painful penile sore suggests chancroid, herpes simplex, herpes zoster, and balanitis. On the other hand, a painless penile sore should suggest chancre, lymphogranuloma venereum, epithelioma, granuloma inguinale, and papilloma.
2. **Is there inguinal adenopathy?** If there is inguinal adenopathy, lymphogranuloma venereum, epithelioma, and chancre should be suspected.

DIAGNOSTIC WORKUP

Routine studies include a smear and culture of material from the sore and a dark field examination. All patients deserve a test for HIV especially if there is risky sexual behavior. A VDRL test should be performed if syphilis is suspected. Many cases require a biopsy of the lesion or a biopsy of the lymph node.

A Frei test will help diagnose lymphogranuloma venereum. A Tzanck test, serologic test, and viral isolation will help diagnose herpes zoster and herpes simplex. There are also serologic tests for lymphogranuloma venereum, if necessary. A lygranum test may help diagnose lymphogranuloma inguinale. Difficult diagnostic problems should be referred to a urologist.

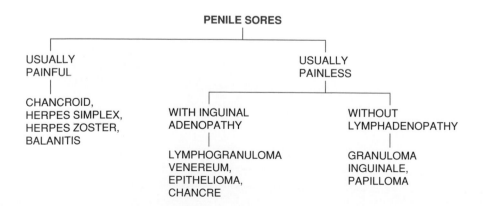

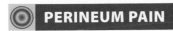

ASK THE FOLLOWING QUESTIONS:

1. **Is there dysuria or a vaginal or urethral discharge?** These findings suggest prostatitis, urethritis, cystitis, bladder calculus, bladder carcinoma, vaginitis, and abscesses of Cowper's glands.
2. **Is there a rectal or anal mass or discharge?** These findings suggest hemorrhoids, perirectal abscess, anal fissure, anal ulcer, rectal carcinoma, and condylomata lata.

DIAGNOSTIC WORKUP

Routine laboratory tests include a CBC, sedimentation rate, urinalysis and urine culture, and a smear and culture of any discharge that is available. If prostatitis is suspected, a serum PSA should be done. An anoscopy and proctoscopy will help diagnose most rectal conditions. Pelvic ultrasound will be helpful in diagnosing endometriosis, ectopic pregnancy, and pelvic appendicitis. Referral to a gynecologist or urologist may be necessary in some cases.

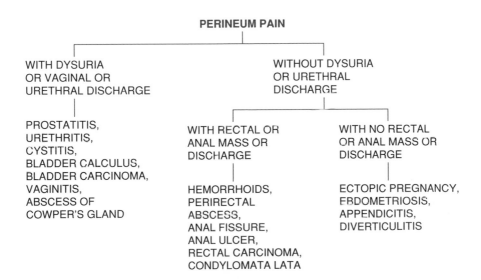

PERINEUM PAIN

WITH DYSURIA OR VAGINAL OR URETHRAL DISCHARGE

PROSTATITIS, URETHRITIS, CYSTITIS, BLADDER CALCULUS, BLADDER CARCINOMA, VAGINITIS, ABSCESS OF COWPER'S GLAND

WITHOUT DYSURIA OR URETHRAL DISCHARGE

WITH RECTAL OR ANAL MASS OR DISCHARGE

HEMORRHOIDS, PERIRECTAL ABSCESS, ANAL FISSURE, ANAL ULCER, RECTAL CARCINOMA, CONDYLOMATA LATA

WITH NO RECTAL OR ANAL MASS OR DISCHARGE

ECTOPIC PREGNANCY, ERDOMETRIOSIS, APPENDICITIS, DIVERTICULITIS

ASK THE FOLLOWING QUESTIONS:

1. **Is there a periorbital or facial rash?** The presence of a periorbital or facial rash should suggest contact dermatitis, angioneurotic edema, trichinosis, and herpes zoster. Remember, herpes zoster is usually unilateral.

2. **Is there a generalized edema?** The presence of generalized edema suggests myxedema, cirrhosis, acute and chronic glomerulonephritis, congestive heart failure, and other disorders.

3. **Is there fever?** The presence of fever suggests acute sinusitis, cavernous sinus thrombosis, orbital cellulitis, meningitis, and neurosyphilis.

4. **What drugs is the patient on?** ACE inhibitors and ARBs may cause angioneurotic edema.

DIAGNOSTIC WORKUP

Routine diagnostic studies include a CBC, sedimentation rate, urinalysis, chemistry panel, thyroid profile, chest x-ray, VDRL test, and x-ray of the sinuses and orbits. If there is fever, a nose and throat culture and blood culture should be done and antibiotics begun without delay. A CT scan of the brain and sinuses probably ought to be done in these cases, but why not get an ear, nose, and throat or neurologic consultation first?

If there is generalized edema, the workup should proceed as outlined on page 144.

Trichinosis can be diagnosed by the skin test, serologic studies, or a muscle biopsy. Superior vena cava syndrome may be diagnosed by a chest x-ray in many cases, but a CT scan of the mediastinum may be necessary.

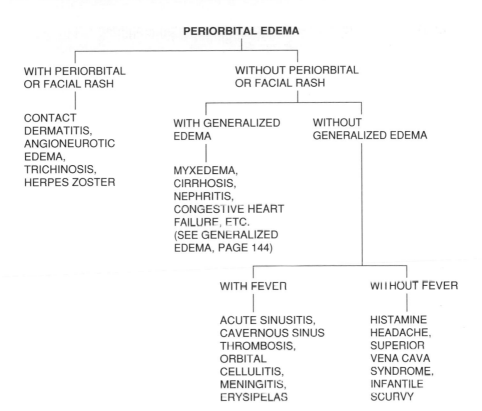

PERIORBITAL EDEMA

WITH PERIORBITAL OR FACIAL RASH

CONTACT DERMATITIS, ANGIONEUROTIC EDEMA, TRICHINOSIS, HERPES ZOSTER

WITHOUT PERIORBITAL OR FACIAL RASH

WITH GENERALIZED EDEMA

MYXEDEMA, CIRRHOSIS, NEPHRITIS, CONGESTIVE HEART FAILURE, ETC. (SEE GENERALIZED EDEMA, PAGE 144)

WITHOUT GENERALIZED EDEMA

WITH FEVER

ACUTE SINUSITIS, CAVERNOUS SINUS THROMBOSIS, ORBITAL CELLULITIS, MENINGITIS, ERYSIPELAS

WITHOUT FEVER

HISTAMINE HEADACHE, SUPERIOR VENA CAVA SYNDROME, INFANTILE SCURVY

Visible peristalsis may be either gastric or intestinal, but it is invariably associated with vomiting and other signs of intestinal obstruction.

In infants with pyloric obstruction, the vomiting is projectile, and the severe dehydration that follows, along with the right upper quadrant mass (a hypertrophied pylorus), helps to make the diagnosis.

In adults with pyloric obstruction, the enlarged stomach with peristaltic waves going downward from left to right and a succussion splash are useful diagnostic signs. A flat plate of the abdomen (demonstrating the dilated stomach) and significant electrolyte alteration of metabolic alkalosis and potassium depletion will help confirm the diagnosis, but an exploratory laparotomy will remove all doubts.

Intestinal peristalsis is also associated with vomiting. The peristalsis is transverse in small intestinal obstruction and vertical in large intestinal obstruction. The abdomen is markedly distended. Once again, a flat plate of the abdomen will confirm the diagnosis.

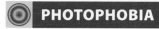

ASK THE FOLLOWING QUESTIONS:

1. **Is there a history of exposure to drugs or toxins?** Quinine, cocaine, atropine, and Apresoline® are just a few of the drugs that may cause photophobia.

2. **Are there abnormalities on the eye examination?** Almost any condition of the eye may cause photophobia, including conjunctivitis, blepharitis, keratitis, iritis, corneal ulcers, and retinitis.

3. **Are there abnormal tonometry readings?** The eye may appear normal, but the tonometry may disclose glaucoma.

4. **Is there nuchal rigidity?** The presence of nuchal rigidity, especially with fever, would suggest meningitis. Without fever or with only a low-grade fever, the presence of nuchal rigidity should suggest subarachnoid hemorrhage.

DIAGNOSTIC WORKUP

A careful eye examination including tonometry and slit lamp examination should be done. A referral to an ophthalmologist may be necessary to accomplish this. If there is nuchal rigidity, a CT scan followed by a spinal tap should be done in conjunction with a neurologic consultation. If there is fever without nuchal rigidity, the workup can proceed as outlined on page 177. A histamine test may be helpful in diagnosing migraine.

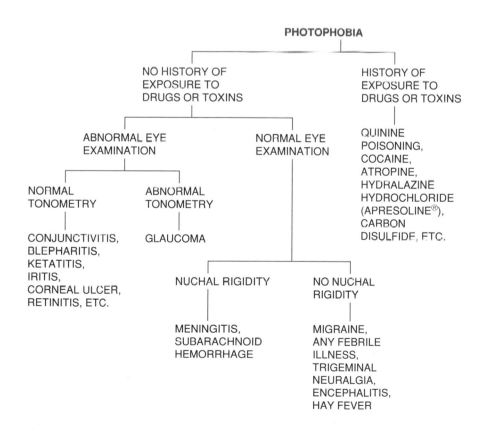

INCREASED

ASK THE FOLLOWING QUESTIONS:

1. **What is the ACTH level?** An increased ACTH in the face of an elevated plasma cortisol suggests a basophilic adenoma of the pituitary or ectopic ACTH producing tumors. A decreased ACTH coupled with an increased plasma cortisol suggests adrenocortical hyperplasia, adenoma or carcinoma.
2. **What are the results of a high-dose dexamethasone suppression test?** If there is suppression, look for adrenal hyperplasia. If no response, look for adrenal adenoma or carcinoma.

DECREASED

ASK THE FOLLOWING QUESTION:

1. **What is the ACTH level?** An increased ACTH coupled with a low plasma cortisol is indicative of adrenal insufficiency, while a decreased ACTH combined with a decreased plasma cortisol suggests hypopituitarism.

DIAGNOSTIC WORKUP

A basophilic adenoma is diagnosed by an MRI of the brain. Further testing for hypopituitarism includes a metapyrapone test, serum growth hormone, FH, LH, and TSH as well as an MRI or CT scan of the brain. A CT scan of the abdomen will help diagnose adrenal hyperplasia, adenoma or carcinoma. An ACTH stimulation test is an excellent test to diagnose adrenal insufficiency but the CT scan of the abdomen is useful as well.

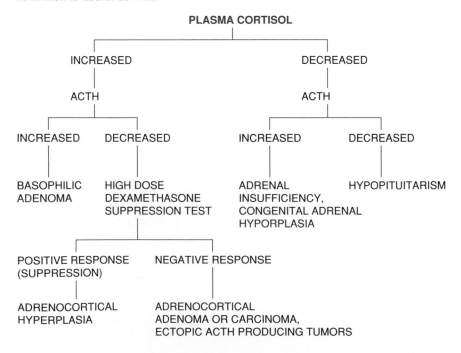

This condition is the passage of gas through the urethra. First, there may be a rectovesical fistula. In these cases, usually there are feces in the urine as well. The fistula results from ruptured diverticulitis, ruptured appendix, or a neoplasm that forms a pelvic abscess that gradually eats its way into the bladder.

Second, there may be a UTI with gas-producing organisms, usually *Escherichia coli*. The patients are usually elderly diabetic females.

Urinalysis shows pus and often blood in both types. The fistula may be diagnosed by an intravenous pyelogram, a barium enema, or cystoscopy. A urine culture may show *E. coli, Enterobacter aerogenes,* or yeasts in those cases without a communicating fistula. A course of antibiotic therapy will usually clear up the UTI and stop the pneumaturia. If it does not, the search should continue for a fistula.

CASE HISTORY

A 36-year-old white female presents for an annual physical, and you are immediately struck by how flushed her face is. You ask about chronic use of alcohol and she assures you that she rarely drinks. Looking through her chart, you find laboratory results that show an increase in hemoglobin and hematocrit. Following the algorithm, you check for clinical signs of dehydration, and there are none. Her oxygen saturation is 96%, so pulmonary fibrosis or emphysema is an unlikely cause. You order a serum erythropoietin and it is normal. You suspect polycythemia vera, but note that she is obese and has purple abdominal striae. You suspect Cushing's syndrome and the plasma cortisol confirms your diagnosis.

ASK THE FOLLOWING QUESTIONS:

1. **What is the plasma volume?** If the plasma volume is decreased, think of dehydration, diuretic use, or other factors.
2. **What is the arterial oxygen saturation?** Decreased oxygen saturation would suggest either emphysema, pulmonary fibrosis, or cardiovascular disorder.
3. **Is the blood erythropoietin level increased?** An increase in the blood erythropoietin would suggest an erythropoietin-secreting tumor such as renal carcinoma or pheochromocytoma. A normal or decreased erythropoietin would point to polycythemia vera, heavy cigarette smoking, or methemoglobinemia.

DIAGNOSTIC WORKUP

In addition to blood gas analysis, blood volume studies, CBC, platelet count, chemistry panel, urinalysis, and sedimentation rate, most patients should have an IVP or CT scan of the abdomen and pulmonary function tests and a chest x-ray. A hematology consult would be wise before undertaking any of the more expensive studies.

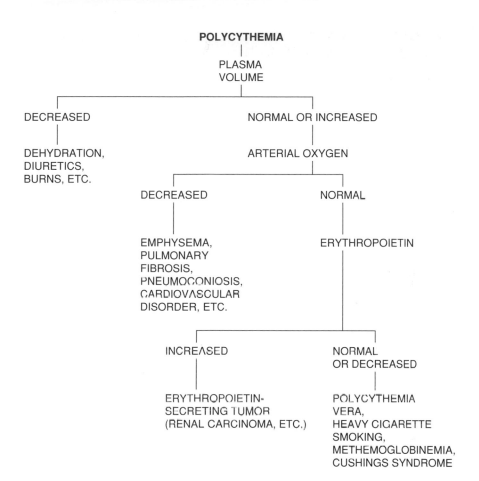

POLYCYTHEMIA
|
PLASMA
VOLUME

DECREASED   NORMAL OR INCREASED

DEHYDRATION,
DIURETICS,
BURNS, ETC.   ARTERIAL OXYGEN

DECREASED   NORMAL

EMPHYSEMA,
PULMONARY
FIBROSIS,
PNEUMOCONIOSIS,
CARDIOVASCULAR
DISORDER, ETC.   ERYTHROPOIETIN

INCREASED   NORMAL
OR DECREASED

ERYTHROPOIETIN-
SECRETING TUMOR
(RENAL CARCINOMA, ETC.)   POLYCYTHEMIA
VERA,
HEAVY CIGARETTE
SMOKING,
METHEMOGLOBINEMIA,
CUSHINGS SYNDROME

POLYDIPSIA

ASK THE FOLLOWING QUESTIONS:

1. **Is there a history of drug ingestion?** Diuretics and arsenic poisoning are among the many causes of excessive thirst.
2. **Is there associated polyphagia and weight loss?** The presence of these symptoms would suggest diabetes mellitus and hyperthyroidism.
3. **Is there massive polyuria?** The presence of massive polyuria suggests diabetes insipidus or psychogenic polydipsia.
4. **Is there mild polyuria?** The presence of mild polyuria should suggest chronic renal failure, renal tubular acidosis, hyperparathyroidism, and febrile illnesses.

DIAGNOSTIC WORKUP

The basic workup includes a CBC, sedimentation rate, urinalysis, 24-hr urine volume, a serum and urine osmolality, a thyroid profile, and x-rays of the skull and long bones.

The diagnosis of hyperparathyroidism may be assisted by ordering a serum parathyroid hormone level. Also, a 24-hr urine collection for calcium may be done to help diagnose this condition. Microscopic examination of the urinary sediment will help diagnose renal disease, as will renal biopsies. If pituitary diabetes insipidus is suspected, a CT scan of the brain and blood tests for serum growth hormone, FSH, LH, ACTH, and TSH may be done. The Hickey–Hare test and monitoring intake and output before and after vasopressin (Pitressin®) will be useful in differentiating pituitary diabetes insipidus from nephrogenic diabetes insipidus. The concentrations of circulating vasopressin may be measured by immunoassay.

An endocrinologist should be consulted before ordering these expensive diagnostic tests.

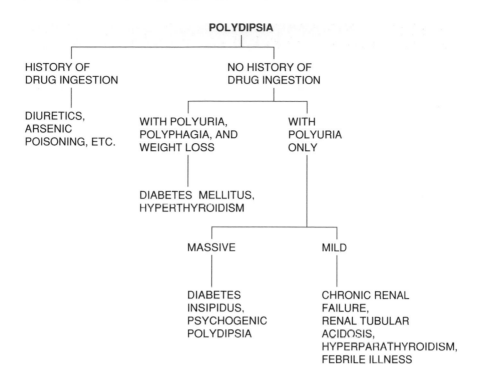

POLYDIPSIA

HISTORY OF
DRUG INGESTION

NO HISTORY OF
DRUG INGESTION

DIURETICS,
ARSENIC
POISONING, ETC.

WITH POLYURIA,
POLYPHAGIA, AND
WEIGHT LOSS

WITH
POLYURIA
ONLY

DIABETES MELLITUS,
HYPERTHYROIDISM

MASSIVE

MILD

DIABETES
INSIPIDUS,
PSYCHOGENIC
POLYDIPSIA

CHRONIC RENAL
FAILURE,
RENAL TUBULAR
ACIDOSIS,
HYPERPARATHYROIDISM,
FEBRILE ILLNESS

POLYPHAGIA

ASK THE FOLLOWING QUESTIONS:

1. **Is there associated polydipsia, polyuria, and weight loss?** The presence of these symptoms would suggest diabetes mellitus or hyperthyroidism.
2. **Is there associated weight gain?** This symptom would indicate that the patient has an insulinoma, Cushing's disease, or idiopathic obesity.
3. **Is there associated anxiety, depression, or other emotional problems?** These symptoms would signal that the polyphagia is related to bulimia, hysteria, or other psychic disorder.
4. **Is there associated diarrhea?** This would suggest that the disorder is related to a malabsorption syndrome, intestinal bypass, or GI fistula.

DIAGNOSTIC WORKUP

The basic workup of polyphagia should include a CBC, sedimentation rate, chemistry panel, thyroid profile, and stool for ovum and parasites.

If diabetes mellitus is suspected, a glucose tolerance test may be done. If Cushing's disease is suspected, a serum-free cortisol should be done. If an insulinoma is suspected, plasma insulin or C-peptide levels may be done, or the patient may be hospitalized for a 72-hr fast with frequent blood sugar determinations. If hyperthyroidism, diabetes mellitus, insulinoma, and intestinal disorders have been ruled out, a referral to a psychiatrist would be indicated.

POLYURIA

ASK THE FOLLOWING QUESTIONS:

1. **Is it transient?** Migraine, asthma, and drugs such as diuretics may produce transient polyuria.

2. **Is it massive?** Massive polyuria is usually due to pituitary or nephrogenic diabetes insipidus and psychogenic polydipsia. It may also be due to diabetes mellitus.

3. **Is there polyphagia and polydipsia?** The presence of polyphagia and polydipsia suggests the possibility of diabetes mellitus and hyperthyroidism.

4. **Is the polyuria mild?** The presence of a mild polyuria suggests chronic nephritis, renal tubular acidosis, hyperparathyroidism, Fanconi's syndrome, and mild diabetes mellitus.

5. **Is there glycosuria?** The presence of glycosuria suggests diabetes mellitus, hyperthyroidism, and Fanconi's syndrome.

DIAGNOSTIC WORKUP

Routine tests include a CBC, sedimentation rate, urinalysis, urine culture and colony count, chemistry panel, thyroid panel, and x-rays of the skull and long bones. The 24-hr intake and output should be measured. A serum and urine osmolality will be helpful, as would a spot urine sodium.

If pituitary diabetes insipidus is suspected, a CT scan of the brain and tests for pituitary hormones should be done. The intake and output before and after Pitressin® may be measured.

If renal disease is suspected, the urinary sediment should be examined microscopically and renal biopsy may be necessary. An endocrinologist and nephrologist should be consulted before undertaking expensive diagnostic tests.

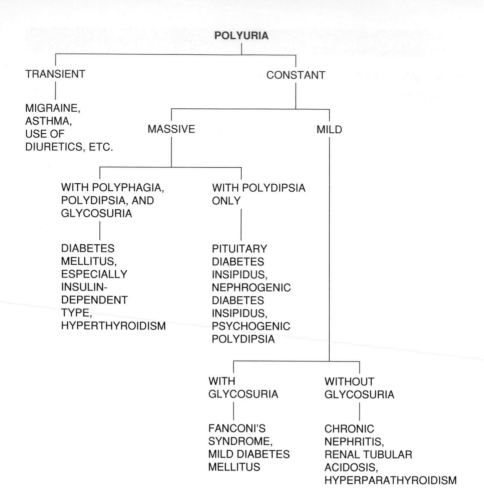

POLYURIA

TRANSIENT

MIGRAINE,
ASTHMA,
USE OF
DIURETICS, ETC.

CONSTANT

MASSIVE

MILD

WITH POLYPHAGIA,
POLYDIPSIA, AND
GLYCOSURIA

DIABETES
MELLITUS,
ESPECIALLY
INSULIN-
DEPENDENT
TYPE,
HYPERTHYROIDISM

WITH POLYDIPSIA
ONLY

PITUITARY
DIABETES
INSIPIDUS,
NEPHROGENIC
DIABETES
INSIPIDUS,
PSYCHOGENIC
POLYDIPSIA

WITH
GLYCOSURIA

FANCONI'S
SYNDROME,
MILD DIABETES
MELLITUS

WITHOUT
GLYCOSURIA

CHRONIC
NEPHRITIS,
RENAL TUBULAR
ACIDOSIS,
HYPERPARATHYROIDISM

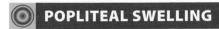

ASK THE FOLLOWING QUESTIONS:

1. **Is it soft or firm?** A soft popliteal swelling may be an abscess, varicose vein, Baker's cyst, popliteal aneurysm, or swollen bursa. A firm popliteal swelling may be an osteosarcoma, periostitis, giant cell tumor, exostoses, lymphadenitis, lipoma, or fibroma.
2. **If the mass is firm, is it connected to the bone?** Masses that are connected to the bone are more likely exostoses, osteosarcomas, periostitis, or giant cell tumors. They may also be a subperiosteal hematoma.
3. **Is there fever?** The presence of fever with a popliteal swelling would suggest an acute abscess.
4. **Is it reducible?** If the popliteal swelling is reducible, a varicose vein is most likely.
5. **Is there associated arthritis of the knee joint?** The presence of associated arthritis of the knee joint suggests a Baker's cyst.
6. **Is it pulsatile?** If the mass is pulsatile, a popliteal aneurysm should be suspected.

DIAGNOSTIC WORKUP

Routine tests include a CBC, sedimentation rate, and x-ray of the knee. If these are negative, MRI or a CT scan of the knee may be ordered, and aspiration of the mass may be undertaken if the mass is not pulsatile or there is no bruit over the mass. However, it is more cost-effective to seek an orthopedic consultation before ordering these tests or undertaking aspiration of the swelling. If the mass is pulsatile, ultrasonography or angiography may be performed. If osteomyelitis is suspected, a bone scan will be helpful.

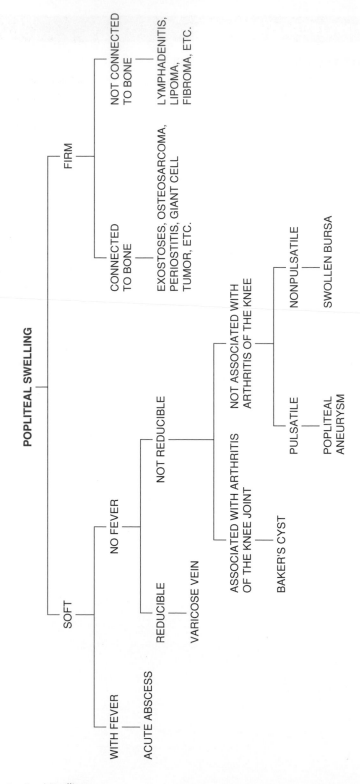

POPLITEAL SWELLING

SOFT

FIRM

WITH FEVER

ACUTE ABSCESS

NO FEVER

REDUCIBLE

VARICOSE VEIN

NOT REDUCIBLE

ASSOCIATED WITH ARTHRITIS
OF THE KNEE JOINT

BAKER'S CYST

NOT ASSOCIATED WITH
ARTHRITIS OF THE KNEE

PULSATILE

POPLITEAL
ANEURYSM

NONPULSATILE

SWOLLEN BURSA

CONNECTED
TO BONE

EXOSTOSES, OSTEOSARCOMA,
PERIOSTITIS, GIANT CELL
TUMOR, ETC.

NOT CONNECTED
TO BONE

LYMPHADENITIS,
LIPOMA,
FIBROMA, ETC.

ASK THE FOLLOWING QUESTIONS:

1. **Is there a history of anabolic steroid ingestion?** Children may take birth control pills early in life, and young boys may want to take anabolic steroids to increase their muscular mass.
2. **Is there headache, papilledema, or other neurologic signs?** These findings would suggest a brain tumor, and a pinealoma is one that should be excluded.
3. **Is there unilateral hyperpigmentation?** This finding suggests McCune–Albright syndrome.
4. **Is there a testicular mass?** The presence of a testicular mass would suggest Leydig cell tumor or hyperplasia.
5. **Is there an adnexal mass?** The presence of an adnexal mass would suggest a granulosa cell tumor or arrhenoblastoma.
6. **Is there an adrenal mass?** The presence of an adrenal mass would suggest adrenocortical hyperplasia or tumor.
7. **Is there masculinization?** This finding would suggest an arrhenoblastoma.
8. **Is there no mass detected on physical examination?** The absence of any mass would suggest constitutional precocious puberty.

DIAGNOSTIC WORKUP

Routine diagnostic studies include a CBC, sedimentation rate, urinalysis, chemistry panel, VDRL test, rapid ACTH test, serum testosterone, dihydrotestosterone, dehydroepiandrosterone, and a flat plate of the abdomen. If a brain tumor is suspected, a CT scan of the brain may be done. If an adrenal tumor is suspected, a CT scan of the abdomen and pelvis may be performed. Pelvic ultrasound or a CT scan of the pelvis may identify an ovarian tumor. Ultrasound may help evaluate a testicular mass. It is best to consult an endocrinologist, urologist, or gynecologist before ordering these expensive diagnostic tests.

PRECOCIOUS PUBERTY

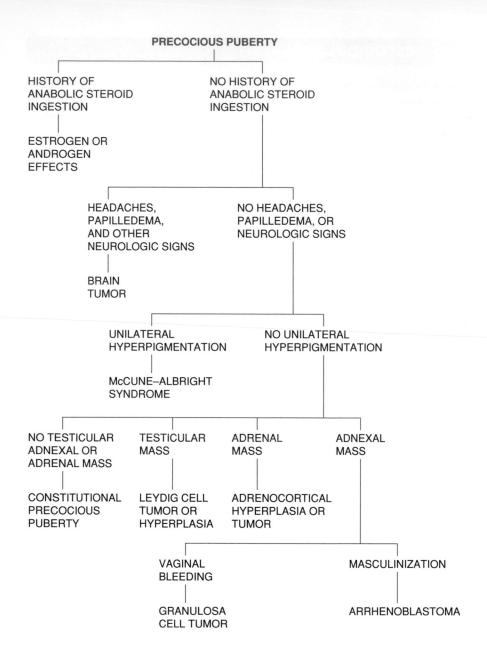

HISTORY OF ANABOLIC STEROID INGESTION

ESTROGEN OR ANDROGEN EFFECTS

NO HISTORY OF ANABOLIC STEROID INGESTION

HEADACHES, PAPILLEDEMA, AND OTHER NEUROLOGIC SIGNS

BRAIN TUMOR

NO HEADACHES, PAPILLEDEMA, OR NEUROLOGIC SIGNS

UNILATERAL HYPERPIGMENTATION

McCUNE–ALBRIGHT SYNDROME

NO UNILATERAL HYPERPIGMENTATION

NO TESTICULAR ADNEXAL OR ADRENAL MASS

CONSTITUTIONAL PRECOCIOUS PUBERTY

TESTICULAR MASS

LEYDIG CELL TUMOR OR HYPERPLASIA

ADRENAL MASS

ADRENOCORTICAL HYPERPLASIA OR TUMOR

ADNEXAL MASS

VAGINAL BLEEDING

GRANULOSA CELL TUMOR

MASCULINIZATION

ARRHENOBLASTOMA

PRECORDIAL THRILL

Because a thrill is essentially a murmur that is bold enough to be felt by the hand placed on the precordium, the differential diagnosis of this sign is the same as for murmurs (page 73). Conditions more often associated with a thrill are ventricular septal defect, pulmonic stenosis, and the combination of the two that is found with tetralogy of Fallot. The diagnostic workup is the same as for murmurs.

PREMENSTRUAL TENSION

This is the emotional tension, insomnia, depression, and irritability associated with the premenstrual week. Somatic sensations associated with this syndrome are similar to pregnancy and include bloating, cramping, tenderness of the breasts, swelling of the hands and feet, and temporary weight gain. The regular association of these symptoms with a certain period of the menstrual cycle makes the diagnosis almost a certainty.

ASK THE FOLLOWING QUESTIONS:

1. **Is there paraplegia or other neurologic signs?** Neurologic findings would suggest spinal cord trauma, tumor or inflammation, multiple sclerosis, and several other disorders.

2. **Is there splenomegaly or lymphadenopathy?** These findings would suggest leukemia and other blood dyscrasias.

3. **Is there African ancestry?** This finding would suggest sickle cell anemia.

4. **Are there abnormalities on urologic examination?** Urethral tumors, traumatic hematomas of the penis, thrombosis of the corpora cavernosa, and prostatism may cause priapism.

DIAGNOSTIC WORKUP

The basic workup includes a CBC, sedimentation rate, urinalysis, urine culture and colony count, sickle cell preparation, coagulation profile, chemistry panel, and serum protein electrophoresis. A urologist should also be consulted.

If there are neurologic signs, MRI of the brain or appropriate level of the spinal cord should probably be done. However, a neurologist should be consulted before ordering these expensive tests. A spinal tap will be helpful in diagnosing multiple sclerosis and central nervous system syphilis.

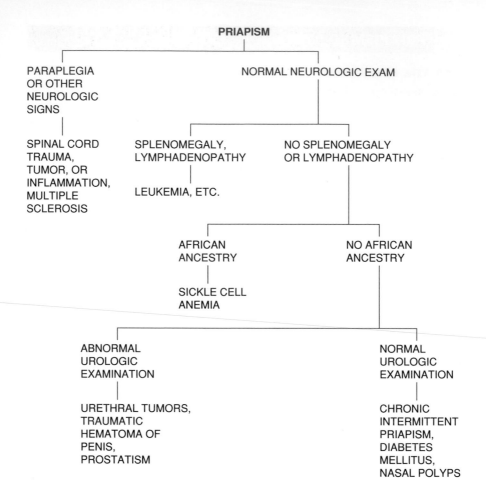

PRIAPISM

PARAPLEGIA OR OTHER NEUROLOGIC SIGNS

SPINAL CORD TRAUMA, TUMOR, OR INFLAMMATION, MULTIPLE SCLEROSIS

NORMAL NEUROLOGIC EXAM

SPLENOMEGALY, LYMPHADENOPATHY

LEUKEMIA, ETC.

NO SPLENOMEGALY OR LYMPHADENOPATHY

AFRICAN ANCESTRY

SICKLE CELL ANEMIA

NO AFRICAN ANCESTRY

ABNORMAL UROLOGIC EXAMINATION

URETHRAL TUMORS, TRAUMATIC HEMATOMA OF PENIS, PROSTATISM

NORMAL UROLOGIC EXAMINATION

CHRONIC INTERMITTENT PRIAPISM, DIABETES MELLITUS, NASAL POLYPS

ASK THE FOLLOWING QUESTIONS:

1. **Are there abnormal liver function tests?** Cirrhosis of the liver and obstructive jaundice are associated with a prolonged prothrombin time.
2. **Is the thrombin time prolonged?** A prolonged prothrombin and thrombin time should make one suspect disseminated intravascular coagulation (DIC), heparin therapy, or policythemia vera.
3. **What is the platelet count?** A decreased platelet count associated with a prolonged prothrombin time is found in acute leukemia and myelophthisic anemia and occasionally DIC.

DIAGNOSTIC WORKUP

Further workup of a patient who presents with a prolonged prothrombin time requires a CBC and platelet count to rule out acute leukemia and polycythemia vera, fibrin split product tests to pick up DIC and a bone marrow examination or liver biopsy.

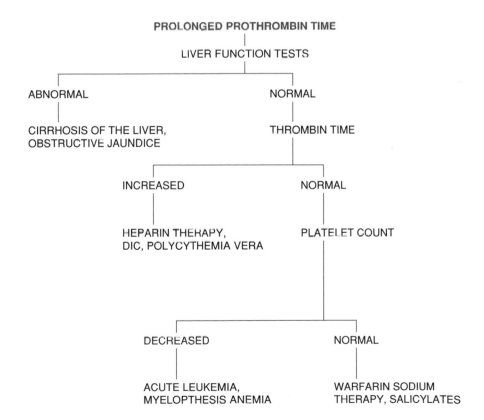

ASK THE FOLLOWING QUESTIONS:

1. **Are there significant numbers of white blood cells (WBCs) in the urine?** This would suggest a UTI. If there are white cell casts or clumps, the infection may be a pyelonephritis. A urine culture and colony count should be ordered. Sterile urine with persistent proteinuria and pyuria may be seen in toxic nephritis.

2. **Are there increased RBCs in the urine?** This would suggest glomerulonephritis, collagen disease, polycystic kidney, tuberculosis, renal calculus, trauma, or neoplasm. The presence of red cell casts would make glomerulonephritis or collagen disease more likely.

3. **Is glucose present in the urine?** This would point to diabetic nephritis or nephrosis.

4. If none of the above associated findings are present, one should look for hypertension, toxemia of pregnancy, fever, cardiac disease, poisoning, orthostatic proteinuria, multiple myeloma, or amyloidosis.

DIAGNOSTIC WORKUP

When faced with a report of protein in the urine, the first thing to do is look at the urine under the microscope. If there are significant numbers of bacteria and WBCs, one only has to order a urine culture and colony count and begin therapy. Recurrent UTIs warrant an IVP and a referral to a urologist, especially in males. If no infection is found, a more thorough workup is warranted, including CBC, chemistry panel, serum protein electrophoresis, ANA, sedimentation rate, urine for Bence Jones protein, Addis count, ASO titer, CRP, and CT scan of the abdomen. A urologist may need to be consulted for cystoscopy and retrograde pyelography. A nephrologist may need to be consulted for renal biopsy and further evaluation.

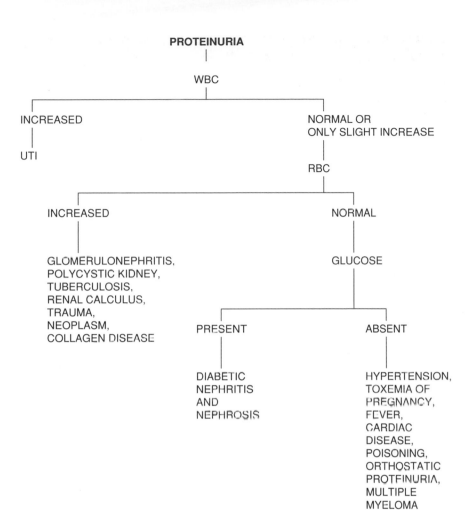

Itching at the anus is almost always due to anal or rectal conditions, the most likely of which is hemorrhoids. If there is frequent passage of bright red blood in the stool along with a painful bowel movement, one should look for an anal fissure. If there is a chronic discharge, one should look for an anal fissure or rectal prolapse. Pinworms must be sought in children. Finally, contact dermatitis and candidiasis are always possible. If candidiasis is the cause, a search for diabetes mellitus should be made.

DIAGNOSTIC WORKUP

If the physical examination is normal, examination with an anoscope is essential. Sigmoidoscopy should also be done but is not adequate to detect hemorrhoids, anal fissures, and fistulas. If these are negative, a trial of antifungal creams (Lotrimin®, etc.) should be given before other expensive diagnostic tests are ordered. A Scotch tape test and stool for ovum and parasites are useful, especially in children.

PRURITUS, GENERALIZED

ASK THE FOLLOWING QUESTIONS:

1. **Is the pruritus associated with a generalized rash?** Almost every generalized rash may be associated with pruritus, but the most common ones are urticaria, dermatitis herpetiformis, eczema, scabies, and pemphigus.
2. **Is there hepatomegaly or jaundice?** The presence of hepatomegaly or jaundice should make one think of obstructive jaundice, hepatitis, metastatic carcinoma to the liver, and biliary cirrhosis. However, almost any form of liver disease may be associated with pruritus.
3. **Is there polyuria, polydipsia, and polyphagia?** These findings would suggest diabetes mellitus, hyperthyroidism, and pregnancy. Pruritus during the first trimester is called pruritus gravidarum of unknown origin.
4. **Is there an unusual odor?** The presence of an unusual odor should bring to mind the possibility of uremia, liver failure, or diabetic acidosis.
5. **Is there plethoric facies?** The presence of plethoric facies suggests polycythemia vera.

DIAGNOSTIC WORKUP

If there is an associated skin rash, microscopic examination of a potassium hydroxide preparation of curetted burrows will be helpful. Additional examinations include Wood's lamp evaluation, a patch test, and skin biopsies. Therapeutic trials for scabies, fungal disease, or other disorders, however, are justified if testing is not economically feasible. Routine laboratory tests for the various systemic diseases that may cause pruritus include a CBC, sedimentation rate, urinalysis, chemistry panel, ANA assay, thyroid profile, and serum protein electrophoresis. Don't forget to order an anti-mitochondrial antibody titer to rule out primary biliary cirrhosis. A bone marrow examination and lymph node biopsy may be useful. A dermatologist, hematologist, or endocrinologist may help solve the diagnostic dilemma. Further workup may include plain films of the chest and abdomen and CT scans of the abdomen and pelvis. A bone scan may be useful in diagnosing metastatic carcinoma. HIV testing may be indicated if the patient has a history of high-risk sexual behavior.

PRURITUS, GENERALIZED

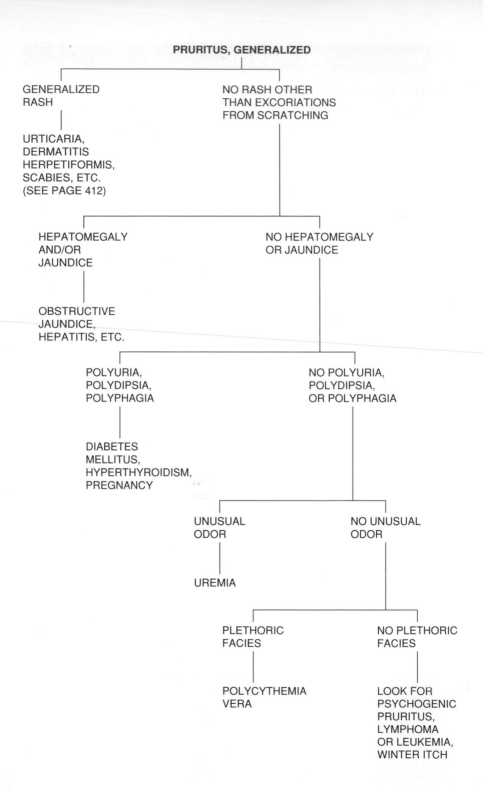

GENERALIZED
RASH

URTICARIA,
DERMATITIS
HERPETIFORMIS,
SCABIES, ETC.
(SEE PAGE 412)

NO RASH OTHER
THAN EXCORIATIONS
FROM SCRATCHING

HEPATOMEGALY
AND/OR
JAUNDICE

OBSTRUCTIVE
JAUNDICE,
HEPATITIS, ETC.

NO HEPATOMEGALY
OR JAUNDICE

POLYURIA,
POLYDIPSIA,
POLYPHAGIA

DIABETES
MELLITUS,
HYPERTHYROIDISM,
PREGNANCY

NO POLYURIA,
POLYDIPSIA,
OR POLYPHAGIA

UNUSUAL
ODOR

UREMIA

NO UNUSUAL
ODOR

PLETHORIC
FACIES

POLYCYTHEMIA
VERA

NO PLETHORIC
FACIES

LOOK FOR
PSYCHOGENIC
PRURITUS,
LYMPHOMA
OR LEUKEMIA,
WINTER ITCH

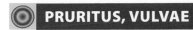

ASK THE FOLLOWING QUESTIONS:

1. **Is there a vaginal discharge?** The presence of a vaginal discharge should suggest candidiasis, trichomoniasis vaginitis, and bacterial vaginitis.
2. **Is there a rash?** The presence of a rash would suggest eczema, herpes simplex, folliculitis, scabies, and tinea infections.
3. **Are there vulval or vaginal lesions?** The presence of a lesion in the vulva or vagina would suggest kraurosis vulvae, leukoplakia or vulval carcinoma, condylomata lata, and condylomata acuminata.

DIAGNOSTIC WORKUP

If there is a discharge, microscopic examination of a potassium hydroxide preparation and saline preparation is necessary. A smear and culture of the discharge should be done for bacteria and fungi. Scrapings of the burrows for scabies may be useful. Skin biopsy may help diagnose the cause of a rash. Lesions should also be biopsied . If senile vaginitis is suspected, serum FSH and estradiol and a Pap smear may help determine if there is estrogen deficiency. A gynecologist should be consulted in all difficult diagnostic problems.

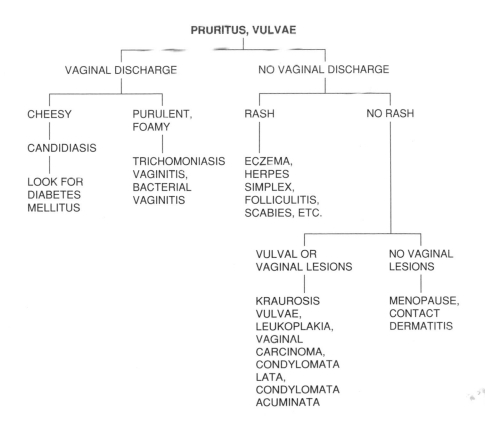

PTOSIS

ASK THE FOLLOWING QUESTIONS:

1. **Are there abnormalities on eye examination?** Pseudoptosis occurs when there is inflammation of the eyelid, cornea, or other ocular structures. Periorbital edema, conjunctivitis, and trachoma are among the many disorders to consider.
2. **Is it intermittent?** Intermittent ptosis would suggest myasthenia gravis, ophthalmoplegic migraine, and transient ischemic attacks.
3. **Is it partial?** The presence of partial ptosis would suggest Horner's syndrome, especially if there is a constricted pupil. However, myotonic dystrophy, myasthenia gravis, and progressive muscular atrophy are just three of the disorders that may present with partial ptosis.
4. **Is there a dilated pupil?** The presence of a dilated pupil, especially with a unilateral ptosis, suggests a ruptured cerebral aneurysm. However, if the dilated pupil is associated with many other neurologic signs, then there are many other conditions to consider.
5. **Is there a constricted pupil?** The presence of a constricted pupil with unilateral complete ptosis would suggest diabetic neuropathy. However, if there is bilateral complete ptosis, chronic progressive external ophthalmoplegia and myasthenia gravis should be considered.
6. **Are there other cranial nerves involved?** The presence of other cranial nerve signs should suggest cavernous sinus thrombosis, cerebral aneurysm, tuberculous meningitis, syphilitic meningitis, Wernicke's encephalopathy, diphtheria, and subdural hematoma.
7. **Are there hyperactive reflexes?** The presence of hyperactive reflexes would suggest syringomyelia, platybasia, brain stem tumors, vertebral basilar occlusion or insufficiency, multiple sclerosis, epidemic encephalitis, and general paresis.
8. **Are there hypoactive reflexes?** The presence of hypoactive reflexes would suggest myotonic dystrophy, tabes dorsalis, and progressive muscular atrophy.

DIAGNOSTIC WORKUP

If there are local conditions responsible for the ptosis, then a smear and culture of the exudate and slit lamp examination or tonometry can be done, or the patient should be referred to an ophthalmologist. If a neurologic disease is suspected, a neurologist should be consulted, especially if the onset is acute.

Routine diagnostic tests include a CBC, sedimentation rate, urinalysis, chemistry panel, glucose tolerance test, ANA, VDRL test, and x-rays of the skull and sinuses. A CT scan or MRI of the brain must be done in most cases. If myasthenia gravis is suspected, a Tensilon test and acetylcholine receptor antibody titer can be done.

If encephalitis, meningitis, central nervous system lues, or multiple sclerosis are suspected, a spinal tap may be useful. Intravenous thiamine is administered in Wernicke's encephalopathy. If Horner's syndrome is suspected, the workup may be found on page 237. If muscular dystrophy is suspected, a 24-hr urine collection for creatinine and creatine and a muscle biopsy may be done. Cerebral angiography will be necessary to diagnose most cerebral aneurysms and cerebral vascular disease, including transient ischemic attacks.

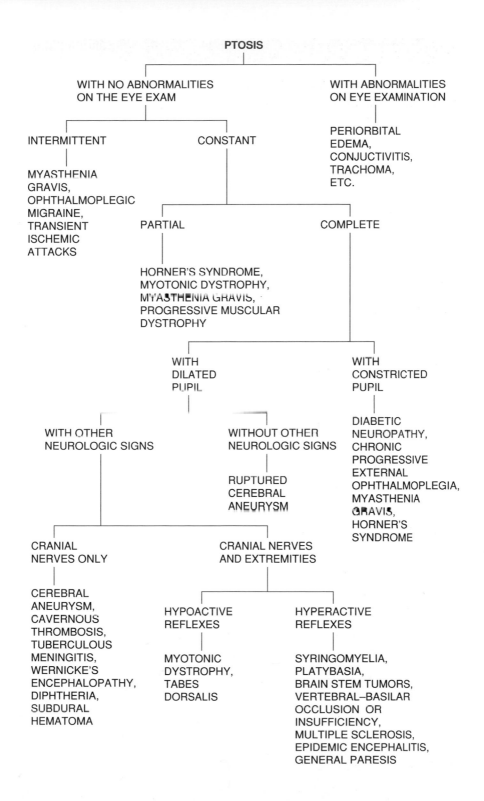

PTOSIS

WITH NO ABNORMALITIES ON THE EYE EXAM

WITH ABNORMALITIES ON EYE EXAMINATION

INTERMITTENT

CONSTANT

PERIORBITAL EDEMA, CONJUCTIVITIS, TRACHOMA, ETC.

MYASTHENIA GRAVIS, OPHTHALMOPLEGIC MIGRAINE, TRANSIENT ISCHEMIC ATTACKS

PARTIAL

COMPLETE

HORNER'S SYNDROME, MYOTONIC DYSTROPHY, MYASTHENIA GRAVIS, PROGRESSIVE MUSCULAR DYSTROPHY

WITH DILATED PUPIL

WITH CONSTRICTED PUPIL

WITH OTHER NEUROLOGIC SIGNS

WITHOUT OTHER NEUROLOGIC SIGNS

DIABETIC NEUROPATHY, CHRONIC PROGRESSIVE EXTERNAL OPHTHALMOPLEGIA, MYASTHENIA GRAVIS, HORNER'S SYNDROME

RUPTURED CEREBRAL ANEURYSM

CRANIAL NERVES ONLY

CRANIAL NERVES AND EXTREMITIES

CEREBRAL ANEURYSM, CAVERNOUS THROMBOSIS, TUBERCULOUS MENINGITIS, WERNICKE'S ENCEPHALOPATHY, DIPHTHERIA, SUBDURAL HEMATOMA

HYPOACTIVE REFLEXES

HYPERACTIVE REFLEXES

MYOTONIC DYSTROPHY, TABES DORSALIS

SYRINGOMYELIA, PLATYBASIA, BRAIN STEM TUMORS, VERTEBRAL–BASILAR OCCLUSION OR INSUFFICIENCY, MULTIPLE SCLEROSIS, EPIDEMIC ENCEPHALITIS, GENERAL PARESIS

⊚ PTYALISM

ASK THE FOLLOWING QUESTIONS:

1. **Is there a history of drug ingestion?** Mercury, iodides, and mouthwash are some of the substances that may cause ptyalism.
2. **Is the oral examination abnormal?** Peritonsillar abscess, carious tooth, ulcerating tumor, herpes simplex, aphthous stomatitis, and ill-fitting dental plates are all conditions that may cause ptyalism. In addition, fracture and dislocation of the jaw may cause ptyalism.
3. **Is it intermittent?** The presence of intermittent ptyalism should suggest myasthenia gravis.
4. **Are there abnormalities on the neurologic examination?** The presence of abnormalities on the neurologic examination should suggest pseudobulbar palsy, bulbar palsy, parkinsonism, dementia, idiocy, rabies, and facial palsies.
5. **Is there atrophy of the tongue?** Atrophy of the tongue will differentiate bulbar palsy from pseudobulbar palsy.

DIAGNOSTIC WORKUP

If there are abnormalities on the examination of the mouth, a referral to a dentist or oral surgeon should be considered. However, many of these conditions can be treated by the family physician. If there are neurologic abnormalities, a referral to a neurologist should be considered before ordering a CT scan or MRI of the brain and other expensive diagnostic tests. In addition to imaging studies, the basic workup of ptyalism might include a spinal tap, nerve conduction velocity studies, EMG, Tensilon tests, and evoked potential studies. A neurologist is in a better position to determine which of these studies is appropriate in any given case.

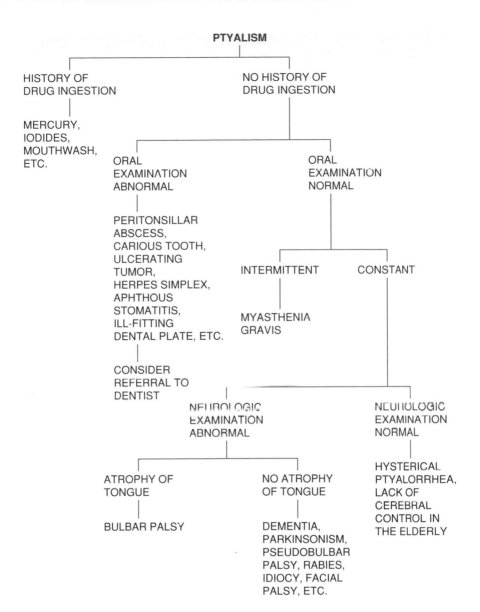

PTYALISM

HISTORY OF
DRUG INGESTION

MERCURY,
IODIDES,
MOUTHWASH,
ETC.

NO HISTORY OF
DRUG INGESTION

ORAL
EXAMINATION
ABNORMAL

PERITONSILLAR
ABSCESS,
CARIOUS TOOTH,
ULCERATING
TUMOR,
HERPES SIMPLEX,
APHTHOUS
STOMATITIS,
ILL-FITTING
DENTAL PLATE, ETC.

CONSIDER
REFERRAL TO
DENTIST

ORAL
EXAMINATION
NORMAL

INTERMITTENT

MYASTHENIA
GRAVIS

CONSTANT

NEUROLOGIC
EXAMINATION
ABNORMAL

ATROPHY OF
TONGUE

BULBAR PALSY

NO ATROPHY
OF TONGUE

DEMENTIA,
PARKINSONISM,
PSEUDOBULBAR
PALSY, RABIES,
IDIOCY, FACIAL
PALSY, ETC.

NEUROLOGIC
EXAMINATION
NORMAL

HYSTERICAL
PTYALORRHEA,
LACK OF
CEREBRAL
CONTROL IN
THE ELDERLY

A pulsatile swelling anywhere is an aneurysm until proven otherwise. However, frequently, there is simply a benign or malignant tumor over a large artery that gives the false impression that the mass is an aneurysm when it is not. In the abdomen, a normal abdominal aorta may be mistaken for an aortic aneurysm, especially in thin patients. In the neck, normal carotid, brachial, or innominate arteries may pulsate vigorously when there is aortic regurgitation. Eggshell cracking along with the pulsation in a mass should suggest an osteosarcoma. A pulsating mass in the right upper quadrant is most likely the enlarged liver due to tricuspid regurgitation or stenosis. The presence of dependent edema and ascites will support the diagnosis. A pulsating tumor of the orbit is most likely a carotid cavernous fistula.

DIAGNOSTIC WORKUP

In cases of suspected abdominal aortic aneurysms, abdominal ultrasound will help differentiate the normal aorta or a tumor from a true aneurysm. When in doubt, CT scan or aortography should be done. It will be necessary before surgery anyway.

All other cases of pulsatile masses suggesting an aneurysm should receive angiography of the artery or arteries supplying the area.

PULSE IRREGULARITY

ASK THE FOLLOWING QUESTIONS:

1. **Is the rate normal, rapid, or slow?** A rapid rate would suggest supraventricular tachycardia, ventricular tachycardia, atrial flutter, and fibrillation. A slow rate would suggest atrioventricular (AV) nodal rhythm, third-degree AV block, sinoatrial block, Wenckebach phenomena, and sick sinus syndrome. A normal rate would suggest atrial and ventricular premature contractions, AV dissociation, bigeminal rhythm, and controlled flutter or fibrillation.
2. **If the rate is rapid, is it regular or irregular?** A rapid regular rate would suggest supraventricular tachycardia or ventricular tachycardia, whereas a rapid irregular rate would suggest atrial flutter or fibrillation.
3. **If the rate is slow, is it regular or irregular?** A slow regular rhythm would suggest AV nodal rhythm, third-degree AV block, or sinoatrial block. A slow irregular rhythm would suggest Wenckebach phenomena or sick sinus syndrome.

DIAGNOSTIC WORKUP

Some physicians will want to refer the patient with a pulse irregularity to a cardiologist at the outset. Other clinicians would rather investigate the patient further.

Routine tests ordered include CBC, sedimentation rate, urinalysis, chemistry panel, serial cardiac enzymes, thyroid profile, ANA test, EKG, and chest x-ray with lateral and anterior oblique views. If there is fever, an ASO titer or streptozyme test should be done to rule out rheumatic fever, and blood cultures should be done to rule out bacterial endocarditis. If the EKG is normal and the symptoms are intermittent, 24-hr Holter monitoring should be done. The patient also can be hospitalized for a few days for telemetry. Newer technology includes using a continuous-loop event recorder to allow monitoring for 2 weeks at a time. Echocardiography will disclose valvular diseases and myocardiopathies. His' bundle studies may be necessary in some cases. Also, angiography and catheterization studies should be considered in difficult cases. Before expensive tests are ordered, it is wise to consult a cardiologist.

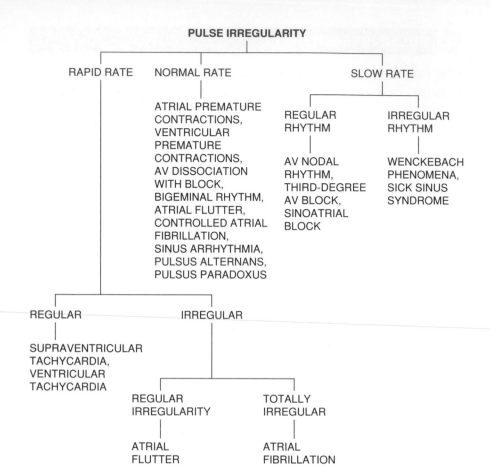

PULSE IRREGULARITY

RAPID RATE

NORMAL RATE

ATRIAL PREMATURE CONTRACTIONS, VENTRICULAR PREMATURE CONTRACTIONS, AV DISSOCIATION WITH BLOCK, BIGEMINAL RHYTHM, ATRIAL FLUTTER, CONTROLLED ATRIAL FIBRILLATION, SINUS ARRHYTHMIA, PULSUS ALTERNANS, PULSUS PARADOXUS

SLOW RATE

REGULAR RHYTHM

AV NODAL RHYTHM, THIRD-DEGREE AV BLOCK, SINOATRIAL BLOCK

IRREGULAR RHYTHM

WENCKEBACH PHENOMENA, SICK SINUS SYNDROME

REGULAR

SUPRAVENTRICULAR TACHYCARDIA, VENTRICULAR TACHYCARDIA

IRREGULAR

REGULAR IRREGULARITY

ATRIAL FLUTTER

TOTALLY IRREGULAR

ATRIAL FIBRILLATION

ASK THE FOLLOWING QUESTIONS:

1. **Is it acute?** Acute reduction of the pulse of an extremity may be due to an arterial embolism, dissecting aneurysm, or fracture of the limb.
2. **Does it involve the upper extremities only?** The upper extremities are involved selectively in the subclavian steal syndrome, Takayasu's disease, a few cases of coarctation of the aorta, congenital anomalies, thoracic outlet syndrome, aneurysm of the arch of the aorta, and supravalvular aortic stenosis.
3. **Is there a history of transient ischemic attacks?** The presence of transient ischemic attacks should suggest subclavian steal syndrome and Takayasu's disease.
4. **Is there hypertension?** The presence of hypertension should suggest coarctation of the aorta.
5. **Does it involve the lower extremities only?** Involvement of the lower extremities only would suggest peripheral arteriosclerosis, Buerger's disease, arteriovenous fistula, and Leriche's syndrome.
6. **Are both the proximal and distal pulses in the lower extremities diminished?** These findings would suggest a Leriche's syndrome.
7. **Does it involve the upper and lower extremities?** Involvement of both the upper and lower extremities would suggest coarctation of the aorta and dissecting aneurysm.

DIAGNOSTIC WORKUP

If the onset is acute, angiography must be done without delay. With a history of trauma, plain films of the involved extremity are essential to rule out fracture. If the onset is gradual, then Doppler studies may be done before angiography. However, angiography will ultimately be necessary in most cases. It is wise to consult a cardiovascular surgeon at the outset. If an arterial embolism is suspected, the source for the embolism must be sought. Serial EKGs and serial cardiac enzymes may disclose an acute myocardial infarction with a mural thrombus. An EKG may disclose auricular fibrillation. Blood cultures may disclose subacute bacterial endocarditis.

PULSES, UNEQUAL

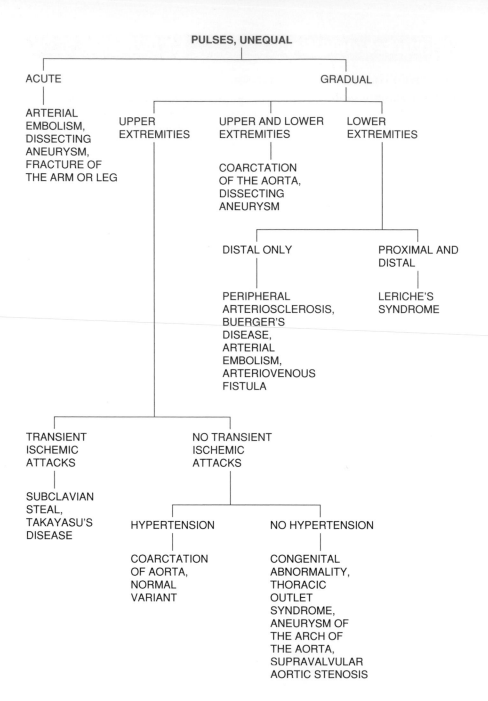

ACUTE

ARTERIAL
EMBOLISM,
DISSECTING
ANEURYSM,
FRACTURE OF
THE ARM OR LEG

GRADUAL

**UPPER
EXTREMITIES**

**UPPER AND LOWER
EXTREMITIES**

COARCTATION
OF THE AORTA,
DISSECTING
ANEURYSM

**LOWER
EXTREMITIES**

DISTAL ONLY

PERIPHERAL
ARTERIOSCLEROSIS,
BUERGER'S
DISEASE,
ARTERIAL
EMBOLISM,
ARTERIOVENOUS
FISTULA

**PROXIMAL AND
DISTAL**

LERICHE'S
SYNDROME

**TRANSIENT
ISCHEMIC
ATTACKS**

SUBCLAVIAN
STEAL,
TAKAYASU'S
DISEASE

**NO TRANSIENT
ISCHEMIC
ATTACKS**

HYPERTENSION

COARCTATION
OF AORTA,
NORMAL
VARIANT

NO HYPERTENSION

CONGENITAL
ABNORMALITY,
THORACIC
OUTLET
SYNDROME,
ANEURYSM OF
THE ARCH OF
THE AORTA,
SUPRAVALVULAR
AORTIC STENOSIS

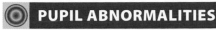

ASK THE FOLLOWING QUESTIONS:

1. **Are both pupils dilated?** The presence of dilated pupils in an otherwise normal subject would suggest drug intoxication such as phenobarbital, marijuana, and PCP. However, the patient may not know that he or she had a concussion recently. Also, glaucoma may cause dilatation of both pupils.

2. **Are both pupils constricted?** The presence of constricted pupils would suggest narcotic intoxication. It should also suggest organophosphate intoxication.

3. **Is one pupil dilated?** The presence of a dilated pupil should suggest oculomotor nerve palsy such as may be due to a ruptured aneurysm or intracranial hematoma. However, if the pupil reacts to light and accommodation, a local condition such as iritis, glaucoma, anisocoria, or irritation of the cervical sympathetic nerves must be considered. If the pupil reacts to accommodation but not to light, then central nervous system syphilis must be suspected. If there is no reaction to light or accommodation, blindness must be considered due to optic nerve lesions.

4. **If one pupil is dilated, does it react to light and accommodation?** This finding would suggest a local condition such as iritis, glaucoma, anisocoria, or irritation of the cervical sympathetic nerves.

5. **Is one pupil constricted?** The presence of a constricted pupil would suggest Horner's syndrome.

6. **Is there ptosis?** The presence of ptosis with a constricted pupil would suggest Horner's syndrome. If there is no ptosis with the constricted pupil, a brain stem lesion such as syringomyelia, tumor, abscess, or encephalitis must be considered.

7. **Is there blindness?** The presence of blindness with a dilated pupil would suggest optic nerve lesions.

DIAGNOSTIC WORKUP

Patients with bilateral dilated or constricted pupils should have a urine drug screen and possibly a blood test for alcohol level. If there is fever or a history of trauma with dilated or constricted pupils or other pupillary abnormalities, a neurologist or neurosurgeon should be consulted immediately before ordering expensive diagnostic tests.

Primary eye conditions can be excluded by tonometry, slit lamp examination, or ophthalmology consultation. Intracranial neoplasms and aneurysms must be excluded by CT scans, MRIs, and possibly angiography. A spinal tap will help diagnose central nervous system lues or multiple sclerosis. VEP studies will help diagnose multiple sclerosis. The workup for Horner's syndrome can be found on page 237.

PUPIL ABNORMALITIES

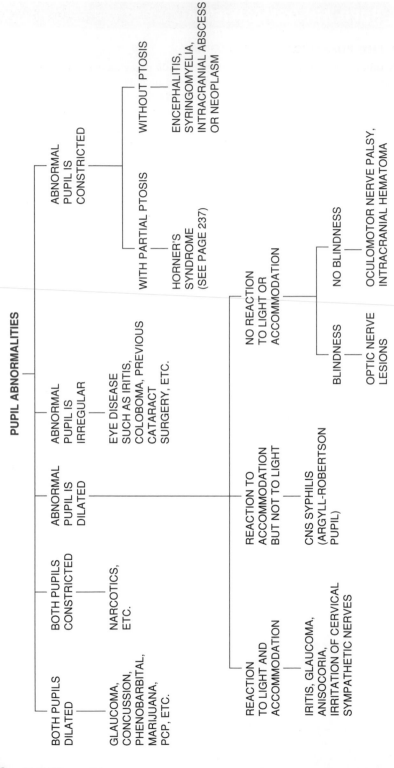

BOTH PUPILS DILATED
— GLAUCOMA, CONCUSSION, PHENOBARBITAL, MARIJUANA, PCP, ETC.

BOTH PUPILS CONSTRICTED
— NARCOTICS, ETC.

ABNORMAL PUPIL IS DILATED
— REACTION TO LIGHT AND ACCOMMODATION
  — IRITIS, GLAUCOMA, ANISOCORIA, IRRITATION OF CERVICAL SYMPATHETIC NERVES
— REACTION TO ACCOMMODATION BUT NOT TO LIGHT
  — CNS SYPHILIS (ARGYLL-ROBERTSON PUPIL)
— NO REACTION TO LIGHT OR ACCOMMODATION
  — BLINDNESS
    — OPTIC NERVE LESIONS
  — NO BLINDNESS
    — OCULOMOTOR NERVE PALSY, INTRACRANIAL HEMATOMA

ABNORMAL PUPIL IS IRREGULAR
— EYE DISEASE SUCH AS IRITIS, COLOBOMA, PREVIOUS CATARACT SURGERY, ETC.

ABNORMAL PUPIL IS CONSTRICTED
— WITH PARTIAL PTOSIS
  — HORNER'S SYNDROME (SEE PAGE 237)
— WITHOUT PTOSIS
  — ENCEPHALITIS, SYRINGOMYELIA, INTRACRANIAL ABSCESS OR NEOPLASM

PURPURA AND ABNORMAL BLEEDING

ASK THE FOLLOWING QUESTIONS:

1. **Is there a petechial rash?** The presence of a petechial rash suggests either a thrombocytopenic purpura, which may be idiopathic or secondary to leukemia, aplastic anemia, collagen disease, or drugs. In addition, petechiae may suggest platelet dysfunction, in which case the platelet count will be normal, or vasculitis, such as from collagen diseases, hereditary telangiectasia, scurvy, or drugs.
2. **Is there ecchymosis or bruises?** The presence of ecchymosis or bruises would suggest hemophilia, Christmas disease, or other major coagulation defects, but it may also be related to platelet disorders or DIC.
3. **If there is a petechial rash, is the platelet count normal?** The presence of a normal platelet count would suggest either thrombocytopathy or vasculitis.
4. **Is there significant mucosal bleeding?** The presence of mucosal bleeding along with ecchymosis and bruises suggests platelet disorders or DIC.

DIAGNOSTIC WORKUP

If a coagulation disorder is suspected, consult a hematologist first. Routine diagnostic studies include a CBC, platelet count, sedimentation rate, blood smear for red cell morphology, urinalysis, chemistry panel, coagulation profile, rheumatoid arthritis factor, ANA test, serum protein electrophoresis, VDRL test, EKG, chest x-ray, and flat plate of the abdomen. The coagulation profile should include a platelet count, a bleeding time, a coagulation time, a partial thromboplastin time, and a prothrombin time.

If there is fever, blood cultures should be done. A bone marrow examination and bone marrow culture may be useful. If DIC is suspected, a fibrinogen assay and estimation of fibrin degradation products should be done. Platelet function may be assessed by clot retraction tests. Spleen and liver scans and bone scans may be needed. A CT scan of the abdomen and pelvis may also be necessary. Skin, muscle, and even kidney biopsies are often done to complete the workup.

It can be seen from the above array of diagnostic tests that a hematologist should be consulted at the outset. Various forms of vasculitis may be confirmed by skin or muscle biopsy.

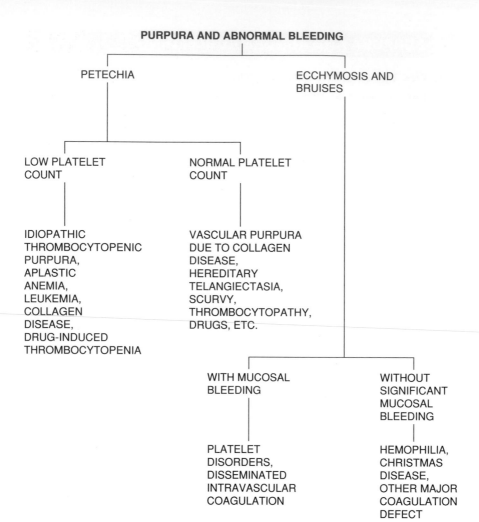

PURPURA AND ABNORMAL BLEEDING

PETECHIA

ECCHYMOSIS AND BRUISES

LOW PLATELET COUNT

NORMAL PLATELET COUNT

IDIOPATHIC THROMBOCYTOPENIC PURPURA, APLASTIC ANEMIA, LEUKEMIA, COLLAGEN DISEASE, DRUG-INDUCED THROMBOCYTOPENIA

VASCULAR PURPURA DUE TO COLLAGEN DISEASE, HEREDITARY TELANGIECTASIA, SCURVY, THROMBOCYTOPATHY, DRUGS, ETC.

WITH MUCOSAL BLEEDING

WITHOUT SIGNIFICANT MUCOSAL BLEEDING

PLATELET DISORDERS, DISSEMINATED INTRAVASCULAR COAGULATION

HEMOPHILIA, CHRISTMAS DISEASE, OTHER MAJOR COAGULATION DEFECT

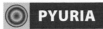

ASK THE FOLLOWING QUESTIONS:

1. **Are there significant RBCs in the urine?** If so, one should consider glomerulonephritis, collagen disease, tuberculosis, neoplasm, trauma, renal calculus, and polycystic kidney disease. If not, the most likely etiology is a UTI.
2. **Are there WBC casts in the urine?** This would make pyelonephritis or interstitial nephritis more likely.
3. **Are there RBC casts in the urine?** This would help differentiate glomerulonephritis and collagen diseases from the other conditions associated with hematuria.

DIAGNOSTIC WORKUP

First, look at the urinary sediment under a microscope. Further workup should include a urine culture and colony count, AFB smear and culture, CBC, sedimentation rate, ANA test, chemistry panel, serum protein electrophoresis, IVP, and a urology consultation. A urologist may do cystoscopy and retrograde pyelography. He may order a CT scan of the abdomen to rule out renal carcinomas and other kidney diseases. A nephrologist may need to be consulted in difficult cases. A urologist should be consulted in all cases of recurrent or persistent pyuria.

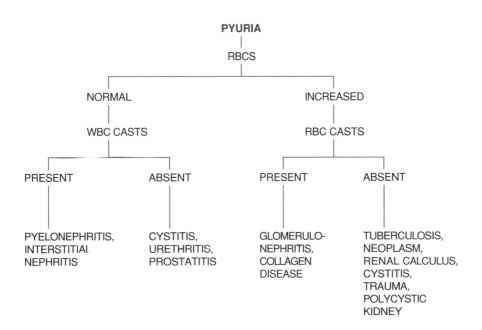

ASK THE FOLLOWING QUESTIONS:

1. **Are they crepitant, sibilant, or sonorous?** Crepitant rales signify congestive heart failure, pneumonia, tuberculosis, pulmonary embolism, adult respiratory distress syndrome, and aspiration pneumonitis. Carcinoma of the lung may also present with crepitant rales. Sibilant or sonorous rales, on the other hand, signify bronchiectasis, asthma, emphysema, pneumoconiosis, and foreign body. Carcinoma of the lung is more likely to be associated with sibilant and sonorous rales than crepitant rales.

2. **Are they focal or diffuse?** Focal crepitant rales may signify pulmonary embolism, lobar pneumonia, or tuberculosis, whereas diffuse crepitant rales are more likely to be associated with congestive heart failure, adult respiratory distress syndrome, and aspiration pneumonitis. Focal sibilant and sonorous rales are more likely to be associated with foreign bodies, bronchiectasis, and carcinoma of the lung, whereas diffuse sibilant and sonorous rales are more likely to be associated with asthma, emphysema, or pneumoconiosis.

3. **Is there associated chest pain?** The presence of crepitant rales with chest pain suggests pulmonary embolism, but it may also be associated with congestive heart failure secondary to an acute myocardial infarction.

4. **Is there cardiomegaly?** The presence of cardiomegaly suggests congestive heart failure or pericardial effusion.

DIAGNOSTIC WORKUP

Routine diagnostic studies include a CBC, sedimentation rate, urinalysis, chemistry panel, ANA titer, VDRL test, chest x-ray, EKG, and pulmonary function test. If sputum can be obtained, a smear and culture of the sputum should be done. Sputum for eosinophils may also be necessary if asthma is suspected.

If congestive heart failure is suspected, a venous pressure and circulation time or BNP should be done. Echocardiography may be done to determine the LVEF. If pulmonary embolism is suspected, a ventilation–perfusion scan and possibly pulmonary angiography may be necessary. Arterial blood gases are also helpful. If tuberculosis is suspected, the appropriate skin tests and AFB culture and guinea pig inoculation may be required. Skin tests and cultures for the various fungi may be useful. Bronchoscopy and biopsy will be helpful in diagnosing carcinoma of the lung. A consultation with a pulmonologist, if not already done, is certainly necessary at this point.

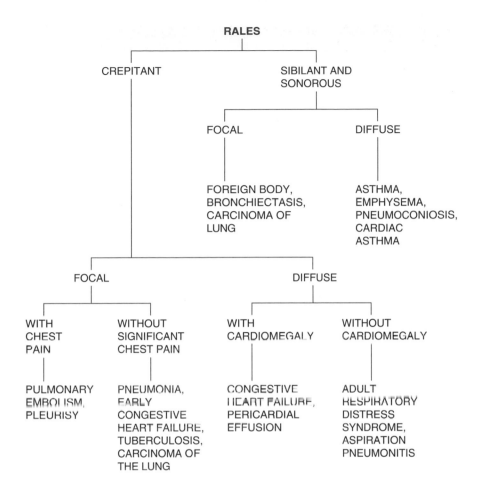

RALES

CREPITANT

SIBILANT AND SONOROUS

FOCAL

FOREIGN BODY, BRONCHIECTASIS, CARCINOMA OF LUNG

DIFFUSE

ASTHMA, EMPHYSEMA, PNEUMOCONIOSIS, CARDIAC ASTHMA

FOCAL

WITH CHEST PAIN

PULMONARY EMBOLISM, PLEURISY

WITHOUT SIGNIFICANT CHEST PAIN

PNEUMONIA, EARLY CONGESTIVE HEART FAILURE, TUBERCULOSIS, CARCINOMA OF THE LUNG

DIFFUSE

WITH CARDIOMEGALY

CONGESTIVE HEART FAILURE, PERICARDIAL EFFUSION

WITHOUT CARDIOMEGALY

ADULT RESPIRATORY DISTRESS SYNDROME, ASPIRATION PNEUMONITIS

ASK THE FOLLOWING QUESTIONS:

1. **Is it focal or diffuse?** Focal rashes suggest dermatophytoses, scabies, actinic dermatitis, herpes zoster, warts, contact dermatitis, erythema nodosum, actinic dermatosis, dyshidrosis, skin tumors, nummular eczema, stasis dermatitis, pyoderma, acne vulgaris, herpes simplex, impetigo, and tuberous sclerosis. Diffuse rashes suggest xanthoma, erythema multiforme, psoriasis, lichen planus, eczema, drug eruptions, dermatitis herpetiformis, secondary syphilis, exfoliative dermatitis, and pemphigus. A diffuse rash also may be due to pityriasis rosea and tinea versicolor.

2. **If diffuse, is it primarily the extremities that are involved?** A diffuse rash that involves primarily the extremities would suggest smallpox and erythema multiforme, eczema, milium, lichen planus, and psoriasis.

3. **If diffuse, does it involve primarily the face and trunk?** A diffuse rash that involves primarily the face and trunk suggests chickenpox, typhoid fever, German measles, pityriasis rosea, tinea versicolor, and pemphigus.

4. **If focal, does it primarily involve the extremities?** A focal rash that involves primarily the extremities suggests dermatophytosis, erythema nodosum, contact dermatitis, warts, discoid lupus, actinic dermatosis, scabies, dyshidrosis, skin tumors, nummular eczema, stasis dermatitis, and pyoderma.

5. **If focal, is it primarily involving the face and head?** A rash that involves primarily the face and head should suggest acne vulgaris, acne rosacea, seborrheic dermatitis, herpes simplex, actinic dermatosis, carcinoma, impetigo, contact dermatitis, Sturge–Weber syndrome, tuberous sclerosis, and tinea capitis.

6. **Is it equally distributed to the trunk and extremities?** A rash that is equally distributed to the trunk and extremities would suggest herpes zoster, neurofibromatosis, scarlet fever, drug eruptions, dermatitis herpetiformis, secondary syphilis, measles, and exfoliative dermatitis.

DIAGNOSTIC WORKUP

Before launching an expensive diagnostic workup, look for systemic symptoms and signs. For example, a rash with bloody diarrhea suggests ulcerative colitis or Crohn's disease. A rash with joint pain would suggest lupus erythematosus or gonorrhea. If there are any exudates, a smear and culture for fungi and routine bacteria should be done. Skin scrapings may be examined microscopically with a saline or potassium hydroxide preparation to rule out scabies and fungi. A Wood's lamp examination is very useful in diagnosing various fungi. All isolated lesions should be biopsied.

Diffuse rashes require routine CBC, sedimentation rate, urinalysis, chemistry panel, ANA test, and VDRL test. If there is fever, blood cultures should probably be done. Skin biopsies in consultation with a dermatologist should be done in a timely fashion. Patch testing and intradermal skin testing should be done when appropriate. A dark field examination may be necessary. GI series, CT scan of the abdomen and barium enemas may be necessary to look for GI neoplasms, Crohn's disease, and ulcerative colitis.

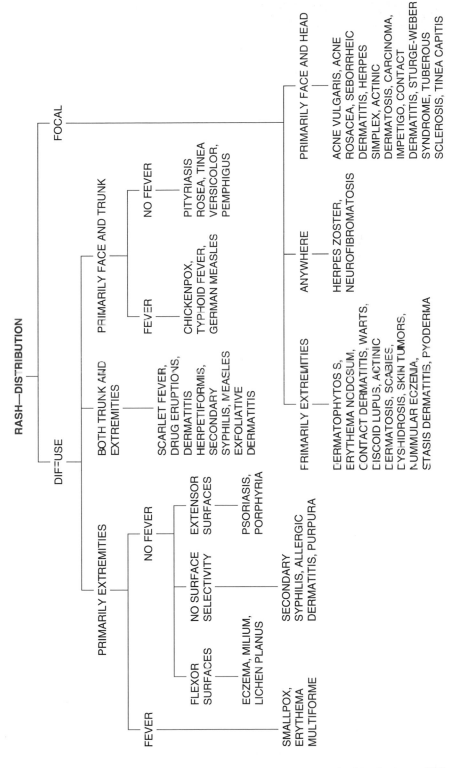

RASH—DISTRIBUTION

DIFFUSE

- PRIMARILY EXTREMITIES
  - FEVER
    - SMALLPOX, ERYTHEMA MULTIFORME
  - NO FEVER
    - FLEXOR SURFACES
      - ECZEMA, MILIUM, LICHEN PLANUS
    - NO SURFACE SELECTIVITY
      - SECONDARY SYPHILIS, ALLERGIC DERMATITIS, PURPURA
    - EXTENSOR SURFACES
      - PSORIASIS, PORPHYRIA
- BOTH TRUNK AND EXTREMITIES
  - SCARLET FEVER, DRUG ERUPTIONS, DERMATITIS HERPETIFORMIS, SECONDARY SYPHILIS, MEASLES EXFOLIATIVE DERMATITIS
- PRIMARILY FACE AND TRUNK
  - FEVER
    - CHICKENPOX, TYPHOID FEVER, GERMAN MEASLES
  - NO FEVER
    - PITYRIASIS ROSEA, TINEA VERSICOLOR, PEMPHIGUS

FOCAL

- PRIMARILY EXTREMITIES
  - DERMATOPHYTOS S, ERYTHEMA NCDCSUM, CONTACT DERMATITIS, WARTS, DISCOID LUPUS, ACTINIC DERMATOSIS, SCABIES, DYSHIDROSIS, SKIN TUMORS, NUMMULAR ECZEMA, STASIS DERMATITIS, PYODERMA
- ANYWHERE
  - HERPES ZOSTER, NEUROFIBROMATOSIS
- PRIMARILY FACE AND HEAD
  - ACNE VULGARIS, ACNE ROSACEA, SEBORRHEIC DERMATITIS, HERPES SIMPLEX, ACTINIC DERMATOSIS, CARCINOMA, IMPETIGO, CONTACT DERMATITIS, STURGE-WEBER SYNDROME, TUBEROUS SCLEROSIS, TINEA CAPITIS

ASK THE FOLLOWING QUESTIONS:

1. **Is the rash macular or papular?** A macular or papular rash would suggest scarlet fever, measles, erythema multiforme, exfoliative dermatitis, pityriasis rosea, eczema, contact dermatitis, secondary syphilis, drug eruption, and actinic dermatoses.

2. **Is the rash pustular?** A pustular rash suggests staphylococcus, scabies, secondary syphilis, acne, folliculitis, and dermatophytosis.

3. **Is the rash vesicular or bullous?** A bullous or vesicular rash would suggest chickenpox, smallpox, dermatitis herpetiformis, contact dermatitis, pemphigus, herpes zoster, bullous impetigo, herpes simplex, dyshidrosis, and nummular eczema. Hand, foot and mouth disease is associated with a vesicular rash of the hands and feet along with a stomatitis. It is caused by a coxsackie virus.

4. **Is the rash scaly?** A scaly rash suggests ichthyosis, psoriasis, lichen planus, neurodermatitis, dermatophytosis, exfoliative dermatitis, and drug eruptions. Seborrheic dermatitis is usually scaly with an erythematous base. Sudden onset of this condition should prompt a search for HIV.

5. **Are there ulcers?** The presence of ulcers in the lesions would suggest basal cell carcinoma, syphilis, lupus erythematosus, diabetic ulcers, ischemic ulcers, pyoderma gangrenosum, and ecthyma.

6. **Is there fever?** The presence of fever suggests scarlet fever, measles, erythema multiforme, exfoliative dermatitis, serum sickness, chickenpox, and smallpox.

7. **Could the rash be complicated by a secondary infection?** Always a good question to ask.

8. **Does it itch?** Pruritis is associated with urticaria, contact dermatitis, and eczema. It is not common with psoriasis, lichen planus and herpes zoster.

DIAGNOSTIC WORKUP

This can be found under Rash—Distribution (page 412).

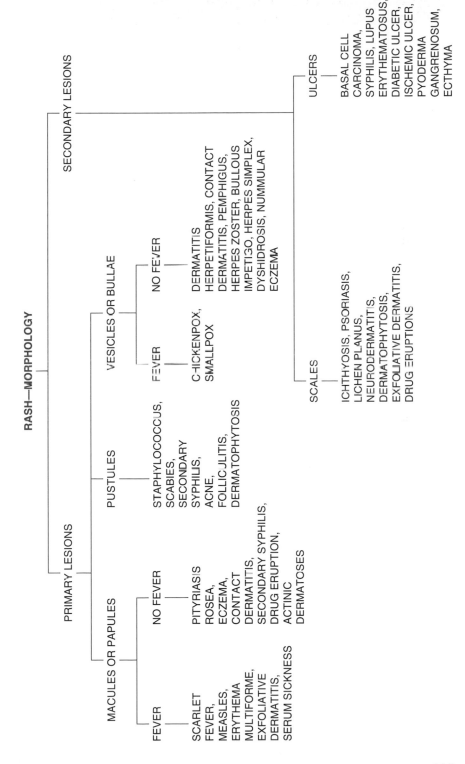

RASH—MORPHOLOGY

PRIMARY LESIONS

MACULES OR PAPULES

FEVER
SCARLET FEVER, MEASLES, ERYTHEMA MULTIFORME, EXFOLIATIVE DERMATITIS, SERUM SICKNESS

NO FEVER
PITYRIASIS ROSEA, ECZEMA, CONTACT DERMATITIS, SECONDARY SYPHILIS, DRUG ERUPTION, ACTINIC DERMATOSES

PUSTULES
STAPHYLOCOCCUS, SCABIES, SECONDARY SYPHILIS, ACNE, FOLLICULITIS, DERMATOPHYTOSIS

VESICLES OR BULLAE

FEVER
CHICKENPOX, SMALLPOX

NO FEVER
DERMATITIS HERPETIFORMIS, CONTACT DERMATITIS, PEMPHIGUS, HERPES ZOSTER, BULLOUS IMPETIGO, HERPES SIMPLEX, DYSHIDROSIS, NUMMULAR ECZEMA

SECONDARY LESIONS

SCALES
ICHTHYOSIS, PSORIASIS, LICHEN PLANUS, NEURODERMATITIS, DERMATOPHYTOSIS, EXFOLIATIVE DERMATITIS, DRUG ERUPTIONS

ULCERS
BASAL CELL CARCINOMA, SYPHILIS, LUPUS ERYTHEMATOSUS, DIABETIC ULCER, ISCHEMIC ULCER, PYODERMA GANGRENOSUM, ECTHYMA

ASK THE FOLLOWING QUESTIONS:

1. **Is there a history of drug ingestion?** Ergotamine, methysergide, and beta-adrenergic receptor blockers are just a few of the drugs that may cause Raynaud's phenomena.
2. **Is there involvement of only one upper extremity?** When there is involvement of only one upper extremity, thoracic outlet syndrome, especially cervical rib, arteriosclerosis of the subclavian artery, and embolism should be considered.
3. **Is there thickening of the skin?** Thickening of the skin should bring to mind scleroderma.
4. **Is there hypertension?** The presence of hypertension might suggest periarteritis nodosa and other collagen diseases, polycythemia vera, macroglobulinemia, cold agglutinins, and sickle-cell anemia.
5. **Are there abnormalities of the blood cells, red cell mass, or serum proteins?** These findings would suggest polycythemia vera, macroglobulinemia, cold agglutinins, and sickle-cell anemia.

DIAGNOSTIC WORKUP

Routine diagnostic studies include a CBC, sedimentation rate, urinalysis, chemistry panel, serum protein electrophoresis, ANA titer, chest x-ray, and EKG.

If macroglobulinemia is suspected, a Sia water test and serum immunoelectrophoresis may be done. If cold agglutinins are suspected, a test for cold agglutinins may be done. A sickle-cell preparation may be necessary if the patient is black. Collagen diseases may be further evaluated by skin and muscle biopsy and esophageal manometry.

Raynaud's phenomena may be demonstrated by immersing the hands in water at a temperature of 10° to 15°C. Whole body exposure to cold is an even better way of demonstrating the actual Raynaud's phenomena. The finding of nail-fold capillary-loop dilation and drop out may also help diagnose Raynaud's phenomena. If scleroderma is suspected, an antisclerodermal antibody titer is done.

Doppler studies and arteriography will rule out subclavian artery occlusions. A rheumatology or neurology consultation may be helpful.

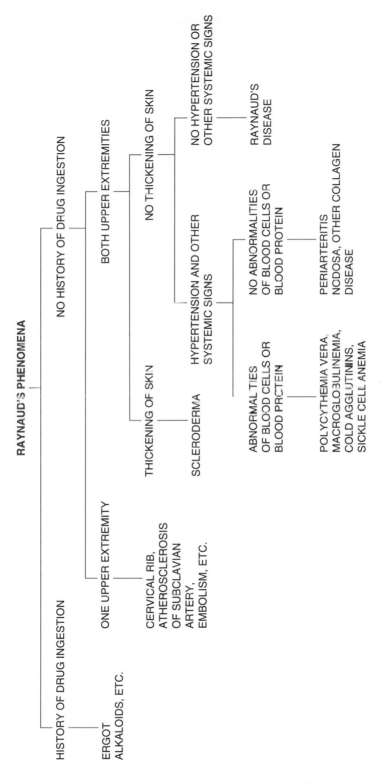

RAYNAUD'S PHENOMENA

HISTORY OF DRUG INGESTION

NO HISTORY OF DRUG INGESTION

ONE UPPER EXTREMITY

BOTH UPPER EXTREMITIES

ERGOT ALKALOIDS, ETC.

CERVICAL RIB, ATHEROSCLEROSIS OF SUBCLAVIAN ARTERY, EMBOLISM, ETC.

THICKENING OF SKIN

NO THICKENING OF SKIN

SCLERODERMA

HYPERTENSION AND OTHER SYSTEMIC SIGNS

NO HYPERTENSION OR OTHER SYSTEMIC SIGNS

ABNORMAL TIES OF BLOOD CELLS OR BLOOD PROTEIN

NO ABNORMALITIES OF BLOOD CELLS OR BLOOD PROTEIN

RAYNAUD'S DISEASE

POLYCYTHEMIA VERA, MACROGLOBULINEMIA, COLD AGGLUTININS, SICKLE CELL ANEMIA

PERIARTERITIS NODOSA, OTHER COLLAGEN DISEASE

ASK THE FOLLOWING QUESTIONS:

1. **Is it severe?** The presence of severe rectal bleeding would suggest ulcerative colitis, amebic dysentery, bacillary dysentery, intussusception, mesenteric thrombosis or embolism, diverticulitis, ischemic colitis, and coagulation disorders.

2. **Is there diarrhea and/or mucus?** The presence of diarrhea with or without mucus would suggest ulcerative colitis, amebic dysentery, or bacillary dysentery.

3. **Are there signs of intestinal obstruction?** The presence of signs of intestinal obstruction would suggest intussusception, mesenteric thrombosis, or embolism.

4. **If the bleeding is mild, is the bleeding mixed well with the stools?** Rectal bleeding that is mixed well with the stools suggests carcinoma of the colon, ulcerative colitis, Crohn's disease, Meckel's diverticulum, diverticulitis, and coagulation disorder.

5. **Are there painful bowel movements?** The presence of painful bowel movements, especially with bright-red bleeding, would suggest anal fissure or thrombosed hemorrhoid.

6. **Is there a rectal mass?** The presence of a rectal mass would suggest a polyp, carcinoma, or internal hemorrhoids.

DIAGNOSTIC WORKUP

Most cases can be diagnosed by anoscopy, sigmoidoscopy, and a barium enema. A stool culture and examination for ovum and parasites should also be done. If the diagnosis is uncertain after these studies, referral to a gastroenterologist should be done for colonoscopy and other diagnostic studies. A CT scan of the abdomen is a lot more expensive than a GI consult. The gastroenterologist may order angiography or small intestinal enteroscopy as well as radioisotope studies.

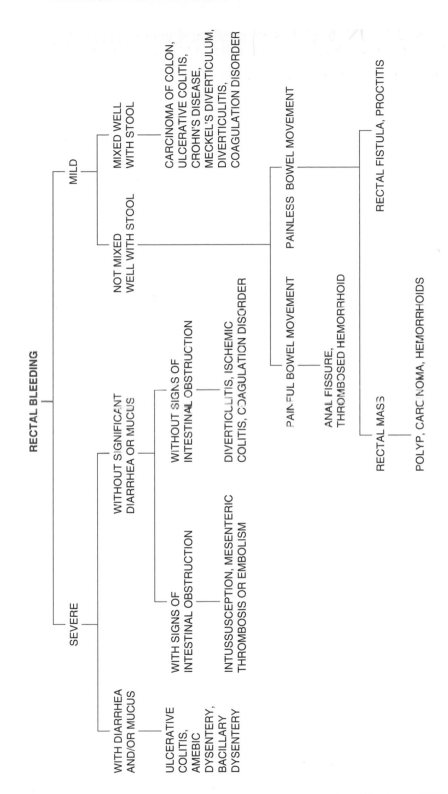

RECTAL BLEEDING

SEVERE

- WITH DIARRHEA AND/OR MUCUS
  - ULCERATIVE COLITIS, AMEBIC DYSENTERY, BACILLARY DYSENTERY
- WITHOUT SIGNIFICANT DIARRHEA OR MUCUS
  - WITH SIGNS OF INTESTINAL OBSTRUCTION
    - INTUSSUSCEPTION, MESENTERIC THROMBOSIS OR EMBOLISM
  - WITHOUT SIGNS OF INTESTINAL OBSTRUCTION
    - DIVERTICULITIS, ISCHEMIC COLITIS, COAGULATION DISORDER

MILD

- NOT MIXED WELL WITH STOOL
  - PAINFUL BOWEL MOVEMENT
    - ANAL FISSURE, THROMBOSED HEMORRHOID
  - PAINLESS BOWEL MOVEMENT
    - RECTAL FISTULA, PROCTITIS
  - RECTAL MASS
    - POLYP, CARCINOMA, HEMORRHOIDS
- MIXED WELL WITH STOOL
  - CARCINOMA OF COLON, ULCERATIVE COLITIS, CROHN'S DISEASE, MECKEL'S DIVERTICULUM, DIVERTICULITIS, COAGULATION DISORDER

ASK THE FOLLOWING QUESTIONS:

1. **Is it mucopurulent or feculent?** A mucopurulent discharge suggests an anal fistula, perirectal abscess, proctitis, anal ulcer, or rectal prolapse. A feculent discharge suggests anal incontinence, internal hemorrhoids, chronic anal fissure, or ulcer.
2. **Is it painful?** Painful discharge suggests a perirectal abscess, proctitis, anal ulcer, or rectal prolapse.
3. **Is there an abnormal neurologic examination?** An abnormal neurologic examination suggests that there is anal incontinence from an upper or lower motor neuron lesion. This may be due to spinal cord trauma, multiple sclerosis, spinal cord tumor, transverse myelitis, and many other disorders.

DIAGNOSTIC WORKUP

Routine laboratory tests include a CBC, sedimentation rate, urinalysis, chemistry panel, and smear and culture of the discharge. A Frei test may be necessary to rule out lymphogranuloma venereum. Sigmoidoscopy, colonoscopy, and a barium enema may be needed in selected cases. A proctologist or gastroenterologist should be consulted in difficult diagnostic problems. If there are abnormalities on the neurologic examination, a neurologist should be consulted.

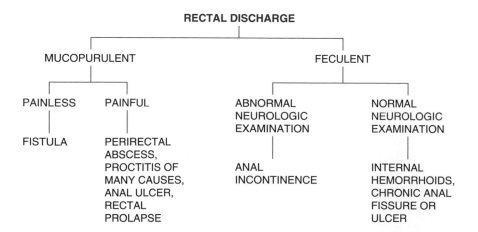

ASK THE FOLLOWING QUESTIONS:

1. **Is it painful?** A painful rectal mass should suggest perirectal abscess, thrombosed hemorrhoid, anal ulcer, ruptured ectopic pregnancy, tubo-ovarian abscess, and pelvic appendix.

2. **Is it soft or cystic?** The presence of a soft or cystic mass would suggest internal hemorrhoids, polyps, intussusception, villous tumor, granular proctitis, ovarian cyst, and blood or pus in the cul-de-sac.

3. **Is it hard?** The presence of a hard lesion would suggest a fecal impaction, foreign body, retroverted uterus, enlarged prostate, malignant deposits in the pouch of Douglas, stricture, and carcinoma.

4. **Is there associated bleeding?** The presence of bleeding should make one suspect carcinoma above all else, but it may be due to internal hemorrhoids, polyps, intussusception, villous tumors, or granular proctitis.

DIAGNOSTIC WORKUP

Routine laboratory tests include a CBC, sedimentation rate, and urinalysis. A smear and culture should be made of any rectal or vaginal discharge. Most cases will be diagnosed by anoscopy and proctoscopy. A pelvic ultrasound and CT scan of the abdomen and pelvis may be useful in evaluating ectopic pregnancy and other gynecologic disorders. Ultrasound of the prostate may also be done to evaluate a prostatic mass. A gynecologist, proctologist, or urologist should be consulted in difficult cases.

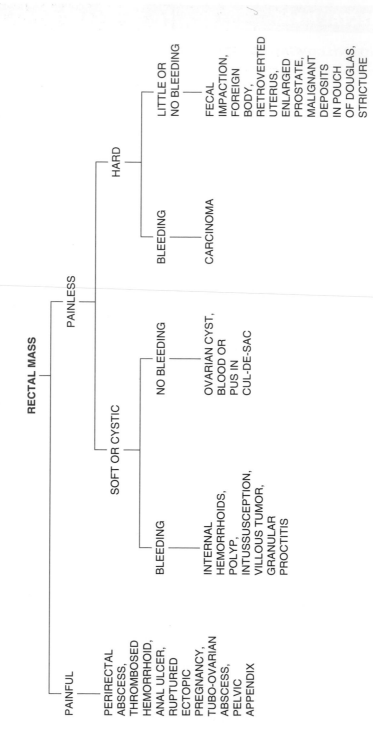

RECTAL MASS

- **PAINFUL**
  - PERIRECTAL ABSCESS, THROMBOSED HEMORRHOID, ANAL ULCER, RUPTURED ECTOPIC PREGNANCY, TUBO-OVARIAN ABSCESS, PELVIC APPENDIX
- **PAINLESS**
  - **SOFT OR CYSTIC**
    - **BLEEDING**
      - INTERNAL HEMORRHOIDS, POLYP, INTUSSUSCEPTION, VILLOUS TUMOR, GRANULAR PROCTITIS
    - **NO BLEEDING**
      - OVARIAN CYST, BLOOD OR PUS IN CUL-DE-SAC
  - **HARD**
    - **BLEEDING**
      - CARCINOMA
    - **LITTLE OR NO BLEEDING**
      - FECAL IMPACTION, FOREIGN BODY, RETROVERTED UTERUS, ENLARGED PROSTATE, MALIGNANT DEPOSITS IN POUCH OF DOUGLAS, STRICTURE

ASK THE FOLLOWING QUESTIONS:

1. **Is there bleeding?** The presence of bleeding with pain suggests an anal fissure, hemorrhoids, carcinoma, rectal prolapse, and intussusception.

2. **Is there a mass?** The presence of rectal pain along with a mass would suggest internal and external hemorrhoids, rectal carcinoma, and perirectal or ischiorectal abscesses. However, in females, masses in the cul-de-sac, such as an acute salpingitis, ectopic pregnancy, or endometriosis, will cause rectal pain. In males, prostatic abscess, foreign bodies, and seminal vesiculitis may cause rectal pain.

3. **Is there a purulent discharge?** Fistula-in-ano, perirectal abscess, ischiorectal abscess, and submucous abscess may cause a purulent discharge.

DIAGNOSTIC WORKUP

Routine diagnostic studies include a CBC, sedimentation rate, urinalysis, chemistry panel, VDRL test, anoscopy, sigmoidoscopy, and barium enema. In females, a pregnancy test and vaginal smear and culture should be done. Ultimately, culdocentesis, pelvic ultrasound, CT scan of the pelvis, and laparoscopy may be necessary, but a gynecologist should be consulted before considering these tests. In males, prostatic massage may yield a urethral discharge for smear and culture. An intravenous pyelogram or cystoscopy with retrograde pyelography may also be helpful.

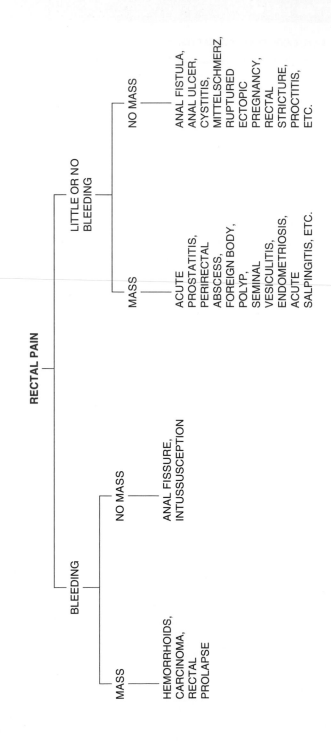

RECTAL PAIN

BLEEDING

MASS
- HEMORRHOIDS, CARCINOMA, RECTAL PROLAPSE

NO MASS
- ANAL FISSURE, INTUSSUSCEPTION

LITTLE OR NO BLEEDING

MASS
- ACUTE PROSTATITIS, PERIRECTAL ABSCESS, FOREIGN BODY, POLYP, SEMINAL VESICULITIS, ENDOMETRIOSIS, ACUTE SALPINGITIS, ETC.

NO MASS
- ANAL FISTULA, ANAL ULCER, CYSTITIS, MITTELSCHMERZ, RUPTURED ECTOPIC PREGNANCY, RECTAL STRICTURE, PROCTITIS, ETC.

ASK THE FOLLOWING QUESTIONS:

1. **Is there dysphagia?** The presence of difficulty swallowing should suggest carcinoma of the esophagus, esophageal strictures, esophageal diverticulum, achalasia, aortic aneurysm, and other mediastinal masses.
2. **Is there significant weight loss?** The presence of significant weight loss suggests carcinoma of the esophagus and esophageal stricture. It is also found in the late stages of achalasia.
3. **Is there heartburn?** Several of the conditions associated with esophageal regurgitation may be accompanied by heartburn, but reflux esophagitis and gastric ulcer are the most common.

DIAGNOSTIC WORKUP

Most disorders will be diagnosed by an upper GI series with an esophagogram and esophagoscopy with a biopsy. A Bernstein test, esophageal pH monitoring, and esophageal manometry may be useful in diagnosing reflux esophagitis. A CBC, serum iron, ferritin, and iron-binding capacity will help diagnose Plummer–Vinson syndrome. An ANA titer and skin biopsy will help diagnose scleroderma. A CT scan of the mediastinum will help diagnose most mediastinal masses, and angiography will be useful in diagnosing an aortic aneurysm.

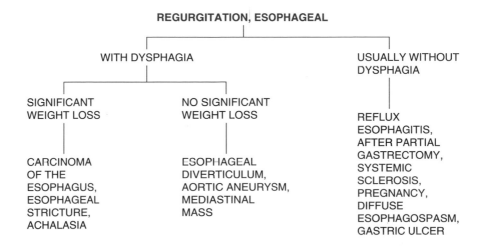

RESPIRATION ABNORMALITIES

ASK THE FOLLOWING QUESTIONS:

1. **Is the respiration rapid?** The presence of rapid respiration indicates dyspnea (page 137), and may be caused by shock, congestive heart failure, asthma, emphysema, and other disorders.
2. **Is the respiration slow?** The presence of slow respiration should suggest diabetes mellitus, alcoholic stupor, uremia, opium poisoning, cerebral concussion, and metabolic acidosis from other causes.
3. **Are the breaths irregular or alternating fast and slow?** This would suggest Cheyne–Stokes respiration or Biot's breathing, and the causes to consider are coma, congestive heart failure, uremia, tuberculosis, bacterial meningitis, typhoid fever, chorea, and many other conditions.
4. **Are the breaths deep or shallow?** The presence of deep respiration should suggest metabolic acidosis due to diabetes mellitus, renal failure, alcoholic stupor, or respiratory alkalosis from salicylate intoxication. The presence of shallow respiration would suggest uremia, opium poisoning, and concussion.

DIAGNOSTIC WORKUP

The basic workup includes a CBC, sedimentation rate, urinalysis, chemistry panel, EKG, chest x-ray, urine drug screen, blood alcohol level, arterial blood gases, and pulmonary function tests. If there is fever, blood cultures, febrile agglutinins, and tuberculin and other skin tests may be ordered. If there is coma, further diagnostic workup may be found on page 88. If there is dyspnea, further diagnostic workup may be found on page 137.

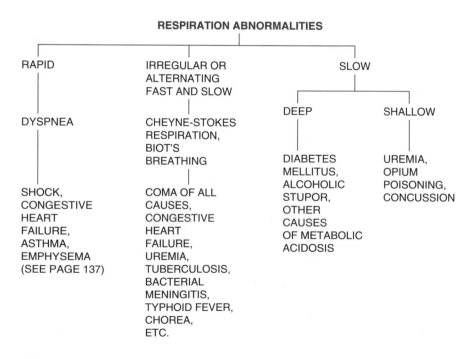

RESPIRATION ABNORMALITIES

ASK THE FOLLOWING QUESTIONS:

1. **Is there a history of drug use?** Many drugs, including barbiturates and benzodiazepines, may cause a restless leg syndrome.
2. **Are there abnormalities on neurologic examination?** Various forms of peripheral neuropathy and multiple sclerosis may be associated with restless leg syndrome. Parkinson's disease may also be associated with the restless leg syndrome.
3. **Is there pallor?** Various types of anemia may be associated with restless leg syndrome also.

DIAGNOSTIC WORKUP

Routine tests include a CBC, sedimentation rate, urinalysis, urine drug screen, chemistry panel, glucose tolerance test, and nerve conduction velocity studies. SSEP studies may be useful in detecting multiple sclerosis. Doppler studies may detect peripheral vascular disease. A pregnancy test should be done on a woman of child-bearing age. A therapeutic trial of a combination of dopa and carbidopa may be useful.

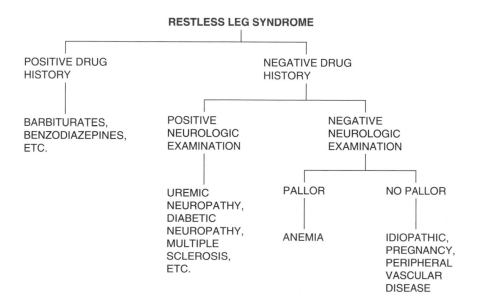

RESTLESS LEG SYNDROME

POSITIVE DRUG HISTORY — BARBITURATES, BENZODIAZEPINES, ETC.

NEGATIVE DRUG HISTORY

POSITIVE NEUROLOGIC EXAMINATION — UREMIC NEUROPATHY, DIABETIC NEUROPATHY, MULTIPLE SCLEROSIS, ETC.

NEGATIVE NEUROLOGIC EXAMINATION

PALLOR — ANEMIA

NO PALLOR — IDIOPATHIC, PREGNANCY, PERIPHERAL VASCULAR DISEASE

RISUS SARDONICUS

ASK THE FOLLOWING QUESTIONS:

1. **Is there a history of recent wound infection or intravenous drug use?** The presence of these findings should suggest tetanus.
2. **Is there a history of psychosis or suicidal ideation?** The presence of these findings should suggest strychnine poisoning and cataplexy.

DIAGNOSTIC WORKUP

Routine diagnostic studies include a CBC, sedimentation rate, urinalysis, urine drug screen, chemistry panel, blood cultures, chest x-ray, and EKG. A careful search for a puncture wound or evidence of frequent intravenous injections should be done and cultures of any exudate obtained. If tetanus has been ruled out, a psychiatrist should be consulted.

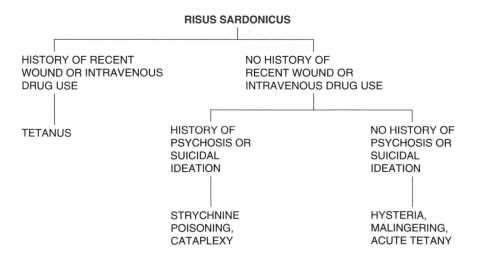

The cause of scalp tenderness is usually obvious when there is dermatitis or inflammatory disorders of the skin such as herpes zoster, pediculosis, tinea capitis, infected sebaceous cyst, and impetigo.

The tenderness is more subtle in temporal arteritis unless there is associated homo-lateral blindness or obvious enlargement of the superficial temporal artery. Tenderness in the occipital area is usually due to occipital major or minor entrapment by the posterior cervical muscles. This is common after flexion–extension injuries of the cervical spine or cervical spondylosis. Referred tenderness from trigeminal neuralgia, sinusitis, otitis media, mastoiditis, and disorders of the teeth may occur. When a patient presents with scalp tenderness, especially at the top of the head, and the physical examination is normal, the diagnosis of psychoneurosis should be entertained.

DIAGNOSTIC WORKUP

When there are obvious skin lesions, cultures, potassium hydroxide preparations, or biopsies will usually establish the diagnosis. A skull x-ray should be done to exclude fracture, rickets, syphilitic periostitis, and primary and secondary tumors of the cranium. A sedimentation rate should be done to exclude temporal arteritis, especially in the elderly. If the physical examination and diagnostic workup are normal and the patient persists with the complaint, a referral to a psychiatrist is in order.

ASK THE FOLLOWING QUESTIONS:

1. **Is there a history of trauma?** Patients with scoliosis and a history of trauma should be suspected of having a thoracic or lumbosacral sprain, fracture, or herniated disk.
2. **Is the neurologic examination abnormal?** Abnormal neurologic findings should suggest poliomyelitis, muscular dystrophy, multiple sclerosis, syringomyelia, Friedreich's ataxia, and many other disorders.
3. **If the neurologic examination is abnormal, are there motor findings only or both sensory and motor findings?** Abnormal motor findings would suggest poliomyelitis or muscular dystrophy, whereas abnormal sensory and motor findings would suggest multiple sclerosis, syringomyelia, and Friedreich's ataxia, among other disorders.
4. **Does the x-ray show bone disease?** Diseases of the bone that may cause scoliosis are Paget's disease, osteoporosis, destructive disease of the vertebrae such as tuberculosis, osteogenesis imperfecta, rickets, congenital hemivertebra, and Klippel–Feil syndrome.
5. **If the x-ray shows bone disease, is the patient a child or an adult?** Children with scoliosis and bone disease may have rickets, osteogenesis imperfecta, congenital hemivertebra, and Klippel–Feil syndrome. Adults with x-ray changes of bone diseases may have Paget's disease, osteoporosis, destructive disease of the vertebrae, and other disorders.
6. **Is one leg shorter than the other?** A short leg would suggest congenital or acquired short-leg syndrome.

DIAGNOSTIC WORKUP

Clinically, the diagnosis of scoliosis can be made by having the patient bend over. In this position, there will be asymmetry in the height of the scapulae (Adam's test). The vast majority of mild cases of scoliosis require only x-rays and watchful expectancy or referral to an orthopedic surgeon. Routine diagnostic workup may include a CBC, sedimentation rate, urinalysis, chemistry panel, arthritis panel with ANA and HLA B27 antigen, tuberculin test, and a spinal survey including both recumbent and upright views. A bone survey may also need to be done. A bone scan may be necessary to detect subtle bone disease. If these tests are negative, the patient should be referred to an orthopedic surgeon. EMG examinations, nerve conduction velocity studies, CT scans, and MRIs may be necessary. Remember, scoliosis is rarely the cause of back pain unless the spinal angulation exceeds 40 degrees.

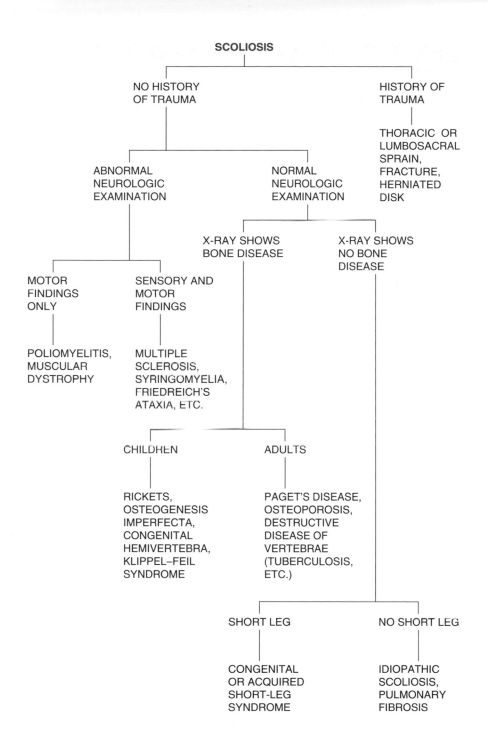

SCOLIOSIS

NO HISTORY
OF TRAUMA

HISTORY OF
TRAUMA

THORACIC OR
LUMBOSACRAL
SPRAIN,
FRACTURE,
HERNIATED
DISK

ABNORMAL
NEUROLOGIC
EXAMINATION

NORMAL
NEUROLOGIC
EXAMINATION

X-RAY SHOWS
BONE DISEASE

X-RAY SHOWS
NO BONE
DISEASE

MOTOR
FINDINGS
ONLY

SENSORY AND
MOTOR
FINDINGS

POLIOMYELITIS,
MUSCULAR
DYSTROPHY

MULTIPLE
SCLEROSIS,
SYRINGOMYELIA,
FRIEDREICH'S
ATAXIA, ETC.

CHILDREN

ADULTS

RICKETS,
OSTEOGENESIS
IMPERFECTA,
CONGENITAL
HEMIVERTEBRA,
KLIPPEL–FEIL
SYNDROME

PAGET'S DISEASE,
OSTEOPOROSIS,
DESTRUCTIVE
DISEASE OF
VERTEBRAE
(TUBERCULOSIS,
ETC.)

SHORT LEG

NO SHORT LEG

CONGENITAL
OR ACQUIRED
SHORT-LEG
SYNDROME

IDIOPATHIC
SCOLIOSIS,
PULMONARY
FIBROSIS

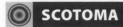

ASK THE FOLLOWING QUESTIONS:

1. **Is it transient?** If the scotomas are transient, then migraine, transient ischemic attacks, and retrobulbar neuritis should be suspected.
2. **Are there abnormalities on the eye examination other than the optic nerve?** On a careful eye examination, the clinician may find corneal opacities, muscae volitantes, cataracts, choroiditis, glaucoma, retinitis, retinal hemorrhage, and detached retina.
3. **Are there other neurologic signs?** The presence of other neurologic signs may suggest multiple sclerosis, carotid artery thrombosis or insufficiency, basilar artery thrombosis or insufficiency, and pseudotumor cerebri, among other disorders.

DIAGNOSTIC WORKUP

This should include a careful eye examination with slit lamp, tonometry, and visual field examinations. If the initial findings suggest an ocular disorder, referral to an ophthalmologist should be made. If the neurologic examination is abnormal, the patient should be referred to a neurologist, rather than ordering expensive tests such as a CT scan, MRI scan, VEP studies, angiography, and spinal fluid examinations.

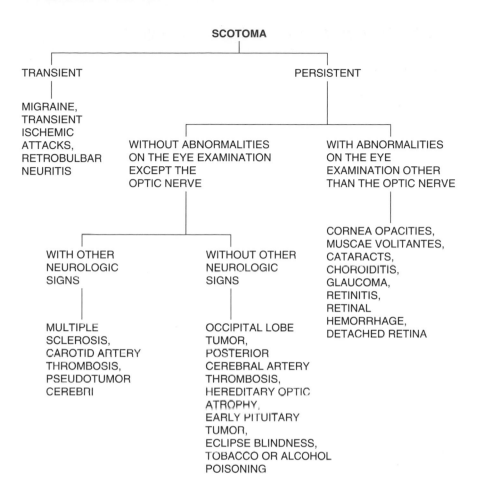

SCOTOMA

TRANSIENT

MIGRAINE,
TRANSIENT
ISCHEMIC
ATTACKS,
RETROBULBAR
NEURITIS

PERSISTENT

WITHOUT ABNORMALITIES
ON THE EYE EXAMINATION
EXCEPT THE
OPTIC NERVE

WITH ABNORMALITIES
ON THE EYE
EXAMINATION OTHER
THAN THE OPTIC NERVE

WITH OTHER
NEUROLOGIC
SIGNS

WITHOUT OTHER
NEUROLOGIC
SIGNS

CORNEA OPACITIES,
MUSCAE VOLITANTES,
CATARACTS,
CHOROIDITIS,
GLAUCOMA,
RETINITIS,
RETINAL
HEMORRHAGE,
DETACHED RETINA

MULTIPLE
SCLEROSIS,
CAROTID ARTERY
THROMBOSIS,
PSEUDOTUMOR
CEREBRI

OCCIPITAL LOBE
TUMOR,
POSTERIOR
CEREBRAL ARTERY
THROMBOSIS,
HEREDITARY OPTIC
ATROPHY,
EARLY PITUITARY
TUMOR,
ECLIPSE BLINDNESS,
TOBACCO OR ALCOHOL
POISONING

⊚ SCROTAL SWELLING

CASE HISTORY

A 32-year-old white male presents at your clinic with a 3-week history of scrotal swelling. Following the algorithm, you note that it is only his left scrotum, so systemic diseases such as congestive heart failure, cirrhosis and nephrosis can be ruled out. It is painless, so it is unlikely that he has torsion of the testicle, or an incarcerated, or strangulated inguinal hernia.

On examination, you find that the mass fails to trans-illuminate ruling out a hydrocele. However, it is reducible, so you suspect a sliding inguinal hernia or varicocele. You would be correct.

ASK THE FOLLOWING QUESTIONS:

1. **Is it diffuse or focal?** Diffuse scrotal swelling would suggest congestive heart failure, nephrosis, uremia, and cirrhosis, as well as focal diseases such as filariasis or bilateral hydrocele. Focal scrotal swelling would suggest a hernia, hydrocele, torsion of the testicle, abscesses, epididymitis, orchitis, varicoceles, and testicular tumors.
2. **If it is diffuse, is there ascites or generalized edema?** The presence of diffuse edema of the scrotum with ascites or generalized edema would suggest congestive heart failure, nephrosis, uremia, or cirrhosis.
3. **If it is focal, is it painful?** The presence of painful scrotal swelling would suggest an incarcerated or strangulated inguinal hernia, torsion of the testicle, a hematoma, orchitis, epididymitis, furuncle, or abscess.
4. **Does it transilluminate?** If the mass transilluminates, it is very likely a hydrocele of the testicle or a spermatocele.
5. **Is it reducible?** If the mass is reducible, it is most likely an inguinal hernia or a varicocele.

DIAGNOSTIC WORKUP

Routine laboratory tests include a CBC, sedimentation rate, urinalysis, urine culture, and urethral smear. If prostatic disease is suspected, a PSA should be ordered. If intestinal obstruction is suspected, a flat plate of the abdomen and lateral decubiti should be ordered. A radionuclide testicular scan with technetium-99m is useful in differentiating between testicular torsion and epididymitis. Scrotal ultrasound may be done to evaluate any kind of testicular or scrotal mass. However, it is much less costly to refer the patient to a urologist.

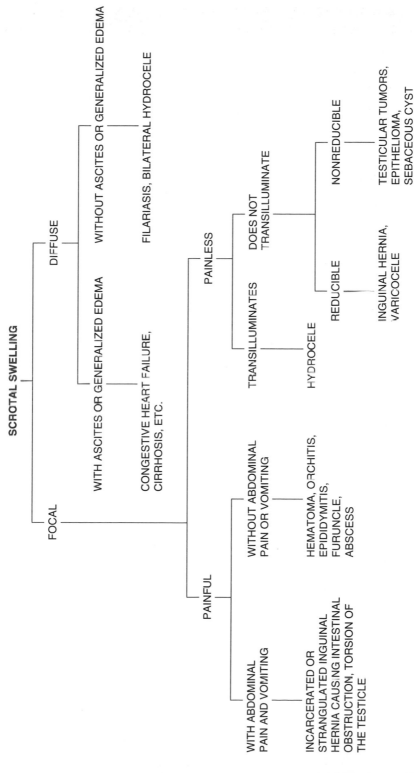

ASK THE FOLLOWING QUESTIONS:

1. **Is it intermittent?** The presence of intermittent sensory changes would suggest a transient ischemic attack, migraine, and epilepsy.
2. **Is there loss of vibratory and position sense only?** The finding of loss of vibratory and position sense only, particularly if it involves all four extremities, would suggest pernicious anemia. If the loss of vibratory and position sense is on one side of the body only, a parietal lobe tumor should be suspected. Diffuse loss of vibratory and position sense only may also be seen in multiple sclerosis, cervical spondylosis, and Friedreich's ataxia.
3. **Is there loss of pain or temperature only?** The presence of loss of pain and temperature on one side of the body is more likely to occur with posterior inferior cerebellar artery occlusions. Rarely, syringomyelia may cause loss of pain and temperature only in the lower extremities if the syringomyelia is in the thoracic cord and in the upper extremities if it is in the cervical cord. Anterior spinal artery occlusions may cause loss of pain and temperature in the lower extremities. Multiple sclerosis can occasionally cause loss of pain and temperature in a diffuse manner.
4. **Is there loss of all modalities together?** If all modalities are lost together on one-half of the body, one should consider thalamic syndrome due to vascular occlusion of the thalamogeniculate artery or its branches. Loss of all modalities in the lower extremities and up to a certain sensory level would probably be due to spinal cord trauma, a space-occupying lesion, or transverse myelitis. However, this condition can also be seen with multiple sclerosis. Loss of all modalities together in the upper extremity may be found in brachial plexus neuropathy or injuries. It may be found with malingering as well. Loss of all modalities in a glove and stocking distribution would suggest peripheral neuropathy. Loss of all modalities in a dermatomal distribution would suggest radiculopathy due to herniated disk, tumor, or arthritic spurs. Platybasia and foramen magnum tumors may cause selective loss of vibratory and position sense in one or more extremities or loss of sensation to all modalities in one or more extremities.

DIAGNOSTIC WORKUP

Routine diagnostic studies include a CBC, sedimentation rate, urinalysis, chemistry panel, ANA, serum protein electrophoresis, VDRL test, chest x-ray, and x-ray of the spine. Findings of a clear-cut sensory loss are a good reason to consult a neurologist at this point. When one is not available, further workup depends on what part of the body is affected.

If only the lower extremities are involved, a CT scan or MRI of the lumbar or thoracic spine may be done. EMG and nerve conduction velocity studies of the lower extremities will complement the diagnostic evaluation.

If both the upper and lower extremities are involved, an MRI of the cervical spine would be the best procedure to perform. A CT scan of the cervical spine is not nearly as precise. EMG examination of the upper and possibly the lower extremities should be done in these cases. Nerve conduction velocity studies may also need to be done.

If the face is involved along with the extremities, a CT scan or MRI of the brain should be done. Skull x-rays are not very useful unless a fracture of the skull is suspected.

Carotid scans, an MRA, and four-vessel angiography are very useful in evaluating cerebral vascular disease. If peripheral neuropathy is suspected, a neuropathy workup (see page 356) should be done. If multiple sclerosis is suspected, a spinal tap and SSEP or VEP studies will assist in the diagnosis. A spinal tap will also be useful in diagnosing central nervous system lues. If pernicious anemia is suspected, a serum B_{12} and folic acid and possibly a Schilling test should be done. Guillain–Barré syndrome is diagnosed by a spinal fluid examination, which will show a markedly elevated spinal fluid protein in the face of a normal cell count.

Entrapment syndromes, such as carpal tunnel syndrome, ulnar nerve entrapment, or tarsal tunnel syndrome are diagnosed by nerve conduction velocity studies.

A wake-and-sleep EEG may diagnose complex partial seizures or parietal lobe seizures. Sometimes, combined myelography and CT scan are better than MRI studies in selected cases.

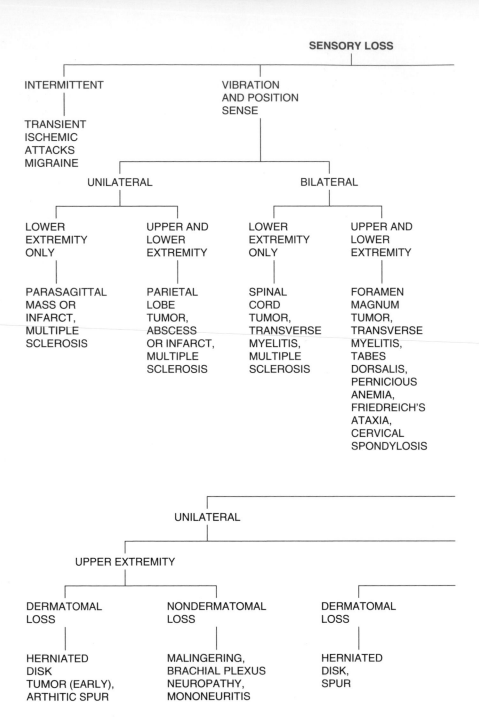

SENSORY LOSS

INTERMITTENT

TRANSIENT
ISCHEMIC
ATTACKS
MIGRAINE

VIBRATION
AND POSITION
SENSE

UNILATERAL

LOWER
EXTREMITY
ONLY

PARASAGITTAL
MASS OR
INFARCT,
MULTIPLE
SCLEROSIS

UPPER AND
LOWER
EXTREMITY

PARIETAL
LOBE
TUMOR,
ABSCESS
OR INFARCT,
MULTIPLE
SCLEROSIS

BILATERAL

LOWER
EXTREMITY
ONLY

SPINAL
CORD
TUMOR,
TRANSVERSE
MYELITIS,
MULTIPLE
SCLEROSIS

UPPER AND
LOWER
EXTREMITY

FORAMEN
MAGNUM
TUMOR,
TRANSVERSE
MYELITIS,
TABES
DORSALIS,
PERNICIOUS
ANEMIA,
FRIEDREICH'S
ATAXIA,
CERVICAL
SPONDYLOSIS

UNILATERAL

UPPER EXTREMITY

DERMATOMAL
LOSS

HERNIATED
DISK
TUMOR (EARLY),
ARTHITIC SPUR

NONDERMATOMAL
LOSS

MALINGERING,
BRACHIAL PLEXUS
NEUROPATHY,
MONONEURITIS

DERMATOMAL
LOSS

HERNIATED
DISK,
SPUR

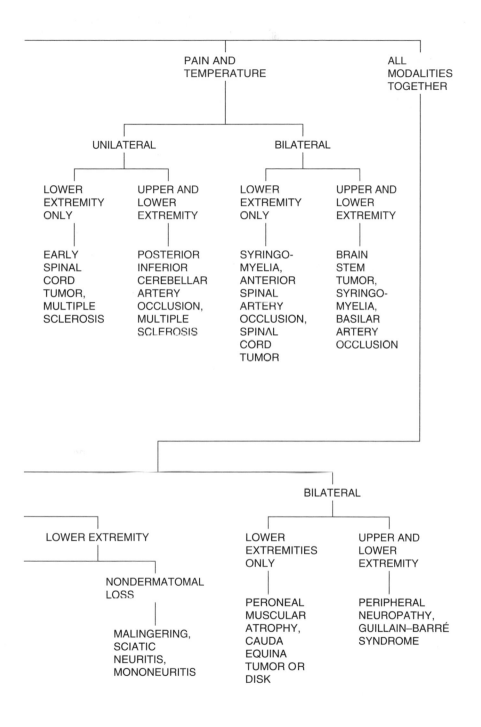

CASE HISTORY

A 29-year-old painter complains of increasing pain in his right shoulder. Following the algorithm, you find that the pain is non-radiating, and is constant. It is not relieved by nitroglycerin. Neurologic examination is within normal limits. There is normal range of motion. Moreover, you find that the pain only occurs on active motion. You suspect subacromial bursitis and a torn rotator cuff and an MRI of the shoulder confirms your suspicion.

ASK THE FOLLOWING QUESTIONS:

1. **Is there significant radiation of pain down the arm?** The presence of significant radiation of pain down the arm would suggest thoracic outlet syndrome, herpes zoster, herniated cervical disk, spinal cord tumor, brachial plexus neuritis, myocardial infarction, sympathetic dystrophy, Pancoast's tumor, and aortic aneurysm.
2. **Is the radiation down the arm transient?** The presence of transient radiation of pain down the arm would suggest coronary insufficiency.
3. **Are there hypoactive reflexes or significant dermatomal loss of sensation in the involved extremity?** These findings would suggest spinal cord tumor, herniated cervical disk, and brachial plexus neuritis, among other disorders.
4. **Is there pain on active motion only?** Pain on active motion only is more frequently found in subacromial bursitis, calcific tendinitis, and torn rotator cuff. Flexing the biceps will cause pain in biceps tendonitis. Acromio-clavicular inflammation is usually traumatic in origin.
5. **Is there pain on both active and passive motion?** This finding would suggest osteoarthritis, rheumatoid arthritis, gout, dislocation of the shoulder, adhesive capsulitis, shoulder–hand syndrome, aseptic bone necrosis, and osteomyelitis.
6. **Is there normal range of motion of the shoulder and normal neurologic examination?** These findings would suggest that the pain is referred from gallbladder disease, pancreatitis, ruptured peptic ulcer, pleurisy, or tuberculosis.
7. **Are there diminished pulses in the involved extremity?** These findings would suggest occlusion of the subclavian artery, thoracic outlet syndrome, or dissecting aneurysm.

DIAGNOSTIC WORKUP

The first thing to do is an x-ray of the shoulder. If this is normal, a trial of conservative therapy may be initiated before ordering an expensive diagnostic workup. If the pain persists, routine diagnostic studies include a CBC, sedimentation rate, urinalysis, chemistry panel, arthritis panel including ANA, x-ray of the shoulder, chest x-ray, and EKG. An MRI of the shoulder may need to be done to rule out a torn rotator cuff. Shoulder arthrography can also be used to diagnose this condition. If there are abnormal neurologic findings, EMG, nerve conduction velocity studies, and MRI of the cervical spine may need to be done. A neurologist should be consulted before ordering these expensive diagnostic tests.

If there are focal trigger points in the bursa or shoulder joints, a therapeutic trial of lidocaine hydrochloride (Xylocaine®) and corticosteroid injections should be done if the x-rays of the shoulder are negative or show only calcific tendinitis.

Stellate ganglion blocks may be diagnostic and therapeutic for sympathetic dystrophy. If there are abnormalities of the brachial or radial pulses, angiography may need to be done. When there is intermittent pain down the arm, an exercise tolerance test may need to be ordered. However, it may be wise to refer the patient to a cardiologist before ordering this test. A gastroenterologist may need to be consulted to rule out cholecystitis, pancreatitis, and peptic ulcer disease.

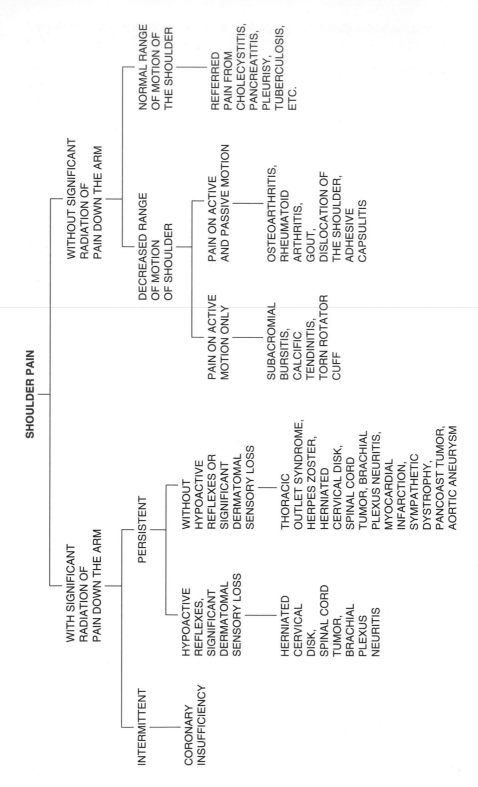

SHOULDER PAIN

INTERMITTENT
- CORONARY INSUFFICIENCY

WITH SIGNIFICANT RADIATION OF PAIN DOWN THE ARM

PERSISTENT

HYPOACTIVE REFLEXES, SIGNIFICANT DERMATOMAL SENSORY LOSS
- HERNIATED CERVICAL DISK, SPINAL CORD TUMOR, BRACHIAL PLEXUS NEURITIS

WITHOUT HYPOACTIVE REFLEXES OR SIGNIFICANT DERMATOMAL SENSORY LOSS
- THORACIC OUTLET SYNDROME, HERPES ZOSTER, HERNIATED CERVICAL DISK, SPINAL CORD TUMOR, BRACHIAL PLEXUS NEURITIS, MYOCARDIAL INFARCTION, SYMPATHETIC DYSTROPHY, PANCOAST TUMOR, AORTIC ANEURYSM

WITHOUT SIGNIFICANT RADIATION OF PAIN DOWN THE ARM

DECREASED RANGE OF MOTION OF SHOULDER

PAIN ON ACTIVE MOTION ONLY
- SUBACROMIAL BURSITIS, CALCIFIC TENDINITIS, TORN ROTATOR CUFF

PAIN ON ACTIVE AND PASSIVE MOTION
- OSTEOARTHRITIS, RHEUMATOID ARTHRITIS, GOUT, DISLOCATION OF THE SHOULDER, ADHESIVE CAPSULITIS

NORMAL RANGE OF MOTION OF THE SHOULDER
- REFERRED PAIN FROM CHOLECYSTITIS, PANCREATITIS, PLEURISY, TUBERCULOSIS, ETC.

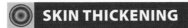

Thickening of the skin is most commonly seen in myxedema and scleroderma. The association of Raynaud's phenomena will help distinguish scleroderma. Thickening of the skin of the lower legs may also be seen in lymphedema, carcinoid syndrome, and vascular insufficiency. Localized thickening in the pretibial area may be seen in hyperthyroidism. Thickening of the skin of the face is seen in Chagas disease and porphyria cutanea tarda.

DIAGNOSTIC WORKUP

In cases of diffuse thickening of the skin, a thyroid profile with T_3, T_4, and TSH should be done. This should also identify hypothyroidism. A positive ANA test with a speckled pattern will help identify scleroderma, but a skin biopsy should also be done. An antisclerodermal antibody titer is also useful if available. Esophageal motility studies will be helpful in early diagnosis. A skin biopsy will help identify many of the other conditions mentioned above. Urine for porphyrins will help identify porphyria.

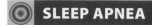

ASK THE FOLLOWING QUESTIONS:

1. **Is there excessive snoring?** Excessive snoring would indicate obstructive sleep apnea from large tonsils, deviated nasal septum, cleft palate, other abnormalities, and obesity.
2. **Is there obesity?** More than 60% of patients with sleep apnea have obesity, and pickwickian syndrome should be considered in these patients, as well as idiopathic obesity.
3. **Are there abnormalities of the neurologic examination?** The presence of neurologic abnormalities should make one think of poliomyelitis, Shy–Drager syndrome, brain stem tumors, and other neurologic disorders.

DIAGNOSTIC WORKUP

The most important diagnostic test is an all-night polygraphic recording (polysomnography). This will differentiate between obstructive and nonobstructive sleep apnea. If obstructive sleep apnea is suspected, a referral should be made to an ear, nose, and throat specialist. If there are abnormalities on the neurologic examination, a neurologic consultation should be sought. If idiopathic nonobstructive sleep apnea is suspected, the patient should be referred to a pulmonologist. A therapeutic trial of continuous positive airway pressure may be done. Some cases should have evaluation for a pituitary tumor, a thyroid profile, and a trial of tricyclic drugs and progesterone.

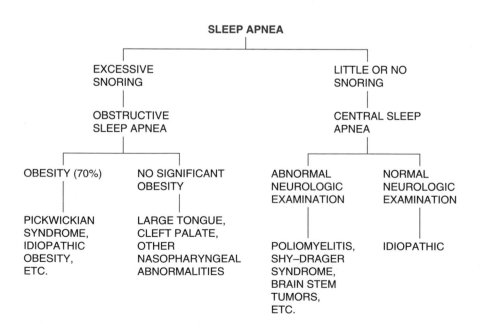

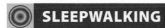

Occasional sleepwalking is normal in children and of no pathologic significance. It is reported in at least 15% of normal children. It should be distinguished from night terrors which occur in stages 3 and 4 of non-REM sleep. When it is frequent, it is a sign of significant emotional disturbances, and a referral to a psychiatrist is in order. Before you make a referral, a wake-and-sleep EEG, preferably with nasopharyngeal electrodes, should be done to exclude partial complex seizures (psychomotor epilepsy).

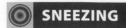

Acute sneezing is often seen in the early stage of the common cold and can be found in almost all URIs. It is also seen in measles and other infectious diseases.

Chronic sneezing is another matter. When environmental irritants, such as tobacco (especially snuff), ammonia, and other irritant gases, have been eliminated, it is almost invariably caused by allergy. The only exception is prolonged repetitive sneezing, which is usually psychological.

DIAGNOSTIC WORKUP

The diagnostic workup is the same as for nasal discharge (page 327). Patients with prolonged repetitive sneezing and a negative workup for allergy should be referred to a psychiatrist.

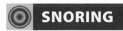

ASK THE FOLLOWING QUESTIONS:

1. **Are there abnormalities on the ear, nose, and throat examination?** A careful ear, nose, and throat examination may disclose hypertrophic tonsils and adenoids, deviated septum, bifid uvula, large floppy palate, and hypertrophic turbinates, among other conditions.
2. **Are there abnormalities on the neurologic examination?** A careful neurologic examination may disclose bulbar palsy, pseudobulbar palsy, myasthenia gravis, and cerebral vascular disease, among other conditions.

DIAGNOSTIC WORKUP

A sleep diary should be kept by the patient and his or her spouse. A tape recording during sleep will be helpful. Polysomnography is the most important diagnostic test. It will often confirm the diagnosis of obstructive sleep apnea. If there are ear, nose, and throat abnormalities, a referral to an ear, nose, and throat specialist should be made. If there are neurologic abnormalities, a referral to a neurologist should be made. A therapeutic trial of continuous positive airway pressure may be useful (see page 444).

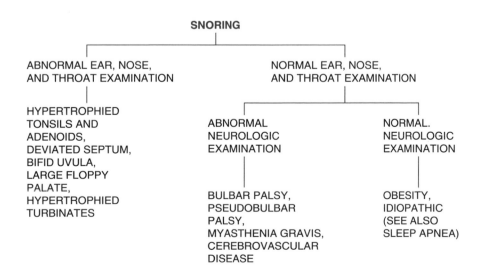

ASK THE FOLLOWING QUESTIONS:

1. **Are there exudates?** This is a key question when evaluating a sore throat. Most cases of sore throat with exudates will be found to have streptococcal pharyngitis. Without exudates, one could still have a streptococcal sore throat, but it is less likely.
2. **Is there a temperature elevation?** A significant elevation of the temperature, with or without exudates, is also characteristic of streptococcal pharyngitis.
3. **Are there enlarged lymph nodes?** If the lymph nodes are enlarged in the peritonsillar area, it is often a sign of streptococcal sore throat, but it certainly is not diagnostic. Interestingly enough, 90% of patients with infectious mononucleosis have posterior cervical adenopathy.
4. **Are there systemic symptoms and signs?** Patients who present with exudative tonsillitis and splenomegaly certainly should be considered to have infectious mononucleosis until proven otherwise. Also, an exudative tonsillitis along with a fever and heart murmur should make one consider rheumatic fever. Systemic symptoms such as dry cough, runny nose, and generalized malaise or fatigue should make one think of a viral URI.

DIAGNOSTIC WORKUP

In a sore throat with typical exudates very suggestive of streptococcal pharyngitis, a throat culture may be all one needs before starting definitive antibiotic therapy. In the more difficult cases, screening for streptococcal antigens (streptozyme test and ASO titer) might be indicated. An ASO titer is particularly important when one suspects rheumatic fever. If the patient's streptococcal sore throat persists, a monospot test and a culture for gonorrhea should be done. Although there are hardly any false-negative monospot tests, there are 10% false positives, and that should be kept in mind. A blood smear for atypical lymphocytes may be helpful, as well as a heterophile antibody titer in those cases.

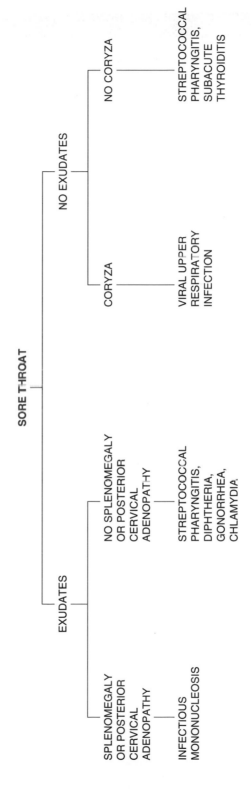

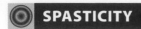
SPASTICITY

Spasticity may arise from pyramidal tract lesions anywhere from the spinal cord to the cerebral cortex. Consequently, the differential diagnosis and workup of this type of spasticity is the same as for hemiplegia (page 223). Spasticity may also be due to extrapyramidal disorders such as parkinsonism. The differential diagnosis and workup of this type of spasticity may be found under Tremor (page 491).

In the stiff-man syndrome, there is persistent muscle rigidity that is often painful and gradually increases over months or years. The cause is unknown, but a hereditary form is known to occur.

These are a group of speech abnormalities that do not fit into the category of aphasia (page 37) or dysarthria (page 131). These are almost always psychogenic in origin. *Stammering speech* is found in emotionally high-strung people and is probably due to psychological trauma in childhood. It is common in left-handed children who were forced to use the right hand. *Lolling speech* is typified by difficulty with consonants. It is more common in mental retardation, but it can be found in otherwise normal persons. *Idioglossia* is a substitution of consonants, making the speech very difficult to understand. It may be associated with high-tone deafness. *Perseveration* means the repetition of a word or sentence. When a patient repeats a word or sentence that he or she just heard, it is called *echolalia*. Both of the last two conditions occur in schizophrenia, but perseveration may occur in organic brain syndrome, especially Korsakoff's psychosis. *Mutism* is often due to schizophrenia or hysteria, but occasionally it is due to total motor aphasia.

SPLENOMEGALY, ACUTE OR SUBACUTE

ASK THE FOLLOWING QUESTIONS:

1. **Is there fever?** The presence of fever should suggest infectious mononucleosis, infectious hepatitis, leptospirosis, acute leukemia, lymphoma, malaria, and bacterial endocarditis, among other things.
2. **Is there a rash?** The presence of a rash should suggest thrombocytopenic purpura, acute leukemia, typhoid fever, septicemia, and lupus erythematosus.
3. **Is there jaundice?** The presence of jaundice should suggest infectious hepatitis, leptospirosis, malaria, hereditary spherocytosis and other hemolytic anemias, and portal vein thrombosis secondary to chronic liver disease.
4. **Is there lymphadenopathy?** The presence of lymphadenopathy should suggest infectious mononucleosis, acute lymphatic leukemia, lymphoma, brucellosis, and reticuloendotheliosis.
5. **Is there a history of trauma?** The presence of a history of trauma would suggest a traumatic rupture of the spleen.

DIAGNOSTIC WORKUP

Routine tests include a CBC, platelet count, sedimentation rate, chemistry panel, febrile agglutinins, serum haptoglobins, ANA test, monospot test, serum protein electrophoresis, tuberculin test, chest x-ray, EKG, and flat plate of the abdomen.

If there is jaundice, a hepatitis profile, red cell fragility test, and blood smear for parasites should be done. If there is fever, serial blood cultures, leptospirosis antibody titer, and smear for malarial parasites should be done. If there is a petechial rash, a coagulation profile should be done. Lymph node biopsies and bone marrow examinations may be necessary. A CT scan of the abdomen and radionuclide scan for liver and spleen size and ratio should be done. The assistance of a hematologist or infectious disease expert should be sought. A surgeon may need to be consulted for an exploratory laparotomy.

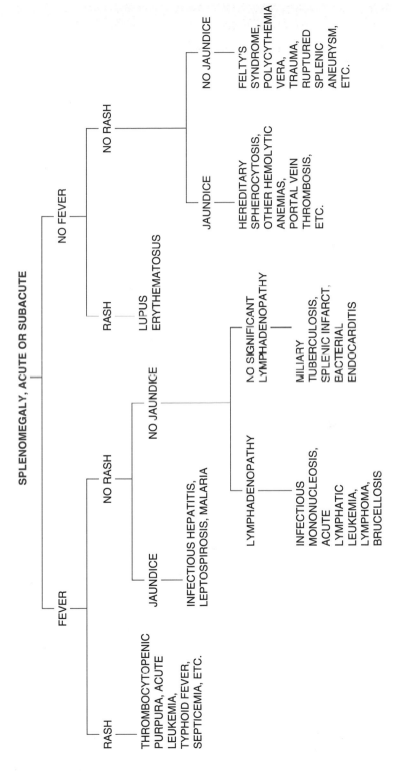

SPLENOMEGALY, ACUTE OR SUBACUTE

FEVER

RASH

THROMBOCYTOPENIC PURPURA, ACUTE LEUKEMIA, TYPHOID FEVER, SEPTICEMIA, ETC.

NO RASH

JAUNDICE

INFECTIOUS HEPATITIS, LEPTOSPIROSIS, MALARIA

NO JAUNDICE

LYMPHADENOPATHY

INFECTIOUS MONONUCLEOSIS, ACUTE LYMPHATIC LEUKEMIA, LYMPHOMA, BRUCELLOSIS

NO SIGNIFICANT LYMPHADENOPATHY

MILIARY TUBERCULOSIS, SPLENIC INFARCT, BACTERIAL ENDOCARDITIS

NO FEVER

RASH

LUPUS ERYTHEMATOSUS

NO RASH

JAUNDICE

HEREDITARY SPHEROCYTOSIS, OTHER HEMOLYTIC ANEMIAS, PORTAL VEIN THROMBOSIS, ETC.

NO JAUNDICE

FELTY'S SYNDROME, POLYCYTHEMIA VERA, TRAUMA, RUPTURED SPLENIC ANEURYSM, ETC.

SPLENOMEGALY, CHRONIC

ASK THE FOLLOWING QUESTIONS:

1. **Is it massive?** Massive splenomegaly is characteristic of Gaucher's disease, chronic myeloid leukemia, kala azar, and agnogenic myeloid metaplasia.
2. **Is there jaundice?** The presence of jaundice with massive splenomegaly would suggest chronic malaria. The presence of jaundice with mild to moderate splenomegaly would suggest alcoholic cirrhosis, chronic hepatitis, and hereditary spherocytosis.
3. **Is there hepatomegaly?** The presence of massive splenomegaly and hepatomegaly is characteristic of Gaucher's disease, chronic myeloid leukemia, kala azar, and agnogenic myeloid metaplasia.
4. **Is there pallor?** The presence of pallor, of course, suggests anemia and that would make one think of hereditary spherocytosis and other hemolytic anemias, collagen disease, and chronic malaria.
5. **Is there lymphadenopathy?** The presence of lymphadenopathy should make one think of chronic lymphatic leukemia, lymphomas, and sarcoidosis.

DIAGNOSTIC WORKUP

The diagnostic workup of chronic splenomegaly is similar to that for acute splenomegaly (page 452). A splenoportogram may be helpful in diagnosing portal vein thrombosis. Angiography may be helpful in diagnosing a splenic aneurysm. A liver biopsy, splenic aspiration and biopsy, and bone marrow biopsy may all be helpful in diagnosing reticuloendothelioses such as Gaucher's disease.

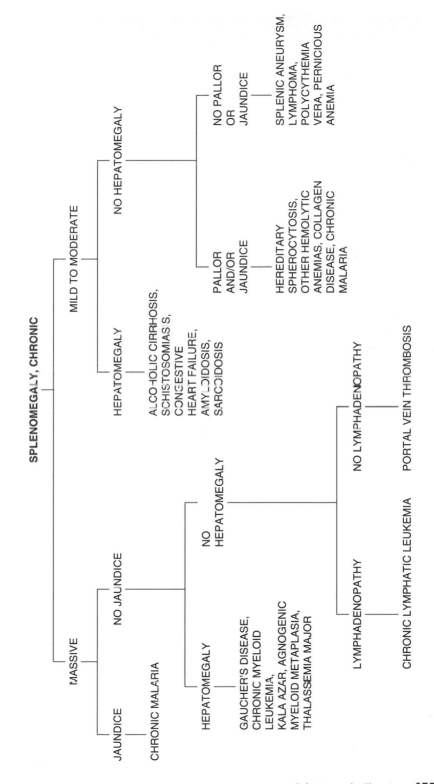

SPLENOMEGALY, CHRONIC

MASSIVE

JAUNDICE — CHRONIC MALARIA

NO JAUNDICE

HEPATOMEGALY — GAUCHER'S DISEASE, CHRONIC MYELOID LEUKEMIA, KALA AZAR, AGNOGENIC MYELOID METAPLASIA, THALASSEMIA MAJOR

NO HEPATOMEGALY

LYMPHADENOPATHY — CHRONIC LYMPHATIC LEUKEMIA

NO LYMPHADENOPATHY — PORTAL VEIN THROMBOSIS

MILD TO MODERATE

HEPATOMEGALY — ALCOHOLIC CIRRHOSIS, SCHISTOSOMIAS S, CONGESTIVE HEART FAILURE, AMYLOIDOSIS, SARCOIDOSIS

NO HEPATOMEGALY

PALLOR AND/OR JAUNDICE — HEREDITARY SPHEROCYTOSIS, OTHER HEMOLYTIC ANEMIAS, COLLAGEN DISEASE, CHRONIC MALARIA

NO PALLOR OR JAUNDICE — SPLENIC ANEURYSM, LYMPHOMA, POLYCYTHEMIA VERA, PERNICIOUS ANEMIA

⊙ SQUINT

Squint simply means the eyes do not line up evenly. In other words, one eye deviates to the left or the right compared to the other. The eyes may be concomitant, in which case the alignment remains the same during extraocular movements, or they may be nonconcomitant, in which case the alignment or amount of deviation changes with movement of the eyes.

Concomitant strabismus is almost always congenital and the result of birth trauma or anoxia. Rather than performing a diagnostic workup, the clinician should simply refer the patient to an ophthalmologist.

Nonconcomitant strabismus is due to paralysis of the extraocular muscles. The differential diagnosis of this disorder is discussed under Diplopia (page 122).

STEATORRHEA

ASK THE FOLLOWING QUESTIONS:

1. **Is the patient a child or an adult?** Children with steatorrhea may have celiac disease, cystic fibrosis, or tropical sprue.
2. **Are there associated respiratory symptoms?** The presence of respiratory symptoms should suggest cystic fibrosis, regardless of whether the patient is an adult or a child.
3. **Is there jaundice?** The presence of jaundice would suggest obstructive jaundice such as that due to biliary cirrhosis and other disorders.
4. **Is there pallor and anemia?** The presence of pallor or anemia suggests malabsorption syndrome, blind loop syndrome, intestinal parasites such as *Diphyllobothrium latum,* scleroderma, amyloidosis, and chronic obstructive jaundice.
5. **Are there signs of systemic disease?** If there are signs of systemic disease, scleroderma, amyloidosis, and cystic fibrosis should be considered.
6. **Is there an abdominal mass?** The presence of an abdominal mass should suggest obstructive jaundice, pancreatic carcinoma, and hemochromatosis. Chronic pancreatitis may also present with an abdominal mass if there is a pseudocyst of the pancreas.

DIAGNOSTIC WORKUP

The basic workup includes a CBC, a blood smear for cell morphology, sedimentation rate, urinalysis, chemistry panel, serum B_{12} and folic acid, serum amylase and lipase, stool for occult blood, ovum and parasites, fat and trypsin, and urine for 5-HIAA.

A sweat test should be done if cystic fibrosis is suspected. A D-xylose absorption test will help differentiate primary diseases of the small intestines. An abnormal yield of labeled carbon dioxide after ingestion of a meal with radioactive ^{14}C-glycocholate will help diagnose bacterial overgrowth. An upper GI series and small bowel follow-through may be helpful. Intubation and analysis of pancreatic secretion of enzymes after pancreozymin or secretin injection will help differentiate pancreatic disorders. A CT scan of the abdomen and endoscopy may be useful. Intestinal biopsy with a Crosby capsule may help differentiate primary intestinal diseases also. Consult a gastroenterologist before ordering many of these expensive diagnostic tests.

A therapeutic trial with pancreatic enzymes, antibiotics, or even a gluten-free diet may also assist in the diagnosis.

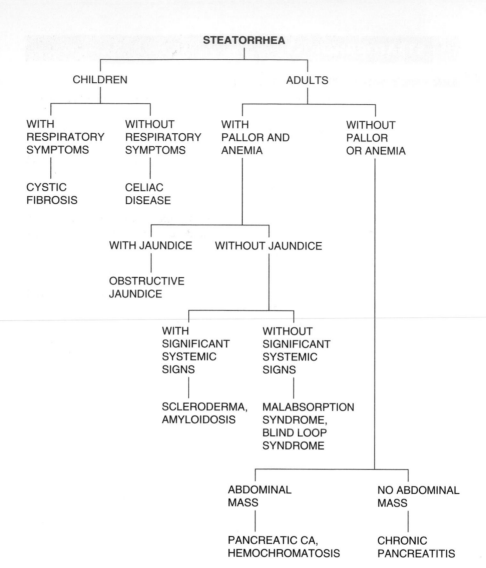

STRANGURY

ASK THE FOLLOWING QUESTIONS:

1. **Is there fever?** The presence of fever suggests acute pyelonephritis or acute prostatitis.
2. **Is there a urethral discharge?** The presence of a urethral discharge is suspicious for urethritis, gonorrhea, or prostatitis.
3. **Is there hematuria?** This makes cystitis, vesicular calculus, vesicular tumor, or tuberculosis very likely.
4. **Is there a pelvic mass?** In this case, one should consider uterine fibroids, ovarian cyst, or tumor pressing on the bladder.
5. If none of the above associated signs is present, one should consider hemorrhoids, anal fissure, tabes dorsalis, or bladder neck obstruction as the most likely cause.

DIAGNOSTIC WORKUP

This will include a CBC, urinalysis, chemistry panel, urine culture, sensitivity and colony count, urethral smear, vaginal smear and culture in females, and cultures for gonorrhea or chlamydia if the history dictates it. If these tests fail to detect the cause, a urologist must be consulted for cystoscopy and intravenous or retrograde pyelography. A vaginal and rectal examination should be done in all cases.

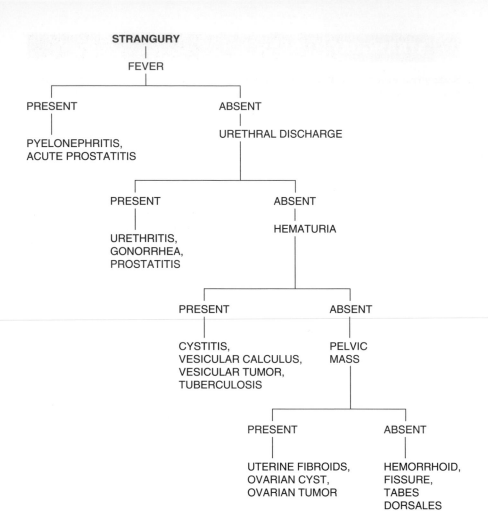

Stress incontinence occurs most commonly in women who have had many pregnancies or who are in menopause. The patient loses control of the bladder when he or she coughs, laughs, or sneezes and consequently leaks small amounts of urine. Nocturia is rare in stress incontinence. There is often an associated cystocele. In postmenopausal women, there is often an atrophic vaginitis due to the deficiency of estrogen. Men occasionally develop stress incontinence following a prostatectomy.

DIAGNOSTIC WORKUP

In most cases, the diagnosis will be obvious. You can ask the patient to cough during a vaginal examination, and the urine will trickle out. If that does not establish the diagnosis, have the patient drink a lot of water and not void until he or she returns to the office. Then you can have him or her cough in the recumbent or erect position, and the urine will be released. This is called a stress test. In the Q-tip test, a Q-tip is inserted in the tip of the urethra, and the patient is asked to cough or strain. The Q-tip will move at least 30 degrees above the horizontal in cases of stress incontinence. A therapeutic trial of local or systemic estrogen may be helpful. For further discussion of incontinence, see page 272.

STRETCH MARKS (STRIAE)

Stretch marks are common in obese patients or during pregnancy, in which case they are of no pathologic significance. However, purple striae of the abdomen, especially when they are associated with moon facies or a buffalo hump, should immediately call to mind Cushing's syndrome. Patients on prolonged corticosteroid therapy also develop purple striae. The workup is the same as for Cushing's syndrome (page 345).

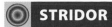

ASK THE FOLLOWING QUESTIONS:

1. **Is the patient an adult or a child?** If the patient is a child, acute epiglottitis, acute laryngotracheitis, foreign body, congenital laryngeal stridor, laryngismus stridulus, and a retropharyngeal abscess should be considered. Diphtheria is rarely found nowadays. If the patient is an adult, myasthenia gravis, bulbar and pseudobulbar palsy, recurrent laryngeal palsy, pharyngitis, laryngotracheitis, carcinoma of the larynx or trachea, angioneurotic edema, foreign bodies, thyroid disorders, and disorders of the mediastinum should be considered.

2. **Is it acute or gradual onset?** The presence of stridor of acute onset would suggest acute epiglottitis, acute pharyngitis, laryngotracheitis, angioneurotic edema, retropharyngeal abscess, laryngismus stridulus, and foreign body.

3. **Is there fever?** The presence of fever would suggest acute laryngotracheitis, diphtheria, subacute thyroiditis, retropharyngeal abscess, and mediastinitis.

4. **Are there abnormalities on the ear, nose, and throat examination?** On ear, nose, and throat examination, the clinician may find pharyngitis, acute epiglottitis, a foreign body, tenderness of the thyroid suggesting thyroiditis, and thyroid masses.

5. **Are there neurologic abnormalities on examination?** Neurologic abnormalities may be found in myasthenia gravis, bulbar and pseudobulbar palsy, bilateral recurrent laryngeal nerve palsy, and comatose states.

DIAGNOSTIC WORKUP

Routine tests may include a CBC; sedimentation rate, smear and culture of material from the nose, throat, and sputum; x-ray of the chest and sinuses; and, in adults, an EKG. In adults, it might also be wise to order a chemistry panel, thyroid profile, and VDRL test, depending on the clinical picture. Direct laryngoscopy can now be done in the office with the fiberoptic laryngoscope. In addition, fiberoptic bronchoscopy may be valuable. A Tensilon test may need to be done. An ear, nose, and throat specialist should be consulted before ordering expensive diagnostic tests. If there are neurologic signs, a neurologist should be consulted.

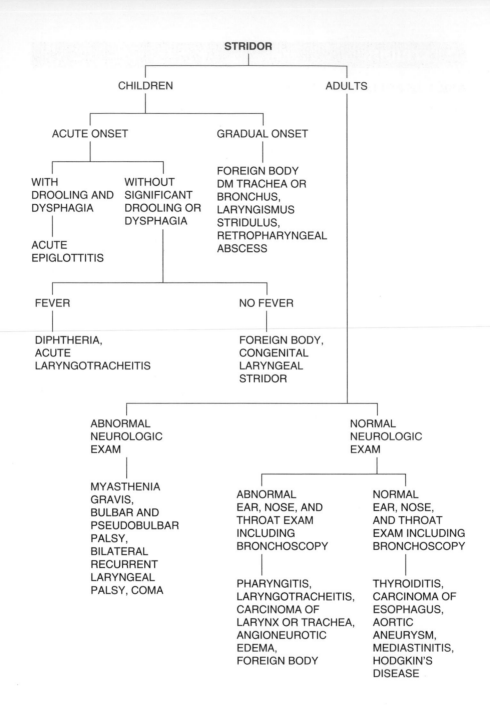

STRIDOR

CHILDREN

ADULTS

ACUTE ONSET

GRADUAL ONSET

WITH DROOLING AND DYSPHAGIA

ACUTE EPIGLOTTITIS

WITHOUT SIGNIFICANT DROOLING OR DYSPHAGIA

FOREIGN BODY DM TRACHEA OR BRONCHUS, LARYNGISMUS STRIDULUS, RETROPHARYNGEAL ABSCESS

FEVER

DIPHTHERIA, ACUTE LARYNGOTRACHEITIS

NO FEVER

FOREIGN BODY, CONGENITAL LARYNGEAL STRIDOR

ABNORMAL NEUROLOGIC EXAM

MYASTHENIA GRAVIS, BULBAR AND PSEUDOBULBAR PALSY, BILATERAL RECURRENT LARYNGEAL PALSY, COMA

NORMAL NEUROLOGIC EXAM

ABNORMAL EAR, NOSE, AND THROAT EXAM INCLUDING BRONCHOSCOPY

PHARYNGITIS, LARYNGOTRACHEITIS, CARCINOMA OF LARYNX OR TRACHEA, ANGIONEUROTIC EDEMA, FOREIGN BODY

NORMAL EAR, NOSE, AND THROAT EXAM INCLUDING BRONCHOSCOPY

THYROIDITIS, CARCINOMA OF ESOPHAGUS, AORTIC ANEURYSM, MEDIASTINITIS, HODGKIN'S DISEASE

STUPOR

ASK THE FOLLOWING QUESTIONS:

1. **Is it intermittent?** Intermittent stupor should suggest epilepsy, chronic illicit drug use, transient ischemic attacks, migraine, and insulinoma.
2. **Is there a positive drug or alcohol history?** This finding would suggest cocaine, barbiturate, alcohol, morphine, LSD, or PCP abuse.
3. **Are there focal neurologic signs?** The presence of focal neurologic signs may mean cerebral vascular disease, advanced brain tumor, cerebral abscess, encephalitis, subdural hematoma, central nervous system lues, Wernicke's encephalopathy, and subarachnoid hemorrhage or meningitis.
4. **Is there nuchal rigidity?** The presence of nuchal rigidity would suggest a subarachnoid hemorrhage or meningitis, but it could occasionally indicate an intracerebral hemorrhage.
5. **Is there a distinguishing odor to the breath?** Besides alcohol, uremia, diabetic acidosis, and liver failure may be suggested by a characteristic odor to the breath.

DIAGNOSTIC WORKUP

Routine tests may include a CBC, sedimentation rate, urinalysis, chemistry panel with electrolytes, arterial blood gas analysis, blood and urine drug and alcohol screen, EEG, and CT scan of the brain. A spinal tap may be done if the CT scan is negative for a space-occupying lesion. A neurologist or neurosurgeon should have been contacted by this time. A cerebral vascular disease may need further investigation, including carotid duplex scan and cerebral angiography.

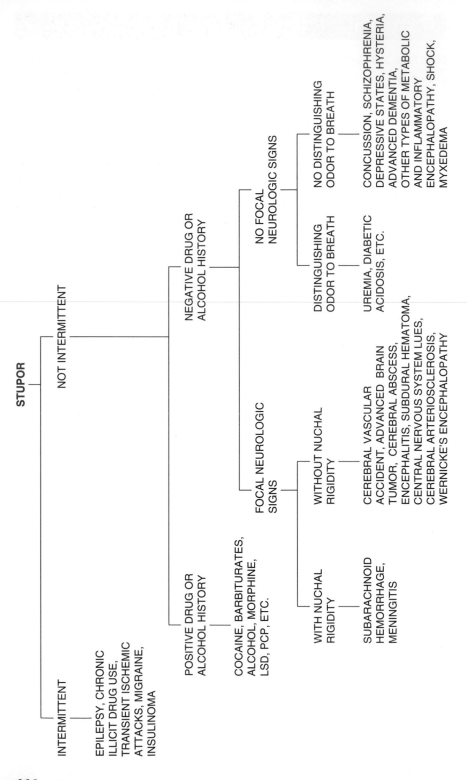

STUPOR

INTERMITTENT
- EPILEPSY, CHRONIC ILLICIT DRUG USE, TRANSIENT ISCHEMIC ATTACKS, MIGRAINE, INSULINOMA

NOT INTERMITTENT

POSITIVE DRUG OR ALCOHOL HISTORY
- COCAINE, BARBITURATES, ALCOHOL, MORPHINE, LSD, PCP, ETC.

NEGATIVE DRUG OR ALCOHOL HISTORY

FOCAL NEUROLOGIC SIGNS

WITH NUCHAL RIGIDITY
- SUBARACHNOID HEMORRHAGE, MENINGITIS

WITHOUT NUCHAL RIGIDITY
- CEREBRAL VASCULAR ACCIDENT, ADVANCED BRAIN TUMOR, CEREBRAL ABSCESS, ENCEPHALITIS, SUBDURAL HEMATOMA, CENTRAL NERVOUS SYSTEM LUES, CEREBRAL ARTERIOSCLEROSIS, WERNICKE'S ENCEPHALOPATHY

NO FOCAL NEUROLOGIC SIGNS

DISTINGUISHING ODOR TO BREATH
- UREMIA, DIABETIC ACIDOSIS, ETC.

NO DISTINGUISHING ODOR TO BREATH
- CONCUSSION, SCHIZOPHRENIA, DEPRESSIVE STATES, HYSTERIA, ADVANCED DEMENTIA, OTHER TYPES OF METABOLIC AND INFLAMMATORY ENCEPHALOPATHY, SHOCK, MYXEDEMA

Most of us have heard these sounds on ourselves after consuming a large quantity of liquid. If they are heard with the stethoscope in a patient with abdominal disturbance, they are of pathologic significance. When there are associated hyperactive and/or high-pitched bowel sounds, intestinal obstruction should be considered. When there are hypoactive bowel sounds, paralytic ileus or peritonitis should be considered.

Succussion sounds coming from the chest are due to hydropneumothorax or hemopneumothorax. The chest x-ray should make the diagnosis obvious. Other rare causes of succussion sounds are acute gastric dilatation, chronic pyloric obstruction, subdiaphragmatic abscess, and pneumoperitoneum. The diagnostic workup will be determined by associated symptoms and signs (vomiting, page 334; abdominal pain, page 1; abdominal mass, page 9).

CASE HISTORY

A 32-year-old white female is brought to your office by her husband who is very concerned about her frequent episodes of fainting during the past 3 months. Following the algorithm, you ask about convulsive movements, incontinence or tongue lacerations following these episodes and there are none of these signs.

Examination shows a normal pulse, no murmurs or cardiomegaly, and the conjunctivae are not pale. Neurologic examination is negative. On further questioning the patient tells you, she gets numbness and tingling of her lips and fingers just before she passes out. The husband confirms that the patient has rapid deep breathing during these attacks confirming your suspicions of hyperventilation syndrome.

ASK THE FOLLOWING QUESTIONS:

1. **Are there convulsive movements or incontinence?** The presence of convulsive movements should suggest convulsions, and the differential diagnosis of this is discussed in page 92. However, convulsive movements can occur with other forms of syncope. A slow recovery phase or Todd's paralysis suggests epilepsy.
2. **Is the pulse slow or absent?** The presence of a slow or absent pulse would suggest heart block, vasovagal syncope, and carotid sinus syncope.
3. **Is the pulse rate normal?** The presence of a normal pulse rate would suggest anemia, aortic stenosis, aortic insufficiency, and cyanotic congenital heart disease.
4. **Is the pulse rate rapid?** The presence of a rapid pulse would suggest the various types of ventricular and supraventricular tachycardias, including auricular fibrillation and flutter, and it should also suggest heat exhaustion or heat stroke.
5. **If the pulse is rapid, is it regular?** The presence of a rapid regular pulse should suggest supraventricular or ventricular tachycardia, heat exhaustion, or heat stroke. Carotid sinus massage can help distinguish supraventricular tachycardia from sinus tachycardia.
6. **Is there a heart murmur?** The presence of a heart murmur should suggest aortic stenosis, aortic insufficiency, and cyanotic congenital heart disease.
7. **Is there pallor?** The presence of pallor should suggest shock or severe anemia and acute bleeding.
8. **Are there focal neurologic signs?** The presence of focal neurologic signs should suggest cerebral vascular insufficiency, hypoglycemia, and transient ischemic attacks.
9. **What drugs is the patient on?** Many antihypertensive drugs are associated with syncope.

DIAGNOSTIC WORKUP

The diagnostic workup includes a CBC, sedimentation rate, urinalysis, chemistry panel, pregnancy test, VDRL test, thyroid profile, glucose tolerance test, EKG, and chest x-ray. Several blood pressure recordings in the recumbent and upright positions should be made. If hypoglycemia is suspected, a 72-hr fast and a tolbutamide tolerance test should be done. The drug history should always be reviewed. A toxicology screen may be helpful. A serum prolactin can be drawn to distinguish hysterical seizures from true epilepsy.

Most cases will require 24-hr Holter monitoring or event Holter monitoring. This may not only pick up heart block and tachyarrhythmias, but also syncope, induced by exercise or the prolonged QT syndrome. In addition, other cardiovascular studies, such as echocardiography and His' bundle studies, may need to be done. Exercise tolerance testing is useful when the syncope seems to be exercise induced. An upright-tilt test is helpful when vasodepressor syncope is suspected, especially when combined with isoproterenol infusion. Signal-averaged EKG can be useful if a ventricular arrhythmia is suspected. If transient ischemic attacks are suspected, a carotid scan and cerebral angiography may be necessary. If the syncopal attacks are thought to be due to epilepsy, a wake-and-sleep EEG may need to be done. A CT scan or MRI of the brain may need to be done.

A cardiologist or neurologist should be consulted before ordering expensive diagnostic tests. A psychiatrist may also need to be consulted.

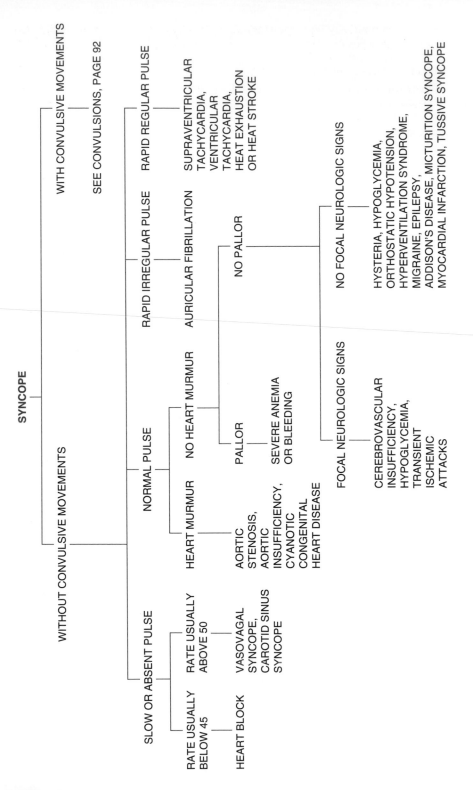

SYNCOPE

WITHOUT CONVULSIVE MOVEMENTS

WITH CONVULSIVE MOVEMENTS

SEE CONVULSIONS, PAGE 92

SLOW OR ABSENT PULSE

NORMAL PULSE

RAPID IRREGULAR PULSE

RAPID REGULAR PULSE

RATE USUALLY BELOW 45

HEART BLOCK

RATE USUALLY ABOVE 50

VASOVAGAL SYNCOPE, CAROTID SINUS SYNCOPE

HEART MURMUR

AORTIC STENOSIS, AORTIC INSUFFICIENCY, CYANOTIC CONGENITAL HEART DISEASE

NO HEART MURMUR

PALLOR

SEVERE ANEMIA OR BLEEDING

NO PALLOR

FOCAL NEUROLOGIC SIGNS

CEREBROVASCULAR INSUFFICIENCY, HYPOGLYCEMIA, TRANSIENT ISCHEMIC ATTACKS

NO FOCAL NEUROLOGIC SIGNS

HYSTERIA, HYPOGLYCEMIA, ORTHOSTATIC HYPOTENSION, HYPERVENTILATION SYNDROME, MIGRAINE, EPILEPSY, ADDISON'S DISEASE, MICTURITION SYNCOPE, MYOCARDIAL INFARCTION, TUSSIVE SYNCOPE

AURICULAR FIBRILLATION

SUPRAVENTRICULAR TACHYCARDIA, VENTRICULAR TACHYCARDIA, HEAT EXHAUSTION OR HEAT STROKE

TACHYCARDIA

ASK THE FOLLOWING QUESTIONS:

1. **Is there a positive alcohol or drug history?** It is well known that alcohol can cause a myocardiopathy. Atropine, caffeine, and many other substances can cause a tachycardia.

2. **Is the heart rate below 160 and/or reduced by carotid sinus massage?** This finding would help confirm the diagnosis of sinus tachycardia and lead to a consideration of fever, thyrotoxicosis, shock, anemia, myocardial infarction, and other disorders as the cause of the tachycardia.

3. **Is there fever?** The presence of fever and tachycardia should make one suspect acute infectious diseases, rheumatic fever, and thyroid storm.

4. **Is there a tremor, neck mass, or systolic hypertension?** These findings suggest thyrotoxicosis.

5. **Is there chest pain?** The presence of chest pain should make one suspect myocardial infarction, pulmonary embolism, and acute pericarditis.

6. **Is there pallor or sweating?** The presence of pallor or sweating should make one think of anemia and shock.

7. **Are there crepitant rales, an enlarged liver, or peripheral edema?** These findings suggest congestive heart failure.

8. **Is there hypotension?** The presence of hypotension should make one think that there may be a pathologic tachycardia such as supraventricular tachycardia, auricular flutter, or auricular fibrillation. Auricular fibrillation is especially likely to be associated with significant hypotension.

9. **Is the rate irregular?** The presence of an irregular heart rate should make one suspect auricular fibrillation, or alternating flutter and fibrillation.

DIAGNOSTIC WORKUP

Routine diagnostic tests should include a CBC, sedimentation rate, urinalysis, chemistry panel, toxicology screen, thyroid profile, ANA titer, VDRL test, chest x-ray, and EKG. If there is fever, then an ASO titer and CRP, febrile agglutinins, and serial blood cultures should be done.

If a myocardial infarction is suspected, serial EKGs and cardiac enzymes need to be ordered. If a pulmonary embolism or infarction is suspected, arterial blood gases and lung scans need to be ordered, and, ultimately, pulmonary angiography may need to be done.

If congestive heart failure is suspected, a venous pressure and circulation time, BNP and possibly pulmonary function studies may be done. Echocardiography may be done to determine the LVEF.

If the tachycardia is paroxysmal, 24-hr Holter monitoring or admission to the hospital for ambulatory telemetry and observation may be necessary. A cardiologist should be consulted. Ultimately, a psychiatrist may need to be consulted also.

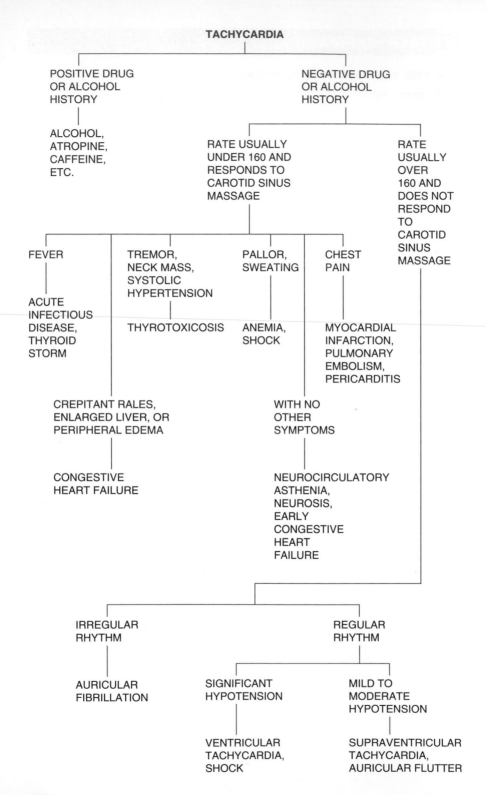

TACHYCARDIA

POSITIVE DRUG OR ALCOHOL HISTORY

ALCOHOL, ATROPINE, CAFFEINE, ETC.

NEGATIVE DRUG OR ALCOHOL HISTORY

RATE USUALLY UNDER 160 AND RESPONDS TO CAROTID SINUS MASSAGE

RATE USUALLY OVER 160 AND DOES NOT RESPOND TO CAROTID SINUS MASSAGE

FEVER

ACUTE INFECTIOUS DISEASE, THYROID STORM

TREMOR, NECK MASS, SYSTOLIC HYPERTENSION

THYROTOXICOSIS

PALLOR, SWEATING

ANEMIA, SHOCK

CHEST PAIN

MYOCARDIAL INFARCTION, PULMONARY EMBOLISM, PERICARDITIS

CREPITANT RALES, ENLARGED LIVER, OR PERIPHERAL EDEMA

CONGESTIVE HEART FAILURE

WITH NO OTHER SYMPTOMS

NEUROCIRCULATORY ASTHENIA, NEUROSIS, EARLY CONGESTIVE HEART FAILURE

IRREGULAR RHYTHM

AURICULAR FIBRILLATION

REGULAR RHYTHM

SIGNIFICANT HYPOTENSION

VENTRICULAR TACHYCARDIA, SHOCK

MILD TO MODERATE HYPOTENSION

SUPRAVENTRICULAR TACHYCARDIA, AURICULAR FLUTTER

ASK THE FOLLOWING QUESTIONS:

1. **Is there distortion of the taste?** Distortion of the taste occurs episodically in uncinate fits of epilepsy and is persistent in hysteria, pregnancy, schizophrenia, glossitis, and jaundice.
2. **If there is distortion, is it constant or intermittent?** If the distortion of the taste is episodic, one should look for uncinate fits of epilepsy.
3. **Is there a positive history of drug or poison ingestion?** This finding should suggest penicillamine, mercury, bismuth, iodine, or bromide toxicity.
4. **Is the ear, nose, and throat or oral examination abnormal?** Abnormalities that may be found on an ear, nose, and throat or oral examination include glossitis, gingivitis, stomatitis, dental caries, rhinitis, and hay fever.
5. **Is the neurologic examination abnormal?** Abnormalities on the neurologic examination may suggest Bell's palsy, temporomandibular joint syndrome, petrositis, and brainstem lesions.

DIAGNOSTIC WORKUP

Routine diagnostic tests include a CBC, sedimentation rate, chemistry panel, urinalysis, urine drug screen, and a chest x-ray. If the ear, nose, and throat or oral examination is revealing, the patient should be referred to an ear, nose, and throat specialist or oral surgeon. If the neurologic examination is abnormal, referral to a neurologist should be considered. A wake-and-sleep EEG with nasopharyngeal electrodes and a CT scan of the brain may be necessary to determine the cause or the diagnosis of uncinate fits. A psychiatrist may need to be consulted if the patient is suspected of a neurosis.

TASTE ABNORMALITIES

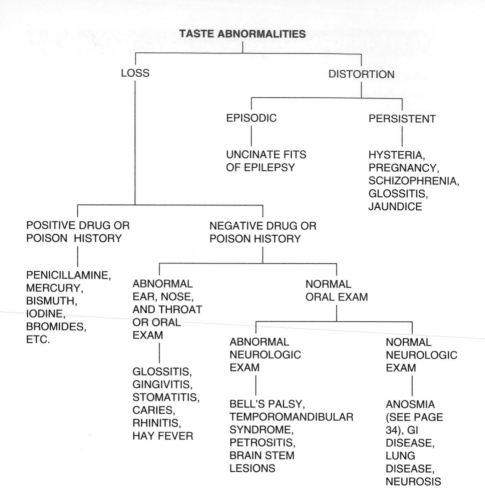

⊙ TESTICULAR ATROPHY

ASK THE FOLLOWING QUESTIONS:

1. **Is it unilateral?** The presence of unilateral atrophy would suggest hernia surgery, previous orchitis from mumps, gonorrhea, syphilis, tuberculosis or elephantiasis, varicocele, hydrocele, and an undescended testicle.
2. **Is there a history of trauma or surgery?** A history of surgery would suggest that the testicular atrophy is related to hernia surgery or surgery for undescended testicle, vasectomy, or prostatectomy. History of trauma may suggest that the patient had an acute orchitis or hemorrhage from trauma.
3. **Is there a history of an infection?** A history of infection would suggest mumps, gonorrhea, syphilis, tuberculosis, or elephantiasis.
4. **Is there a loss of secondary sex characteristics?** These findings would suggest Klinefelter's syndrome.
5. **Is there an enlarged liver?** The presence of an enlarged liver or other signs of hepatic dysfunction would suggest cirrhosis or hemochromatosis.
6. **Are there abnormal neurologic findings?** The presence of abnormal neurologic findings would suggest myotonia atrophica.

DIAGNOSTIC WORKUP

Unilateral testicular atrophy usually requires no workup as long as there are no complaints of sexual infertility or impotence. A smear and culture of any urethral discharge should be done. Sometimes, prostatic massage may be necessary to obtain a good specimen.

The workup of bilateral testicular atrophy may include a serum testosterone, FSH, urine gonadotrophins, and chromosome studies to rule out Klinefelter's syndrome; liver function tests and liver biopsy to rule out cirrhosis and hemochromatosis; and EMG and muscle biopsies to rule out myotonia atrophica. A testicular biopsy may be necessary ultimately. A urologist will be consulted long before most of these tests would be performed.

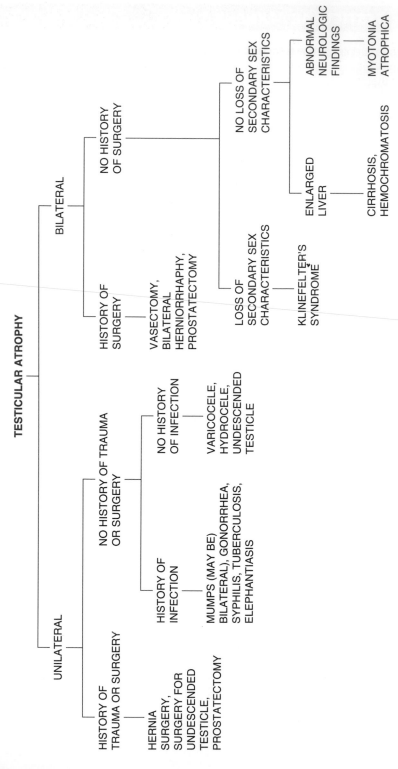

TESTICULAR ATROPHY

UNILATERAL

HISTORY OF TRAUMA OR SURGERY

HERNIA SURGERY, SURGERY FOR UNDESCENDED TESTICLE, PROSTATECTOMY

NO HISTORY OF TRAUMA OR SURGERY

HISTORY OF INFECTION

MUMPS (MAY BE) BILATERAL), GONORRHEA, SYPHILIS, TUBERCULOSIS, ELEPHANTIASIS

NO HISTORY OF INFECTION

VARICOCELE, HYDROCELE, UNDESCENDED TESTICLE

BILATERAL

HISTORY OF SURGERY

VASECTOMY, BILATERAL HERNIORRHAPHY, PROSTATECTOMY

NO HISTORY OF SURGERY

LOSS OF SECONDARY SEX CHARACTERISTICS

KLINEFELTER'S SYNDROME

NO LOSS OF SECONDARY SEX CHARACTERISTICS

ENLARGED LIVER

CIRRHOSIS, HEMOCHROMATOSIS

ABNORMAL NEUROLOGIC FINDINGS

MYOTONIA ATROPHICA

⊚ TESTICULAR PAIN

It is rare for pain in the testicle to occur without a mass. Therefore, the algorithmic diagnosis is essentially the same as that of testicular swelling (page 478). Keep in mind that there are cases of orchitis, epididymitis, and torsion not associated with testicular swelling. Also, in cases of renal colic (nephrolithiasis, etc.) and herniated lumbar disk, pain may be referred to the testicle.

TESTICULAR SWELLING

ASK THE FOLLOWING QUESTIONS:

1. **Is there pain or tenderness of the testicle?** The presence of pain or tenderness should suggest torsion of the testicle, orchitis, epididymitis, and a strangulated inguinal hernia.
2. **Is the testicle retracted or does elevation of the testicle aggravate the pain?** These findings would suggest torsion of the testicle. An absent cremasteric reflex should also suggest torsion.
3. **Does the swelling transilluminate?** If the swelling transilluminates, the mass or swelling is most likely a hydrocele or spermatocele.
4. **Is the swelling reducible?** If the swelling is reducible, the mass is probably an inguinal hernia or varicocele. A mass that does not reduce could still be an incarcerated inguinal hernia.

DIAGNOSTIC WORKUP

A CBC, sedimentation rate, urinalysis, chemistry panel, and VDRL test should be done routinely. If a tumor of the testicle is suspected, 24-hr urine gonadotrophins and alpha-fetoprotein levels may be ordered. If there is a urethral discharge, a smear and culture for gonorrhea and chlamydia should be done. If a hernia is strongly suspected, a general surgeon should be consulted. Testicular scans with technetium-99m and ultrasonography will help distinguish torsion of the testicle from orchitis or epididymitis. Scrotal ultrasound may also be useful in differentiating a hematoma, abscess, or rupture from orchitis. It may also be helpful in evaluating testicular tumors. CT scan of the abdomen and pelvis may be necessary to rule out metastasis.

The expense of some or all of these tests may be avoided by consulting a urologist early in the diagnostic workup.

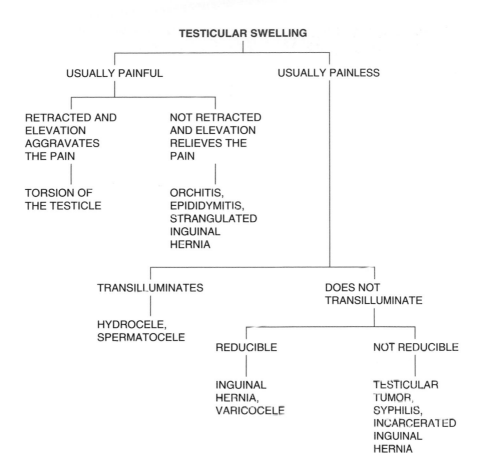

ASK THE FOLLOWING QUESTIONS:

1. **Is there a positive drug or alcohol history?** Alcohol, amitriptyline, diuretics, and many other drugs may cause excessive thirst.
2. **Is there fever?** The presence of fever would make one suspect an infectious disease (see page 177).
3. **Is there pallor or shock?** Pallor or shock should make one think of GI bleeding, ruptured ectopic pregnancy, trauma, and other disorders associated with anemia or shock.
4. **Is there significant polyuria?** Polyuria that is either significant or massive would suggest diabetes insipidus, diabetes mellitus, or thyrotoxicosis. Mild or insignificant polyuria may be due to hypercalcemia, hyperparathyroidism, and excessive salt intake.

DIAGNOSTIC WORKUP

Routine tests include a CBC, sedimentation rate, urinalysis, chemistry panel, thyroid panel, glucose tolerance test, blood alcohol level, and 24-hr urine collection for sodium, potassium, and calcium. If pituitary diabetes insipidus is suspected, a CT scan of the brain, the Hickey–Hare test, and a vasopressin (Pitressin®) injection test may need to be done. If hyperparathyroidism is suspected, a serum parathyroid hormone assay and x-rays of the skull and long bones may be done. A consultation with an endocrinologist may be necessary.

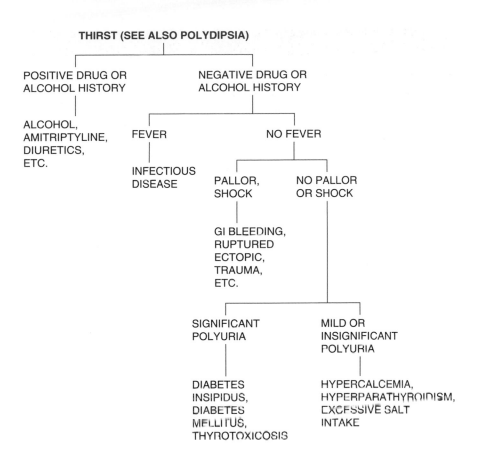

THIRST (SEE ALSO POLYDIPSIA)

POSITIVE DRUG OR ALCOHOL HISTORY

NEGATIVE DRUG OR ALCOHOL HISTORY

ALCOHOL, AMITRIPTYLINE, DIURETICS, ETC.

FEVER

NO FEVER

INFECTIOUS DISEASE

PALLOR, SHOCK

NO PALLOR OR SHOCK

GI BLEEDING, RUPTURED ECTOPIC, TRAUMA, ETC.

SIGNIFICANT POLYURIA

MILD OR INSIGNIFICANT POLYURIA

DIABETES INSIPIDUS, DIABETES MELLITUS, THYROTOXICOSIS

HYPERCALCEMIA, HYPERPARATHYROIDISM, EXCESSIVE SALT INTAKE

THROMBOCYTOPENIA

ASK THE FOLLOWING QUESTIONS:

1. **What is the WBC count?** Thrombocytopenia with a high white count suggests leukemia or myeloid metaplasia. Thrombocytopenia with a normal white count suggests idiopathic thrombocytopenic purpura or drug reaction. Thrombocytopenia with a low white count suggests lupus erythematosus, aplastic anemia, myelofibrosis, drugs, myelophthisic anemia, or pernicious anemia.
2. **What is the ANA?** A positive ANA in the face of thrombocytopenia and a low white count suggests lupus erythematosus.

DIAGNOSTIC WORKUP

The diagnostic workup should include a CBC, blood smear, sedimentation rate, urinalysis, serum B_{12}, chemistry panel, ANA, serum haptoglobins, red cell survival, liver spleen scan, CT scan of the abdomen, and a hematology consult for bone marrow study.

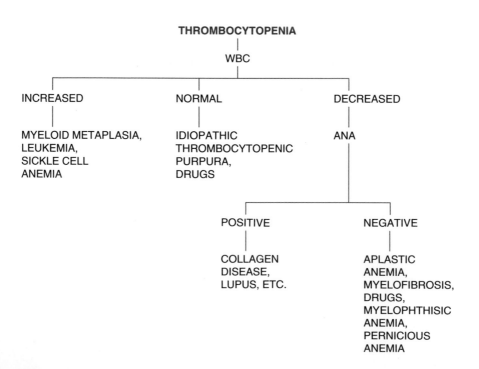

ASK THE FOLLOWING QUESTIONS:

1. **Is it focal or diffuse?** Focal masses in the thyroid include thyroglossal cyst, toxic adenoma, colloid cyst, Riedel's struma, nontoxic adenoma, and malignancies.
2. **Is there movement with protrusion of the tongue?** This is a typical finding in cases of thyroglossal cyst.
3. **If focal, are there signs of thyrotoxicosis?** The presence of thyrotoxicosis and a focal mass suggest toxic adenoma.
4. **If diffuse, are there signs of thyrotoxicosis?** Diffuse thyroid enlargement with thyrotoxicosis indicates Graves' disease.
5. **Is it tender?** The presence of a tender enlarged thyroid suggests subacute thyroiditis and Hashimoto's thyroiditis.

DIAGNOSTIC WORKUP

Routine tests include a CBC, sedimentation rate, urinalysis, thyroid profile with a TSH immunoassay, chemistry panel, chest x-ray, and EKG. Thyroid antibodies may be tested if Hashimoto's thyroiditis is suspected.

The most important study is a thyroid technetium-99m or iodine-123 uptake and scan. If the results of these are abnormal, then an endocrinologist or general surgeon should be consulted to assist in the interpretation. If the scan indicates a cold nodule, ultrasonography may be done to determine whether the nodule is cystic or solid. If it is cystic, generally it can be aspirated and followed. If it is solid, a biopsy or aspiration and biopsy should be undertaken. If there are malignant cells or at least suspicious cells for malignancy, surgery should be done. If the scan reveals a hot nodule and there is clinical and laboratory evidence of thyrotoxicosis, the patient should be treated with radioactive iodine or surgery. If the scan shows diffuse uptake of radioactive materials and there is clinical thyrotoxicosis, the patient also may be treated with radioactive iodine or surgery.

THYROID ENLARGEMENT

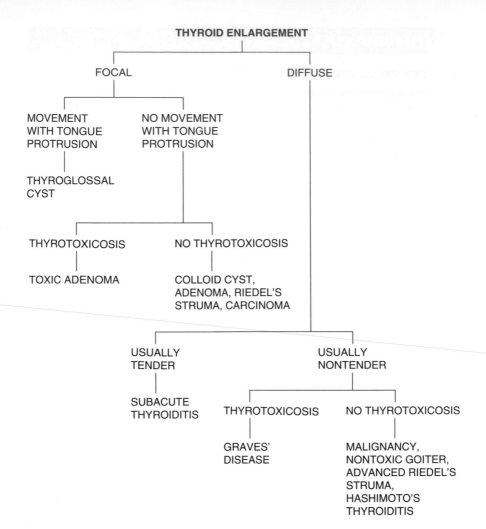

FOCAL

DIFFUSE

MOVEMENT
WITH TONGUE
PROTRUSION

NO MOVEMENT
WITH TONGUE
PROTRUSION

THYROGLOSSAL
CYST

THYROTOXICOSIS

NO THYROTOXICOSIS

TOXIC ADENOMA

COLLOID CYST,
ADENOMA, RIEDEL'S
STRUMA, CARCINOMA

USUALLY
TENDER

USUALLY
NONTENDER

SUBACUTE
THYROIDITIS

THYROTOXICOSIS

NO THYROTOXICOSIS

GRAVES'
DISEASE

MALIGNANCY,
NONTOXIC GOITER,
ADVANCED RIEDEL'S
STRUMA,
HASHIMOTO'S
THYROIDITIS

ASK THE FOLLOWING QUESTIONS:

1. **Is it subjective or objective?** Objective tinnitus is unusual, but it may indicate glomus tumors, arteriovenous malformations, carotid stenosis, aneurysms, anemia, a patent eustachian tube, or myoclonus. Objective tinnitus means that both the patient and the examiner can hear the noises.
2. **If it is subjective, is it unilateral or bilateral?** Unilateral subjective tinnitus is more likely to be associated with a more serious disorder such as Ménière's disease, acoustic neuroma, cholesteatoma, or vascular disease. Since von Recklinghausen disease is associated with acoustic neuromas, look for café au lait spots.
3. **Is there a history of trauma?** A history of trauma would suggest that the tinnitus is due to whiplash, concussion, or trauma to the middle or inner ear.
4. **Is there a history of the use of ototoxic drugs?** Drugs that may cause tinnitus include aminoglycosides, tetracyclines, clindamycin, caffeine, and the tricyclic antidepressants. Aspirin and quinine may also be associated with tinnitus.
5. **Are there abnormalities found on the ear examination?** Abnormalities on the ear examination include cerumen, otitis externa, otitis media, mastoiditis, and cholesteatomas. The tympanic membrane may be red in cases of glomus tumors.
6. **Is there vertigo and deafness?** The presence of vertigo with deafness should suggest Ménière's disease, acoustic neuroma, and cholesteatoma, as well as multiple sclerosis, basilar artery insufficiency, and brainstem tumors.
7. **Are there other neurologic signs?** The presence of other neurologic signs along with vertigo and deafness would suggest multiple sclerosis, advanced acoustic neuroma, basilar artery occlusion or insufficiency, brainstem tumors, and central nervous system syphilis.

DIAGNOSTIC WORKUP

The basic workup includes a CBC, sedimentation rate, urinalysis, chemistry panel, thyroid profile, VDRL test, audiometry, caloric tests (electronystagmography), and x-rays of the mastoids and petrous bones. Specialized audiometry may be performed, such as impedance audiometry, Békésy audiometry, and BSEP studies.

If an acoustic neuroma is strongly suspected, CT scans with iodine infusion or instillation of 4 cc of oxygen in the subarachnoid space would be indicated. Gadolinium-enhanced MRI may also diagnose an early acoustic neuroma. Angiography and venography may help diagnose objective tinnitus. A spinal tap may be helpful in diagnosing multiple sclerosis and central nervous system syphilis. A glucose tolerance test may be indicated to rule out diabetes mellitus.

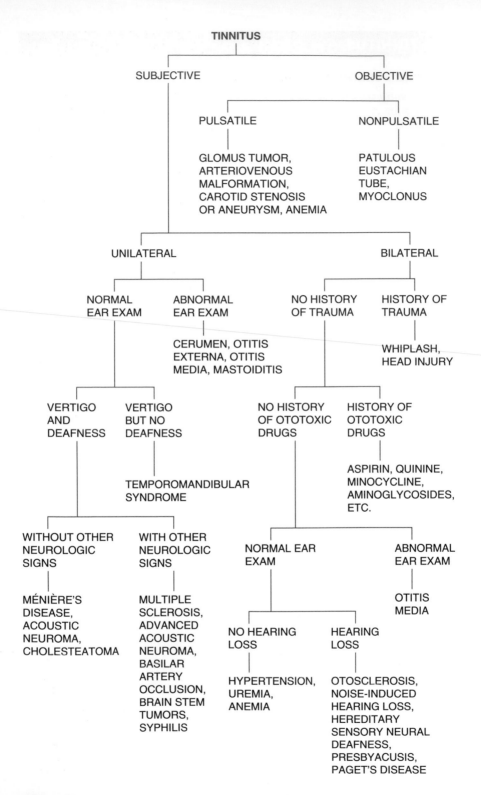

ASK THE FOLLOWING QUESTIONS:

1. **Is it painful?** Painful swellings of the tongue include trauma, burns, herpes simplex, pemphigus, erythema bullosum, carcinoma, Ludwig's angina, angioneurotic edema, bee stings, and hemorrhage due to coagulation disorders.
2. **Is the mass or swelling focal or diffuse?** Focal masses include trauma, herpes simplex, pemphigus, erythema bullosum, carcinoma, angioma, fibroma, lipoma, mucus cyst, papilloma, or syphilitic gumma. Diffuse masses include Ludwig's angina, angioneurotic edema, bee sting, hemorrhage, myxedema, acromegaly, cretinism, mongolism, primary amyloidosis, diffuse lymphoma, and riboflavin deficiency.

DIAGNOSTIC WORKUP

Focal lesions of the tongue should be referred to an oral surgeon or dermatologist for biopsy or excision. Diffuse enlargement or swellings require a workup including CBC, sedimentation rate, urinalysis, chemistry panel, thyroid panel, VDRL test, and ANA titer. If a coagulation disorder is suspected, a coagulation profile may be done. If a vitamin deficiency is suspected, a therapeutic trial of vitamins is indicated. If amyloidosis is suspected, a biopsy may be done. Other disorders may require biopsy also. A trial of antibiotics or corticosteroids may be necessary.

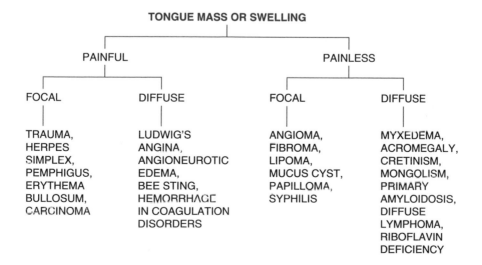

TONGUE MASS OR SWELLING

PAINFUL — FOCAL: TRAUMA, HERPES SIMPLEX, PEMPHIGUS, ERYTHEMA BULLOSUM, CARCINOMA

PAINFUL — DIFFUSE: LUDWIG'S ANGINA, ANGIONEUROTIC EDEMA, BEE STING, HEMORRHAGE IN COAGULATION DISORDERS

PAINLESS — FOCAL: ANGIOMA, FIBROMA, LIPOMA, MUCUS CYST, PAPILLOMA, SYPHILIS

PAINLESS — DIFFUSE: MYXEDEMA, ACROMEGALY, CRETINISM, MONGOLISM, PRIMARY AMYLOIDOSIS, DIFFUSE LYMPHOMA, RIBOFLAVIN DEFICIENCY

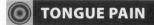

Pain in the tongue is rarely an isolated symptom. There is usually a focal or diffuse inflammation of the tongue or an ulcerating lesion. Diffuse inflammation is found in antibiotic glossitis, glossitis of avitaminosis (pernicious anemia), aphthous stomatitis, thrush, streptococcal glossitis, and acute diffuse glossitis. Focal lesions include cuts and ulcerations from trauma, such as the bitten tongue or burned tongue (hot pizza, etc.), or injury from a sharp tooth or jagged dental plate. Other painful focal lesions are carcinoma, tuberculosis, syphilis (often painless), and herpes simplex ulcers. When the tongue is completely normal, trigeminal neuralgia, polymyositis, trichinosis, and calculus of the submaxillary gland should be considered.

DIAGNOSTIC WORKUP

Most lesions will respond to conservative treatment and time. In patients with signs of systemic disease and vitamin deficiency, the workup includes serum B_{12} and folate level, upper GI series, ANA, and *Trichinella* antibody titer. Focal lesions that persist should command a referral to a dentist or oral surgeon.

TONGUE ULCERS

Ulcerations of the tongue are most commonly due to aphthous stomatitis (canker sore), but they may appear in various stages of syphilis, in herpes zoster, as a result of repetitive trauma from a sharp or carious tooth, in tuberculosis, and in carcinoma. The chancre of primary syphilis rarely causes severe pain, so this will often distinguish the lesion from the others. To differentiate the other causes, a smear and culture and, ultimately, a biopsy must be done. Most physicians will find referral to a dentist or oral surgeon is the best course of action when the ulcer persists.

As physicians, we often neglect inspection of the teeth. We seem to expect the dentist to do this part of the examination for us. Multiple cavities are found in diabetes mellitus, pernicious anemia, and multiparous women. Separation of the teeth may be a clue to hypopituitarism, whereas teeth that taper to a thin edge are typical of the screwdriver appearance of Hutchinson teeth in congenital syphilis. Who has not heard of the dramatic gum hypertrophy associated with phenytoin use in epileptic children? In scurvy, the gums become swollen, and the teeth get loose, drop out, or become misaligned. In dental ectodermal dysplasia, the teeth may be partially or completely absent, and, at times, there is no evidence of enamel formation. The dark blue line positioned where the gums meet the teeth is a sign of lead intoxication.

Mothers frequently complain that their children grind their teeth, but this is rarely of pathologic significance. Of course, it may be a sign of malocclusion and temporomandibular joint syndrome, especially in adults.

Yellow teeth are a sign that a child has been affected by tetracyclines either *in utero* or early childhood.

TREMOR

CASE HISTORY

You are asked to see a 46-year-old white female because of increasing tremor of her hands for the past year. Following the algorithm, you ask about weight loss, palpitations, and sweating, and she has none of these symptoms.

On your examination, there is no tremor at rest and the tremor is most pronounced on finger to nose testing bilaterally. There are no other neurologic signs, so you rule out multiple sclerosis, hereditary and neoplastic diseases of the cerebellum. On further questioning, you find that her mother has a similar condition, so you suspect familial or essential tremor. You would be correct.

ASK THE FOLLOWING QUESTIONS:

1. **When does the tremor occur?** Intention tremor, which means that the tremor occurs on movement, would suggest that the patient is suffering from a familial or senile tremor or multiple sclerosis, Wilson's disease, or hereditary familial ataxia. It also may suggest alcoholism. Nothing is more dramatic than the intention tremor of alcohol withdrawal. A tremor occurring at rest would suggest Parkinson's disease or manganese poisoning. A fine tremor of the outstretched hands, which is sometimes described as *tension tremor*, would suggest hyperthyroidism.

2. **The next question to ask is whether there are associated neurologic findings.** A tremor with long tract findings, such as hyperactive reflexes or Babinski's sign, would suggest multiple sclerosis, whereas a fairly symmetrical tremor with no long tract signs or other neurologic findings would suggest a familial or senile tremor. A tremor with mental deterioration would suggest Wilson's disease.

3. **Are there associated systemic findings?** If the patient has tachycardia and an enlarged thyroid, one should consider hyperthyroidism. However, simply tachycardia alone might indicate that the patient is very sensitive to caffeine. Kayser–Fleischer ring and enlarged liver would suggest Wilson's disease. An enlarged liver alone would suggest alcoholism.

DIAGNOSTIC WORKUP

Certainly a thyroid profile should be done on all cases that present with a tremor alone. In addition, blood tests for serum copper and ceruloplasmin should be done when Wilson's disease is suspected. A drug and alcohol screen should also be done. If multiple sclerosis, Wilson's disease, or a cerebellar tumor is suspected, a CT scan or MRI of the brain should be done. When there is doubt as to whether the tremor is a resting or active tremor, an EMG may be done to separate the two. Most patients presenting with a mild intention tremor that is symmetrical and not associated with other neurologic findings will probably have familial or senile tremor, and the response to beta-blockers can be determined.

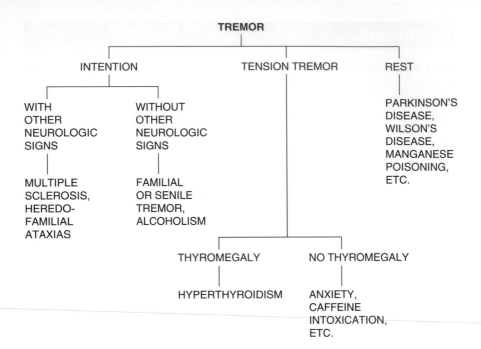

TREMOR

INTENTION

WITH OTHER NEUROLOGIC SIGNS

MULTIPLE SCLEROSIS, HEREDO-FAMILIAL ATAXIAS

WITHOUT OTHER NEUROLOGIC SIGNS

FAMILIAL OR SENILE TREMOR, ALCOHOLISM

TENSION TREMOR

THYROMEGALY

HYPERTHYROIDISM

NO THYROMEGALY

ANXIETY, CAFFEINE INTOXICATION, ETC.

REST

PARKINSON'S DISEASE, WILSON'S DISEASE, MANGANESE POISONING, ETC.

TRISMUS

True trismus or lockjaw is found in tetanus, rabies, and trichinosis. In strychnine poisoning, it is a late development, as the twitchings and convulsions are well established before it appears. Intermittent trismus may be found in epilepsy and cataplexy. Trismus may be simulated by impacted wisdom teeth, temporomandibular joint syndrome, scleroderma, and malingering or hysteria. The diagnostic workup will be obvious in cases of true trismus. Cases not associated with a systemic disease should have an EEG and x-rays of the teeth and temporomandibular joints. A referral to a dental specialist is often in order.

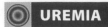

ASK THE FOLLOWING QUESTIONS:

1. **What is the BUN/creatinine ratio?** If this ratio is 20:1 or greater, one should look for pre-renal azotemia. Confirmation with a serum and urine osmolality will be helpful. If this ratio is 10:1 or less, one should look for renal diseases or obstructive uropathy.
2. **Is the bladder enlarged, or is there significant residual urine?** These findings point to obstructive uropathy, particularly bladder neck obstruction. If these findings are absent, the cause of the uremia is most likely renal disease in cases in which the BUN/creatinine ratio is 10:1 or less.
3. **What drugs is the patient on?** ACE inhibitors, diuretics and NSAIDs can cause renal failure.

DIAGNOSTIC WORKUP

Two things to do at the outset are a microscopic examination of the urine and renal and bladder ultrasound. Further workup should include a CBC, urinalysis, urine culture and colony count, serum and urine osmolality, chemistry panel, sedimentation rate, arterial blood gas analysis, blood volume, cystoscopy and retrograde pyelography, a nephrology consult, and a urology consult. Additional studies include abdominal CT scans and a renal biopsy.

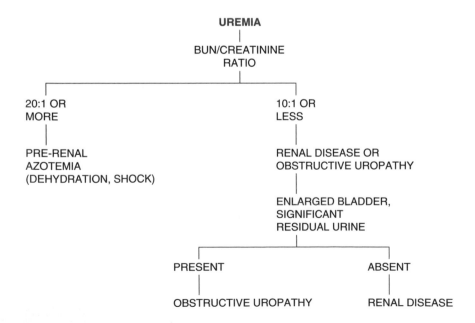

Most cases of urethral discharge in both males and females are due to gonorrhea or *Chlamydia trachomatis*. When the smear and culture are negative for gonorrhea, a course of tetracycline can be given as a therapeutic trial to diagnose *Chlamydia* infection. Alternatively, the urine can be cultured for chlamydia. Recently, DNA probe testing and rapid antigen testing of the urine have become available for gonorrhea and chlamydia. If there are joint pains or uveitis, look for Reiter's syndrome. Other etiologies for nongonococcal urethritis are *Ureaplasma genitalium* and *Trichomonas vaginalis*. Alert the laboratory in advance if these organisms are suspected because they may require special culture media for isolation. A prostate examination should always be done in males, as acute and chronic prostatitis are common causes of urethral discharge. In teenagers, a urethral discharge may develop in prolonged abstinence or excessive masturbation. Rarer causes of urethral discharge are syphilis, tuberculosis, foreign body, and herpes. Carcinoma of the urethra is extremely rare. Anyone with a urethral discharge needs a VDRL and HIV antibody titer. Sexual partners should be tested as well.

URINE COLOR CHANGES

Red urine may be due to hematuria (page 219), hemoglobinuria (hemolytic anemia), myoglobinuria (muscle trauma, myocardial infarction), and coproporphyria or uroporphyria (porphyria). Phenazopyridine hydrochloride (Pyridium®) also colors the urine red or orange. Ingestion of large amounts of beets will also color the urine red. Brown urine is usually due to hepatitis or obstructive jaundice, but myoglobin and melanuria may also color the urine brown. Black urine is found in malignant melanoma. Porphyrins may also color the urine black. In alkaptonuria, the urine turns black on standing. Green or blue urine may be found in patients taking methylene blue, indigo carmine, or indigo blue. *Pseudomonas aeruginosa* infection may turn urine green also. The key to the diagnostic workup is to send the urine to the laboratory for complete analysis and culture. Most of the conditions listed above will have another symptom that will offer additional keys to the diagnostic workup using these pages.

ASK THE FOLLOWING QUESTIONS:

1. **Is it purulent?** A purulent vaginal discharge suggests nonspecific bacterial vaginitis and gonorrhea. In contrast, the discharge of bacterial vaginitis is white and has a fishy odor.
2. **Is it frothy and yellow?** This type of discharge is very often due to trichomoniasis vaginitis.
3. **Is it cheesy and associated with itching?** These findings suggest candidiasis vaginitis.
4. **Is it watery and bloodstained?** This type of discharge suggests carcinoma of the cervix or endometrium, polyps, hydatidiform mole, and chronic cervicitis. If a frankly bloody discharge is noted, consult the differential diagnosis discussed on page 316.
5. **Is it offensive smelling?** An offensive smelling discharge would suggest foreign body in the vagina.
6. **Is there inflammation of the cervix?** The presence of cervical inflammation would suggest chronic cervicitis and gonorrhea.

DIAGNOSTIC WORKUP

The most important test is microscopic examination of a saline and potassium hydroxide preparation. This will diagnose most cases of trichomoniasis and candidiasis. *Gardnerella vaginalis* can be diagnosed if clue cells are found, and the pH of the discharge will be greater than 4.7. If this is unrevealing, a Gram stain for gonorrhea and cultures for trichomoniasis, candidiasis, chlamydia, *G. vaginalis*, and gonorrhea may be done. Recently, DNA probe or rapid antigen testing of urine may be used to diagnose gonorrhea or chlamydia. If the results of these tests are negative, look for pinworms. A Pap smear should be done to rule out malignancy. Polyps or inflamed areas of the cervix should be biopsied. Colposcopy may help further differentiate a cervical lesion. A dilation and curettage may be necessary to diagnose endometrial carcinoma and hydatidiform mole. Occasionally, pelvic ultrasound and CT scans are necessary. However, before ordering these expensive diagnostic tests, a gynecologist should be consulted. Patients with documented evidence of gonorrhea should have a VDRL test and HIV testing. A therapeutic trial of tetracycline or metronidazole may be successful in bacterial vaginitis.

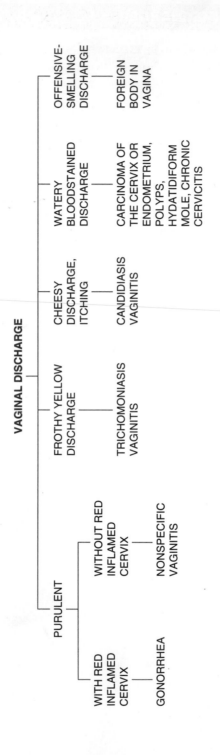

VAGINAL DISCHARGE

PURULENT

WITH RED INFLAMED CERVIX — GONORRHEA

WITHOUT RED INFLAMED CERVIX — NONSPECIFIC VAGINITIS

FROTHY YELLOW DISCHARGE — TRICHOMONIASIS VAGINITIS

CHEESY DISCHARGE, ITCHING — CANDIDIASIS VAGINITIS

WATERY BLOODSTAINED DISCHARGE — CARCINOMA OF THE CERVIX OR ENDOMETRIUM, POLYPS, HYDATIDIFORM MOLE, CHRONIC CERVICITIS

OFFENSIVE-SMELLING DISCHARGE — FOREIGN BODY IN VAGINA

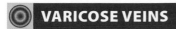

Varicose veins are common in the lower extremities and are usually not a sign of other disease. Varicose veins of the rectum are called hemorrhoids and can be a sign of cirrhosis of the liver or portal vein obstruction from other causes. Distention of the abdominal veins may be due to cirrhosis of the liver, thrombosis of the inferior vena cava, or distention of the abdomen due to a large tumor (e.g., ovarian cyst), ascites, or massive hepatic or splenic enlargement. Varicose veins of the thorax and upper extremities are seen in mediastinal malignancies (primary or metastatic), thoracic aortic aneurysms, and chronic fibrous mediastinitis.

DIAGNOSTIC WORKUP

Obviously, a liver profile will be important. Chest x-rays and a flat plate of the abdomen should be routine. When these fail to identify a lesion—and even when they do identify a lesion—it is often necessary to get a CT scan of the thorax or abdomen. Exploratory surgery may be necessary to establish a tissue diagnosis, as biopsy may be dangerous.

VULVAL OR VAGINAL MASS

ASK THE FOLLOWING QUESTIONS:

1. **Is it tender?** A tender vulval or vaginal mass would suggest vulvitis, hematoma, acute bartholinitis, or urethral caruncle.
2. **Is it reducible?** A reducible vulval or vaginal mass would suggest pudendal hernia, varicocele, cystocele, rectocele, and uterine prolapse.
3. **Is the rectal examination abnormal?** The rectal examination will be abnormal when there is an impacted feces or rectal carcinoma.

DIAGNOSTIC WORKUP

Referral to a gynecologist or urologist can obviate an expensive diagnostic workup in most cases. However, a primary care physician may wish to treat acute bartholinitis or vulvitis. A culture and sensitivity is the only procedure required in those cases.

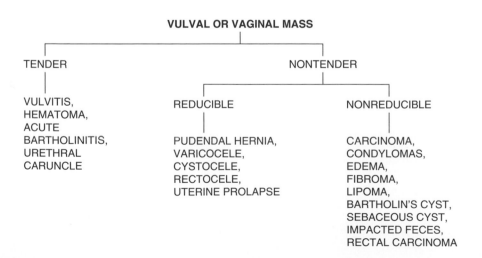

VULVAL OR VAGINAL MASS

TENDER

VULVITIS, HEMATOMA, ACUTE BARTHOLINITIS, URETHRAL CARUNCLE

NONTENDER

REDUCIBLE

PUDENDAL HERNIA, VARICOCELE, CYSTOCELE, RECTOCELE, UTERINE PROLAPSE

NONREDUCIBLE

CARCINOMA, CONDYLOMAS, EDEMA, FIBROMA, LIPOMA, BARTHOLIN'S CYST, SEBACEOUS CYST, IMPACTED FECES, RECTAL CARCINOMA

ASK THE FOLLOWING QUESTIONS:

1. **Is the lesion or are the surrounding lymph nodes tender?** The presence of tenderness of the lesion or the surrounding lymph nodes would suggest chancroid, lymphogranuloma venereum, herpes genitalis, and carcinoma. On the other hand, if the lesions or the surrounding lymph nodes are nontender, chancre, yaws, condyloma latum, and lupus should be suspected.
2. **Is there only itching and erythema?** Look for candidiasis or pinworms.

DIAGNOSTIC WORKUP

The workup includes a CBC, sedimentation rate, urinalysis, and VDRL test. A smear and culture of material from the ulceration should be done. A dark field examination may also be necessary. The Frei test may diagnose lymphogranuloma venereum, but a serologic test for this disorder may also be ordered. Biopsy may be ultimately necessary. It is wise to enlist the help of a urologist or gynecologist in difficult cases.

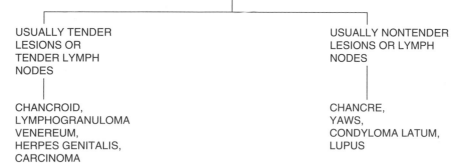

VULVAL OR VAGINAL ULCERATIONS

USUALLY TENDER LESIONS OR TENDER LYMPH NODES

CHANCROID, LYMPHOGRANULOMA VENEREUM, HERPES GENITALIS, CARCINOMA

USUALLY NONTENDER LESIONS OR LYMPH NODES

CHANCRE, YAWS, CONDYLOMA LATUM, LUPUS

ASK THE FOLLOWING QUESTIONS:

1. **Is there fever?** The presence of fever would suggest an infectious disease, such as tuberculosis, AIDS, brucellosis, and typhoid fever, but collagen diseases and neoplasms should not be forgotten.
2. **Is there anorexia?** The presence of anorexia may be related to a febrile process, but if there is no fever one should consider the possibility of Addison's disease, anorexia nervosa, Simmonds' disease, drug abuse, poisoning such as arsenic poisoning, scurvy, malabsorption syndrome, uremia, and liver failure. There may also be a neoplasm.
3. **Is there lymphadenopathy?** The presence of generalized lymphadenopathy should suggest leukemia, sarcoidosis, and lymphoma, as well as infectious disease processes.
4. **Is there an abdominal mass?** An abdominal mass may be an enlarged spleen, a pancreatic carcinoma, an enlarged liver, or renal mass. These masses would suggest disease of those organs. The mass also may be a carcinoma of the stomach or intestine.
5. **Is there hyperpigmentation?** The presence of hyperpigmentation would suggest Addison's disease.
6. **Is the appetite normal or increased?** The presence of a normal or increased appetite in the presence of weight loss should suggest hyperthyroidism and diabetes mellitus. The patient also may be taking thyroid hormone medication in increased quantities.
7. **Is the thyroid gland enlarged?** The presence of an enlarged thyroid would suggest hyperthyroidism. One should also look for a focal thyroid mass which might be a toxic adenoma.
8. **Is the chest x-ray abnormal?** Abnormalities found on x-ray that may induce weight loss are carcinoma of the lung, tuberculosis, congestive heart failure, pulmonary emphysema, and fibrosis.
9. **Is there a history of risky sexual behavior?** This should always prompt the consideration of the possibility of AIDS.

DIAGNOSTIC WORKUP

Routine diagnostic studies include a CBC, sedimentation rate, urinalysis, chemistry panel, thyroid panel, serum amylase and lipase, febrile agglutinins, tuberculin test, ANA titer, serum protein electrophoresis, serum B_{12} and folic acid, chest x-ray, EKG, and a flat plate of the abdomen. An HIV antibody titer needs to be done in selected clinical circumstances.

A stool for fat, trypsin, occult blood, and ovum and parasites should be done. Further tests for steatorrhea are listed on page 457. If these tests are within normal limits or are unrevealing, it is best to refer the patient to a gastroenterologist or oncologist for further evaluation. Sometimes, clinical clues suggest the need for an endocrinologist or psychiatrist as well. However, if the primary care physician wishes to proceed further, he may order an upper GI series and esophagogram, a small bowel series, barium enema, and a sigmoidoscopic examination. A CT scan of the abdomen and pelvis may be useful, but it is an expensive procedure.

Twenty-four-hour urine collection for free cortisol or rapid ACTH stimulation test will diagnose Addison's disease. Quantitative stool fat and D-xylose absorption or a simple glucose tolerance test will diagnose some cases of malabsorption syndrome. Endoscopic procedures, including laparoscopy and even an exploratory laparotomy, have their place in the diagnostic workup. However, it is always best to enlist the help of specialists before considering these procedures, even if one is located in an isolated community. If a trial of a nutritional supplement halts the weight loss, depression is most likely the cause.

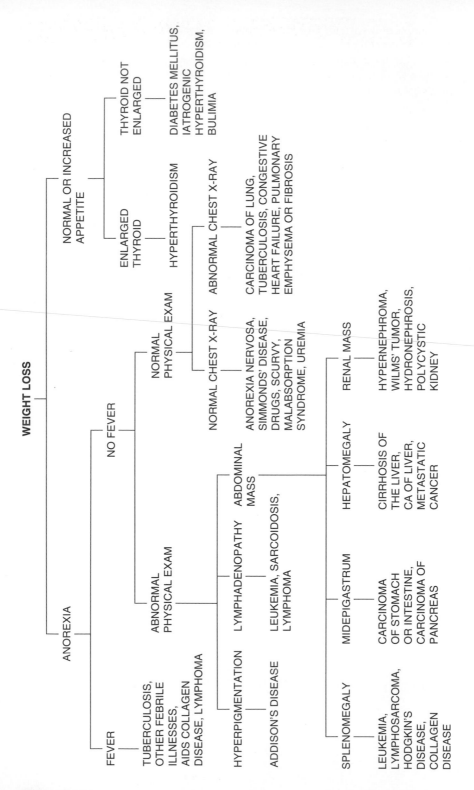

WEIGHT LOSS

- **ANOREXIA**
  - **FEVER**
    - TUBERCULOSIS, OTHER FEBRILE ILLNESSES, AIDS COLLAGEN DISEASE, LYMPHOMA
  - **NO FEVER**
    - **ABNORMAL PHYSICAL EXAM**
      - **HYPERPIGMENTATION**
        - ADDISON'S DISEASE
      - **LYMPHADENOPATHY**
        - LEUKEMIA, SARCOIDOSIS, LYMPHOMA
      - **ABDOMINAL MASS**
        - **SPLENOMEGALY**
          - LEUKEMIA, LYMPHOSARCOMA, HODGKIN'S DISEASE, COLLAGEN DISEASE
        - **MIDEPIGASTRUM**
          - CARCINOMA OF STOMACH OR INTESTINE, CARCINOMA OF PANCREAS
        - **HEPATOMEGALY**
          - CIRRHOSIS OF THE LIVER, CA OF LIVER, METASTATIC CANCER
        - **RENAL MASS**
          - HYPERNEPHROMA, WILMS' TUMOR, HYDRONEPHROSIS, POLYCYSTIC KIDNEY
    - **NORMAL PHYSICAL EXAM**
      - **NORMAL CHEST X-RAY**
        - ANOREXIA NERVOSA, SIMMONDS' DISEASE, DRUGS, SCURVY, MALABSORPTION SYNDROME, UREMIA
      - **ABNORMAL CHEST X-RAY**
        - CARCINOMA OF LUNG, TUBERCULOSIS, CONGESTIVE HEART FAILURE, PULMONARY EMPHYSEMA OR FIBROSIS
- **NORMAL OR INCREASED APPETITE**
  - **ENLARGED THYROID**
    - HYPERTHYROIDISM
  - **THYROID NOT ENLARGED**
    - DIABETES MELLITUS, IATROGENIC HYPERTHYROIDISM, BULIMIA

Wheezing is classically due to bronchial asthma, but there is a danger in jumping to that conclusion because it occurs in a few other conditions as well. The wheezing of bronchial asthma is heard primarily on expiration, whereas the wheezing of tracheal or laryngeal obstruction is heard on inspiration, such as tracheobronchitis in children. The wheezing of cardiac asthma (in congestive heart failure with acute pulmonary edema) is associated with pink, frothy sputum, whereas the sputum of bronchial asthma is thick and tenacious. Acute infectious bronchitis may simulate bronchial asthma, but the response to epinephrine is poor. This is true also of pulmonary emphysema, but the history will usually differentiate this condition from bronchial asthma. A foreign body may often be distinguished because the wheezing is unilateral. Look for occupational causes of asthma such as methane exposure and animal dander.

DIAGNOSTIC WORKUP

The CBC, sedimentation rate, BNP, serum alpha-1 trypsin deficiency, sweat test chest x-ray, EKG, sputum analysis and culture, and pulmonary function testing will usually assist with the clinical diagnosis. Hereditary angioneurotic edema may be diagnosed by a deficiency of C1 esterase inhibitor. Bronchoscopy may also be needed, especially when there is hemoptysis (see page 225).

Suggested Orders for the Workup of Common Symptoms

The author wants to emphasize that these orders are only suggestions and not meant to be just automatically copied onto the order sheet in the hospital or office. Rather, the clinician should select the orders most appropriate, á la carte to fit the individual patient.

These orders are divided into those that can be cost effective for the primary care provider without the help of a consultant and those that should be ordered only after consultation with a specialist. It is almost always cheaper to consult a specialist before ordering a CT scan, MRIs and other expensive diagnostic tests. For example, you should not order an MRI of the brain in a patient with headache and no focal neurologic signs, without consulting a neurologist first.

Abdominal Pain, Acute

A. Initial Workup
1. CBC
2. Urinalysis
3. Chemistry panel
4. Sedimentation rate
5. Serum amylase and lipase
6. Pregnancy test
7. Flat plate of abdomen and upright
8. Chest x-ray
9. ECG

B. Expanded Workup
1. Consultation with a surgeon or gastroenterologist
2. Gall bladder ultrasonography
3. HIDA scan
4. CT scan of the abdomen with contrast
5. Lateral decubitus films
6. Serial cardiac enzymes
7. Peritoneal tap
8. Double enema
9. Gastroscopy
10. Laparoscopy
11. Gallium scan
12. Exploratory laparotomy

Abdominal Pain, Chronic

A. Initial Workup
1. CBC
2. Sedimentation rate
3. Chemistry panel
4. Urinalysis
5. Urine culture and colony count
6. Serum amylase and lipase
7. Pregnancy test
8. Stool for occult blood X3
9. Stool for ovum and parasites
10. Stool for *Giardia* antigen

11. Abdominal film series
12. Chest x-ray
13. ECG
14. Therapeutic trial of antibiotics, amebicides, or anthelmintics

B. Expanded Workup
1. Gastroenterology consult
2. CT scan of abdomen and pelvis
3. Barium enema
4. Upper GI series and esophagram
5. Small bowel series
6. Gall bladder ultrasonography
7. IVP
8. Esophagoscopy gastroscopy
9. Colonoscopy
10. Gallium or indium scan
11. Mesenteric angiography
12. Lymphangiography
13. Exploratory laparotomy

Back Pain

A. Initial Workup
1. CBC
2. Urinalysis
3. Sedimentation rate
4. Chemistry panel
5. Radiographs of thoracic or lumbar spine

B. Expanded Workup
1. Orthopedic or neurology consult
2. CT scan or MRI of spine
3. EMG and NCV of lower extremities
4. Bone scan
5. HLA-B27 antigen
6. RA test
7. ANA
8. PSA (in men)

9. Serum protein electrophoresis
10. Gynecology consult
11. CT scan of abdomen and pelvis
12. Ultrasonography of pelvis
13. Aortography
14. Urine culture and colony count
15. Therapeutic trail of NSAIDs
16. Trigger point injections or nerve blocks

Blurred Vision and Blindness

1. Ophthalmology consult
2. Visual acuity
3. Visual field examination
4. Tonometry
5. Slit lamp examination
6. Carotid duplex scan
7. Sedimentation rate and VDRL
8. Neurology consult
9. CT scan or MRI of the brain
10. MRA
11. Spinal fluid analysis
12. Cerebral angiography
13. Pituitary function studies
14. Uveitis workup

Breast Mass

A. Initial Workup

1. CBC
2. Sedimentation rate
3. Culture of discharge
4. Mammography
5. Ultrasonography
6. Surgical consult

B. Expanded Workup

1. Aspiration of cystic fluid
2. Biopsy
3. Serum prolactin
4. Pregnancy test
5. Skull x-ray or CT scan of brain
6. Serum FSH and LH
7. Endocrinology consult

Cardiac Arrhythmia

A. Initial Workup

1. CBC
2. Sedimentation rate
3. CRP
4. ASO titer
5. Chemistry panel
6. Urinalysis
7. Serial cardiac enzymes
8. Troponins
9. D-dimer
10. Thyroid profile
11. ECG

12. Chest x-ray
13. BNP

B. Expanded Workup

1. Cardiology consult
2. Echocardiography
3. Holter monitoring
4. Arterial blood gases
5. Spirometry
6. Blood cultures
7. 24-hr urine catecholamines
8. Exercise tolerance test
9. Cardiac catheterization and angiocardiography

Chest Pain

A. Initial Workup

1. CBC
2. Sedimentation rate
3. Chemistry panel
4. Urinalysis
5. Serial cardiac enzymes
6. Troponins
7. D-dimer
8. BNP
9. Serial ECGs
10. Sputum smear and culture
11. Arterial blood gases
12. Chest x-ray
13. Response to nitroglycerin
14. Response to lidocaine viscus

B. Expanded Workup

1. Cardiology consult
2. Ventilation–perfusion scan
3. Spiral CT scan of chest
4. Thallium-201 scan
5. Echocardiography
6. 24-hr Holter monitoring
7. Exercise tolerance test
8. Cardiac catheterization and coronary angiography
9. Gastroenterology consult
10. Esophagoscopy and gastroscopy
11. Gall bladder ultrasonography
12. Bernstein test
13. Trigger point injection

Coma

1. CBC
2. Sedimentation rate
3. Chemistry panel
4. Urinalysis
5. Urine drug screen
6. Arterial blood gases
7. Blood ammonia level
8. Serum and urine osmolality
9. IV dextrose or glucogen IM

10. IV thiamine
11. Neurology consult
12. CT scan of brain
13. Spinal fluid analysis
14. Blood lead level
15. EEG
16. MRI of brain
17. Urine porphobilinogen
18. Trial of naloxone IV
19. Trial of benzodiazepine antagonist

Constipation

A. Initial Workup
1. CBC
2. Chemistry panel
3. Plain films of abdomen
4. Urinalysis
5. Stool for occult blood X3
6. Stool for ovum and parasites
7. Quantitative stool fat
8. Thyroid profile
9. PTH
10. PSA
11. Glucose tolerance test
12. Anoscopy and sigmoidoscopy
13. Barium enema
14. VDRL

B. Expanded Workup
1. Gastroenterology consult
2. Colonoscopy
3. Pelvic ultrasonography
4. Endocrinology consult
5. Psychiatric consult
6. Neurology consult
7. Therapeutic trial of Metamucil or stool softener

Convulsions

A. Initial Workup
1. CBC
2. Sedimentation rate
3. Chemistry panel
4. Urinalysis
5. Urine drug screen
6. VDRL
7. CT scan
8. Spinal fluid analysis
9. EEG, wake and sleep

B. Expanded Workup
1. Neurology consult
2. MRI of brain
3. Carotid duplex scan
4. ANA
5. HIV antibody titer
6. Stool for ovum and parasites
7. Serum protein electrophoresis

8. Therapeutic trial of anti-convulsants

Cough

A. Initial Workup
1. Withdrawal of all medications if possible
2. CBC
3. Sedimentation rate
4. Chemistry panel
5. Sputum smear and culture
6. AFB smear and culture
7. Cold agglutinins
8. Influenza rapid screen test
9. Chest x-ray
10. *Legionella* culture
11. Tuberculin test
12. Therapeutic trial of antibiotics or antihistamines

B. Expanded Workup
1. Pulmonary consult
2. Spirometry
3. Arterial blood gases
4. Echocardiography
5. Bronchoscopy
6. CT scan of chest
7. Fungal skin tests and cultures
8. ECG
9. Kveim test
10. ANA
11. Alpha-1 antitrypsin test
12. Allergy skin test
13. 24-hr sputum volume
14. Sputum for eosinophils
15. Bronchography
16. Sweat test

Depression
1. CBC
2. Sedimentation rate
3. Chemistry panel
4. VDRL
5. Thyroid profile
6. Urinalysis
7. Urine drug screen
8. Eliminate as many medications as possible
9. Serum cortisol
10. Serum FSH
11. Serum estradiol
12. Therapeutic trial of estrogen if menopause is suspected
13. Psychiatric consult
14. Endocrinology consult
15. EEG
16. CT scan of brain
17. MRI of brain

Diarrhea, Acute

1. CBC
2. Sedimentation rate
3. Chemistry panel
4. Electrolytes
5. Stool for occult blood
6. Stool for smear and culture
7. Stool for leucocytes
8. Stool for ovum and parasites
9. Stool for *Giardia* antigen
10. Stool for *Clostridia difficile* toxin
11. Sigmoidoscopy
12. Barium enema
13. Gastroenterology consult

Diarrhea, Chronic

A. Initial Workup

1. CBC
2. Sedimentation rate
3. Chemistry panel
4. Electrolytes
5. VDRL
6. HIV antibody titer
7. Urinalysis
8. Stool for occult blood X3
9. Stool for ovum and parasites
10. Stool smear and culture
11. Stool for *Giardia* antigen
12. Stool for *C. difficile* toxin
13. Sigmoidoscopy
14. Barium enema
15. Therapeutic trial of metronidazole

B. Expanded Workup

1. Gastroenterology consult
2. Colonoscopy
3. Thyroid profile
4. Lactose tolerance test
5. Urine 5-HIAA
6. D-xylose absorption test
7. Serum gastrin
8. Stool for quantitative fat and trypsin
9. Stool volume after fasting
10. Upper GI series and small bowel follow through
11. CT scan of abdomen
12. Neurology consult and search for anal sphincter incompetence

Dizziness

A. Initial Workup

1. CBC
2. Sedimentation rate
3. Chemistry panel
4. Urinalysis

5. VDRL
6. Audiogram
7. Caloric testing
8. EKG
9. X-ray of skull and mastoids

B. Expanded Workup

1. Neurology consult
2. ENT consult
3. CT scan of brain
4. MRI of brain
5. EEG
6. Electronystagmography
7. Cardiology consult
8. ECG
9. Holter monitoring
10. Carotid duplex scan
11. MRA
12. Spinal fluid analysis
13. 24-hr blood pressure monitoring
14. Tilt table test
15. 5-hr glucose tolerance test
16. 72-hr fast with glucose monitoring
17. Plasma insulin and C-peptide

Dyspnea

A. Initial Workup

1. CBC
2. Chemistry panel
3. Sedimentation rate
4. BNP
5. D-dimer
6. Urinalysis
7. Arterial blood gas analysis
8. Chest x-ray
9. EKG
10. Serial cardiac enzymes
11. Troponins
12. Spirometry

B. Expanded Workup

1. Cardiology consult
2. Echocardiography
3. Ventilation–perfusion scan
4. Spiral CT scan of the chest
5. Sputum smear and culture
6. Sputum for eosinophils
7. Pulmonary consult
8. Cardiac catheterization and angiocardiography
9. Bronchoscopy
10. Trial of diuretics
11. Trial of epinephrine

Dysuria

A. Initial Workup

1. CBC
2. Sedimentation rate

3. Chemistry panel
4. Urinalysis with microscopic
5. Urine culture and colony count
6. Urethral smear and culture
7. Vaginal smear and culture
8. Prostatic massage and examination of exudates.

B. Expanded Workup
1. Urology consult
2. Gynecology consult
3. Pelvic ultrasonography
4. CT scan of abdomen and pelvis
5. IVP and cystogram
6. Cystoscopy and retrograde pyelography
7. Cultures for *Neisseria gonorrhea, Chlamydia,* and *Mycobacterium tuberculosis*
8. Therapeutic trial of ciprofloxacin or sulfonamides

Earache

A. Initial Workup
1. CBC
2. Sedimentation rate
3. Culture and sensitivity of exudates
4. Tympanogram
5. Audiogram
6. Radiographs of mastoids and petrous bones
7. Rapid strep test

B. Expanded Workup
1. ENT consult
2. CT scan of brain
3. MRI of brain
4. Neurology consult
5. Trial of antibiotics

Edema

A. Initial Workup
1. CBC
2. Sedimentation rate
3. Chemistry panel
4. Urinalysis
5. Serum protein electrophoresis
6. Thyroid profile
7. Serum and urine osmolality
8. Addis count
9. ANA
10. BNP
11. D-dimer
12. ECG
13. Chest x-ray
14. 24-hr urine protein

B. Expanded Workup
1. Cardiology consult
2. Echocardiography
3. Pulmonary function studies
4. CT scan of chest
5. CT scan of abdomen and pelvis
6. Venous ultrasonography
7. Lymphangiography
8. Muscle biopsy
9. Trial of diuretics

Extremity Pain, Lower

A. Initial Workup
1. CBC
2. Sedimentation rate
3. Chemistry panel
4. VDRL
5. D-dimer
6. ANA, RA
7. Radiography of extremities and joints
8. Venous ultrasonography
9. Ankle/brachial index
10. X-ray of lumbosacral spine
11. Bone scan

B. Expanded Workup
1. Orthopedic consult
2. Neurology consult
3. CT scan or MRI of lumbar spine
4. EMG and NCV of lower extremities
5. Femoral angiography
6. Contrast venography
7. Synovial fluid analysis and culture
8. Trigger point injection
9. Nerve blocks
10. Epidural blocks

Extremity Pain, Upper

A. Initial Workup
1. CBC
2. Sedimentation rate
3. Chemistry panel
4. VDRL
5. ANA
6. RA
7. Urinalysis
8. Radiographs of the extremity and joints
9. X-ray of cervical spine
10. Chest x-ray
11. Bone scan
12. ECG

B. Expanded Workup
1. Orthopedic consult
2. Neurology consult
3. CT scan of extremity and joints
4. MRI of shoulder
5. MRI of cervical spine
6. EMG and NCV of upper extremities
7. Exercise tolerance test
8. Stellate ganglion block
9. Trigger point injections
10. Nerve blocks
11. Venography
12. Angiography

Eye Pain
1. CBC
2. Sedimentation rate
3. Visual acuity
4. Tonometry
5. Slit lamp examination
6. Fluorescein dye test for foreign body or corneal abrasion
7. Culture and sensitivity of exudate
8. Trail of sumatriptan
9. Ophthalmology consult
10. Trial of corticosteroids

Failure to Thrive

A. Initial Workup
1. CBC
2. Sedimentation rate
3. Chemistry panel
4. Serum protein electrophoresis
5. Thyroid profile
6. Liver profile
7. Sweat test
8. Stool for quantitative fat
9. Stool for ovum and parasites
10. Chest x-ray
11. ECG
12. Skeletal survey for bone age

B. Expanded Workup
1. Endocrinology consult
2. CT scan of brain
3. Serum growth hormone analysis
4. Chromosome analysis
5. Somatomedin C
6. Overnight dexamethasone suppression test
7. Bone scan

Fatigue

A. Initial Workup
1. CBC
2. Sedimentation rate
3. Chemistry panel

4. Electrolytes
5. VDRL
6. HIV antibody titer
7. ANA
8. RA antibody titer
9. Urinalysis
10. Urine culture and colony count
11. Thyroid profile
12. Serum cortisol
13. Monospot test
14. PPD, intermediate
15. EKG
16. Response to vitamins and corrective diet
17. Psychometric testing
18. Therapeutic trial of thyroid medication
19. Therapeutic trial of hormone replacement therapy.

B. Expanded Workup
1. Endocrinology consult
2. Infectious disease consult
3. Rheumatology consult
4. Discontinue all medications if possible
5. Drug screen
6. 5-hr glucose tolerance test
7. Lyme disease serology
8. Febrile agglutinins
9. Brucellin antibody titer
10. Skeletal survey
11. Bone scan
12. Stool for ovum and parasites
13. Muscles biopsy
14. CT scan of abdomen and chest
15. Acetylcholine receptor antibody titer

Fever of Unknown Origin

A. Initial Workup
1. CBC
2. Sedimentation rate
3. Chemistry panel
4. VDRL
5. HIV antibody titer
6. ANA
7. RA titer
8. Lyme disease antibody titer
9. Febrile agglutinins
10. Brucellin antibody titer
11. PPD, intermediate
12. Urinalysis
13. Urine culture and colony count
14. Chest x-ray
15. Blood cultures
16. ASO titer
17. CRP
18. Monospot test

B. Expanded Workup
1. Infectious disease consult
2. Culture of all available body fluids
3. CSF analysis and culture
4. CT scan of chest, abdomen and pelvis
5. Bone scan
6. Gallium or indium scan
7. Pelvic ultrasonography
8. Echocardiography
9. Fibrin test
10. Urine for etiocholanolone
11. Urine for porphobilinogen
12. Oncology consult

Frequency of Urination

A. Initial Workup
1. CBC
2. Sedimentation rate
3. Chemistry panel
4. Urinalysis and microscopic
5. Urine culture and colony count
6. Flat plate of abdomen

B. Expanded Workup
1. Ultrasonography of bladder and pelvis
2. Pregnancy test
3. Urology consult
4. CT scan of abdomen and pelvis
5. Prostatic message and microscopic
6. Catheterize for residual urine
7. Urine culture for anaerobic organisms
8. AFB urine smear and culture
9. IVP
10. Cystoscopy and retrograde pyelography
11. Endocrinology consult
12. Plasma ADH
13. Hickey–Hare test
14. CT scan of brain
15. Serum PTH
16. Psychiatric consult
17. Trial of antibiotics

Headache

A. Initial Work
1. CBC
2. Sedimentation rate
3. Chemistry panel
4. VDRL
5. Urinalysis
6. Radiographs of sinuses
7. Radiographs of cervical spine
8. Visual acuity
9. Tonometry

10. Therapeutic trial of sumatriptan
11. Histamine test

B. Expanded Workup
1. Neurology consult
2. Ophthalmology consult
3. CT scan or MRI of brain
4. Therapeutic trial of beta-blockers
5. Trigger point injections
6. Occipital nerve block
7. Spinal fluid analysis
8. Psychiatric consult

Heartburn

A. Initial Workup
1. CBC
2. Urinalysis
3. Sedimentation rate
4. Chemistry panel
5. Stool for occult blood X3
6. *Helicobacter pylori* antibody titer
7. Upper GI series and esophagram
8. Therapeutic trial of lidocaine viscus
9. Therapeutic trial of proton pump inhibitors
10. Bernstein test

B. Expanded Workup
1. Gastroenterology consult
2. Esophagoscopy, gastroscopy and biopsy
3. Cardiology consult
4. Exercise tolerance test
5. Gallbladder ultrasonography
6. Esophageal manometry
7. Esophageal pH monitoring

Hematemesis

1. CBC
2. Chemistry panel
3. Urinalysis
4. Coagulation profile
5. Type and cross match four units of blood
6. Gastroenterology consult
7. Esophagoscopy, gastroscopy and duodenoscopy
8. Ultrasonography for esophageal varices
9. CT scan of abdomen and chest

Hematuria

A. Initial Workup
1. CBC
2. Chemistry panel

3. Sedimentation rate
4. Urinalysis with microscopic
5. Urine culture and colony count
6. Strain all urine for stones
7. ASO titer
8. Flat plate of abdomen
9. Renal ultrasonography
10. PPD, intermediate

B. **Expanded Workup**
1. Urology consult
2. Nephrology consult
3. CT scan of abdomen and pelvis
4. IVP
5. Cystoscopy and retrograde pyelography
6. Urine culture for anaerobic organism
7. Urine for AFB culture
8. Renal angiography
9. MRI
10. Renal biopsy

Hemoptysis

A. **Initial Workup**
1. CBC
2. Sedimentation rate
3. Chemistry panel
4. Urinalysis
5. Sputum smear and culture
6. D-dimer
7. Arterial blood gases
8. Chest x-ray
9. ECG
10. Pulmonary function studies

B. **Expanded Workup**
1. Pulmonary consult
2. Spiral CT scan of chest
3. Ventilation/perfusion scan
4. Bronchoscopy
5. Cardiology consult
6. Echocardiography
7. Coagulation profile
8. MRI of chest
9. Needle biopsy of lesions

Hip Pain

A. **Initial Workup**
1. CBC
2. Sedimentation rate
3. Chemistry panel
4. Urinalysis
5. RA test
6. ANA test
7. Radiograph of both hips
8. Radiograph of lumbosacral spine

9. Bursal or hip injection of lidocaine
10. Trigger point injections

B. **Expanded Workup**
1. Orthopedic consult
2. Neurology consult
3. CT scan of hips
4. CT scan of lumbosacral spine
5. MRI of lumbosacral spine
6. Bone scan
7. Serum protein electrophoresis
8. PSA
9. EMG and nerve conduction studies

Hoarseness

A. **Initial Workup**
1. CBC
2. Sedimentation rate
3. Chemistry panel
4. Urinalysis
5. Throat culture
6. Rapid strep test
7. Viral antigen test for influenza
8. Sputum culture
9. Chest x-ray
10. X-ray of sinuses

B. **Expanded Workup**
1. ENT consult
2. Fiberoptic laryngoscopy
3. CT scans of chest, neck and mediastinum
4. Thyroid profile
5. AFB smear and culture
6. Acetylcholine receptor antibody titer
7. Tensilon test
8. MRI of the chest
9. Neurology consult
10. Esophagram
11. Esophageal pH monitoring
12. Allergy skin testing
13. Therapeutic trial of antibiotics
14. Therapeutic trial of antihistamines
15. Therapeutic trial of corticosteroids

Hypertension

A. **Initial Workup**
1. CBC
2. Sedimentation rate
3. Chemistry panel
4. Serial electrolytes
5. Urinalysis with microscopic
6. Urine culture and colony count
7. ANA

8. ECG
9. Chest x-ray
10. Plain abdominal films
11. Ankle/brachial index

B. Expanded Workup
1. Nephrology consult
2. CT scan of abdomen
3. Spiral CT angiography or MRA
4. Plasma renin and aldosterone and potassium after salt loading
5. 24-hr urine cortisol
6. Plasma and 24-hr urine metanephrine or catecholamines
7. Chest MRI
8. Renal ultrasound
9. Renal angiography

Indigestion

A. Initial Workup
1. CBC
2. Chemistry panel
3. Sedimentation rate
4. Urinalysis
5. Upper GI series and esophagram
6. Gall bladder ultrasonography
7. Stool for occult blood X3
8. Serum B_{12} and folic acid

B. Expanded Workup
1. Gastroenterology consult
2. Withhold as many drugs as possible
3. Avoid alcohol and caffeine
4. Therapeutic trial of proton pump inhibitors
5. Thyroid profile
6. Hepatitis profile
7. Esophagoscopy, gastroscopy and duodenoscopy
8. Bernstein test
9. CT scan of abdomen
10. Esophageal manometry
11. Quantitative stool fat
12. D-xylose absorption test

Jaundice

A. Initial Workup
1. CBC
2. Sedimentation rate
3. Chemistry panel
4. Hepatitis profile
5. Urinalysis
6. Serum haptoglobins
7. Chest x-ray
8. Flat plate of abdomen
9. Ultrasonography of gall bladder

10. Serum amylase and lipase
11. Stool for occult blood X3

B. Expanded Workup
1. Gastroenterology consult
2. CT scan of abdomen
3. Upper GI series
4. ERCP
5. Antimitochondrial antibodies
6. Febrile agglutinins
7. Monospot test
8. Leptospirosis antibody titer
9. Stool for ovum and parasites
10. Serum iron and iron-binding capacity
11. Blood smear for parasites
12. ANA
13. Smooth muscle antibody titer
14. HIV antibody titer
15. Liver biopsy
16. Steroid whitewash
17. Peritoneoscopy
18. Exploratory laparotomy

Joint Pain or Swelling

A. Initial Workup
1. CBC
2. Sedimentation rate
3. Chemistry panel
4. Urinalysis
5. RA titer
6. ANA
7. CRP
8. ASO titer
9. Radiographs of involved joints
10. Synovial fluid analysis and culture
11. Therapeutic trial of colchicine or NSAIDs
12. Therapeutic trial of intra-articular steroids

B. Expanded Workup
1. Orthopedic consult
2. Rheumatology consult
3. MRI of joint
4. Bone scan
5. Arthroscopy
6. Arthrography
7. Gonococcal antibody titer
8. Coagulation profile
9. VDRL
10. Serologic test for Lyme disease
11. Monospot test
12. Sickle cell prep
13. HLA-B27 antigen
14. Urine for homogentisic acid

Melena

A. **Initial Workup**
1. CBC
2. Sedimentation rate
3. Chemistry panel
4. Urinalysis
5. Stool for occult blood X3
6. Stool for ovum and parasites
7. Upper GI series and esophagram
8. Immunoglobulin G-serologic test for *H. pylori*
9. Coagulation profile

B. **Expanded Workup**
1. Gastroenterology consult
2. Esophagoscopy, gastroscopy, and duodenoscopy
3. Small bowel series
4. Liver function tests
5. Fluorescein string test
6. Nuclear scan after intravenous injection of chromium-tagged red cells
7. Ultrasonography of esophageal varies and portal venous system
8. Mesenteric angiography
9. Exploratory laparotomy

Memory Loss

A. **Initial Workup**
1. CBC
2. Sedimentation
3. Chemistry panel
4. Urinalysis
5. VDRL
6. Serum B_{12} and folate
7. Thyroid profile
8. HIV antibody titer
9. Drug screen
10. Withhold as many medications as possible, preferably one at a time
11. Therapeutic trial of vitamin B complex
12. Therapeutic trial of hormone replacement therapy

B. **Expanded Workup**
1. Neurology consult
2. MRI of brain
3. Wake and sleep EEG
4. Psychometric testings
5. Spinal fluid analysis
6. Radionuclide cisternography
7. Therapeutic trial of removal of spinal fluid
8. Psychiatric consult

Nausea and Vomiting

A. **Initial Workup**
1. CBC
2. Sedimentation rate
3. Chemistry panel
4. Urinalysis
5. Drug screen
6. Blood lead level
7. Pregnancy test
8. Electrolytes
9. Serum amylase and lipase
10. Gall bladder ultrasonography
11. Flat plate of abdomen
12. Chest x-ray
13. Stool for occult blood X3
14. Stool smear and culture
15. Stool for ovum and parasites

B. **Expanded Workup**
1. Gastroenterology consult
2. Esophagoscopy, gastroscopy, duodenoscopy, ERCP
3. HIDA scan
4. Small bowel series
5. CT scan of abdomen
6. Neurology consult
7. Ophthalmology consult
8. Psychiatric consult

Neck Pain

A. **Initial Workup**
1. CBC
2. Sedimentation rate
3. Chemistry panel
4. Urinalysis
5. Arthritis panel
6. Plain films of the cervical spine
7. Chest x-ray
8. ECG
9. Thyroid profile

B. **Expanded Workup**
1. Neurology consult
2. MRI of the cervical spine
3. MRI of the neck
4. Trigger point injections
5. Nerve blocks
6. Facet injections
7. Therapeutic trial of NSAIDs

Obesity

A. **Initial Workup**
1. CBC
2. Sedimentation rate
3. Chemistry panel
4. Urinalysis
5. Thyroid profile including TSH
6. 72-hr fast with glucose monitoring

B. Expanded Workup
1. Endocrinology consult
2. CT scan of brain and abdomen
3. Serum cortisol
4. Plasma insulin
5. C-peptide
6. Chromosomal analysis
7. Psychiatric consult

Palpitations

A. Initial Workup
1. CBC
2. Sedimentation rate
3. Chemistry panel
4. Urinalysis
5. ASO titer
6. CRP
7. BNP
8. Thyroid profile
9. ECG
10. Chest x-ray
11. Drug screen
12. Avoid caffeine, alcohol and nicotine
13. Discontinue all unnecessary drugs if possible, preferably one at a time

B. Expanded Workup
1. Cardiology consult
2. Echocardiography
3. Holter monitoring
4. Exercise tolerance test
5. 24-hr urine metanephrines or catecholamines
6. Spirometry
7. Arterial blood gas analysis
8. Coronary angiography
9. Therapeutic trial of diuretics
10. Therapeutic trial of beta-blockers.

Paresthesias of the Lower Extremities

A. Initial Workup
1. CBC
2. Sedimentation rate
3. Chemistry panel
4. Urinalysis
5. VDRL
6. Arthritis panel
7. Serum B_{12} and folic acid
8. Radiographs of lumbosacral spine
9. Glucose tolerance test
10. ANA
11. Therapeutic trial of vitamin B_{12} injections
12. Therapeutic trial of vitamin B complex

B. Expanded Workup
1. Neurology consult
2. MRI of lumbar spine
3. EMG and NCV
4. Blood lead level
5. Urine for porphobilinogen
6. Quantitative urine thiamine, niacin and pyridoxine after loading
7. Serum protein electrophoresis
8. Blood viscosity
9. HIV antibody titer
10. Lymph node biopsy
11. Kveim test
12. Muscle biopsy

Paresthesias of the Upper Extremity

A. Initial Workup
1. CBC
2. Sedimentation rate
3. Chemistry panel
4. Urinalysis
5. ANA
6. Radiographs of the cervical spine and chest
7. Serum B_{12} and folic acid
8. VDRL
9. Serum protein electrophoresis

B. Expanded Workup
1. Neurology consult
2. EMG and NCV
3. MRI of the cervical spine
4. MRI of the brain
5. MRI of the neck
6. Carotid duplex scan
7. ECG
8. Exercise tolerance test
9. Therapeutic trial of vitamin B complex
10. Therapeutic trial of shoulder halter or cervical collar
11. Stellate ganglion block
12. Nerve blocks.

Penile Sores
1. CBC
2. Chemistry
3. Sedimentation rate
4. Smear and culture of exudates
5. Dark field examination
6. Frei test
7. Biopsy of lesion
8. Tzanck test
9. Lymph node biopsy
10. Serologic test for lymphogran-uloma venereum
11. HIV antibody titer
12. Urology consult

13. Dermatology consult
14. Fluorescent treponema pallidum antibody
15. Therapeutic trial of acyclovir
16. Therapeutic trial of penicillin
17. Therapeutic trial of other antibiotics

Rash

A. Initial Workup
1. CBC
2. Sedimentation
3. Chemistry panel
4. Urinalysis
5. VDRL
6. Routine smear and culture of exudates
7. Microscopic examination of KOH preparation for fungi and scabies
8. Wood's lamp examination
9. ANA
10. Therapeutic trial of local anti-biotics
11. Therapeutic trial of anti-fungal preparations
12. Therapeutic trial of scabicides
13. Therapeutic trial of corticos-teroids
14. Stool for occult blood X3

B. Expanded Workup
1. Dermatology consult
2. Skin biopsy
3. Patch tests
4. RAST
5. Intradermal allergy skin testing
6. Blood cultures
7. Lyme disease serology
8. Weil–Felix reaction
9. Dark-field examination
10. Gastroenterology consult
11. Barium enema
12. Muscle biopsy
13. Coagulation profile
14. Blood smear for parasites

Rectal Bleeding

A. Initial Workup
1. CBC
2. Chemistry panel
3. Sedimentation rate
4. Urinalysis
5. Stool for occult blood X3
6. Anoscopy
7. Sigmoidoscopy
8. Barium enema

9. Stool culture
10. Stool for ovum and parasites

B. Expanded Workup
1. Gastroenterology consult
2. Colonoscopy
3. CT scan of abdomen and pelvis
4. Coagulation profile
5. Mesenteric angiography
6. Upper GI series
7. Gastroscopy and duodenoscopy
8. Nuclear scan after intravenous chromium ragged red cells
9. Small bowel series
10. Frei test

Red Eye

A. Initial Workup
1. CBC
2. Sedimentation rate
3. Chemistry panel
4. Urinalysis
5. Smear and culture of exudates
6. Fluorescein dye test for foreign body or corneal abrasions
7. Check for urethral discharge
8. Nose and throat culture
9. X-ray of sinuses
10. Tonometry
11. Slit lamp examination
12. Smear of exudates for eosinophils
13. Visual acuity
14. Trial of antibiotic drops

B. Expanded Workup
1. Ophthalmology consult
2. CT scan of brain and sinuses
3. MRI of brain
4. Refraction
5. Uveitis workup (as ordered by ophthalmologist)
6. Allergy skin testing
7. HLA typing

Scrotal Swelling
1. CBC
2. Sedimentation rate
3. Chemistry panel
4. Urinalysis
5. PSA
6. Smear and culture of prostatic exudates
7. Urine culture and colony count
8. Ultrasonography of scrotum
9. Radionuclide scan of testicle
10. Testicular biopsy
11. Flat plate of abdomen

Shoulder Pain

A. Initial Workup
1. CBC
2. Sedimentation rate
3. Chemistry panel
4. Arthritis panel
5. X-ray of shoulder
6. Radiograph of chest
7. Radiograph of cervical spine
8. Trigger point injection
9. Lidocaine injection of bursa or shoulder joint

B. Expanded Workup
1. Orthopedic consult
2. MRI of shoulder
3. Neurology Consult
4. MRI of cervical spine
5. Gall bladder ultrasonography
6. Exercise tolerance test
7. Arthrogram
8. Arthroscopy
9. EMG and NCV studies

Sore Throat
1. CBC
2. Sedimentation rate
3. Chemistry panel
4. Urinalysis
5. Nose and throat culture
6. Urinalysis
7. ASO titer or streptozyme
8. Monospot test
9. Culture for Neisseria gonorrhea
10. Culture for diphtheria bacilli
11. Thyroid panel
12. ENT consult

Syncope

A. Initial Workup
1. CBC
2. Sedimentation rate
3. Chemistry panel
4. Urinalysis
5. Urine drug screen
6. Thyroid profile
7. Glucose tolerance test
8. C-peptide or plasma insulin
9. ECG
10. Chest x-ray
11. Several blood pressure readings in recumbent and upright positions
12. Tilt table test

B. Expanded Workup
1. Cardiology consult
2. Holter monitoring
3. Echocardiography
4. Neurology consult
5. EEG
6. MRI and MRA of brain
7. Carotid duplex scan
8. Ambulatory EEG monitoring
9. Hospitalization for telemetry and video monitoring
10. Psychiatric consult
11. Trial of anticonvulsants

Tremor
1. CBC
2. Sedimentation rate
3. Chemistry panel
4. Urinalysis
5. Urine drug screen
6. Blood alcohol level
7. Thyroid profile
8. Serum copper and ceruloplasmin
9. Liver function tests
10. Neurology consult
11. MRI of brain
12. EEG
13. Spinal fluid analysis

Vaginal Bleeding

A. Initial Workup
1. Vaginal and rectovaginal examination and Pap smear
2. CBC
3. Sedimentation rate
4. Chemistry panel
5. Urinalysis
6. Pregnancy test
7. Serum iron and iron-binding capacity
8. Thyroid profile
9. Coagulation profile
10. ANA
11. Flat plate of abdomen
12. Pelvic ultrasonography
13. Vaginal smear and culture
14. DNA probe or rapid antigen testing for gonorrhea and chlamydia

B. Expanded Workup
1. Gynecology consult
2. CT scan of abdomen and pelvis
3. Laparoscopy
4. VDRL
5. HIV antibody titer
6. Endometrial biopsy
7. D & C
8. Trail of cyclic progesterone
9. Endocrinology consult
10. CA-125 test

Vaginal Discharge

A. Initial Workup
1. CBC
2. Sedimentation rate
3. Urinalysis
4. Urine culture and colony count
5. DNA probe or rapid antigen testing of urine for gonorrhea and chlamydia
6. Microscopic examination of saline and KOH preparations of discharge
7. Endocervical smear and culture
8. Search for clue cells in exudates
9. Pap smear
10. Culture for *Candida*
11. VDRL

B. Expanded Workup
1. Gynecology consult
2. Pelvic ultrasonography
3. FTA-ABS
4. HIV antibody titer
5. CT scan of abdomen and pelvis
6. D & C

Weight Loss

A. Initial Workup
1. CBC
2. Sedimentation rate
3. Chemistry panel
4. Urinalysis
5. Thyroid profile
6. Serum amylase and lipase
7. ANA
8. RA test
9. Tuberculin test
10. Febrile agglutinins
11. Serum protein electrophoresis
12. Stool for quantitative fat
13. HIV antibody titer
14. Chest x-ray
15. Flat plate of abdomen
16. Stool for occult blood X3

B. Expanded Workup
1. Gastroenterology consult
2. Upper GI series
3. Small bowel series
4. Barium enema
5. CT scan of abdomen and pelvis
6. Stool for ovum and parasites
7. Urine 5-HIAA
8. Endocrinology consult
9. Plasma cortisol
10. Rapid ACTH stimulation test
11. Serum growth hormone
12. Serum FSH, LH
13. Exploratory laparotomy

The Laboratory Workup of Disease

A

Abortion, threatened: Serum B–human chorionic gonadotropin (hCG), serum progesterone levels, urine, hCG, pregnanediol, sonogram

Achalasia: Barium swallow, mecholyl test, esophagoscopy, and esophageal manometry

Acoustic neuroma: Skull x-ray, computed tomography (CT) scan, posterior fossa myelogram, magnetic resonance imaging (MRI)

Acquired Immunodeficiency Syndrome (AIDS): Human immunodeficiency virus (HIV) antibody titer, enzyme linked immunosorbent assay (ELISA), western blot, viral load, CD4 count

Acromegaly: Skull x-ray, CT scan, serum growth hormone, MRI

Actinomycosis: Smear for sulfur granules, culture skin lesions

Addison disease: Serum cortisol before and after corticotrophin, CT scan of abdomen, metyrapone test

Adrenogenital syndrome: Serum cortisol, hydroxyprogesterone, 11-deoxycortisol, urine 17-ketosteroids and pregnanetriol, dexamethasone suppression test, CT scan of the abdomen

Adult respiratory distress syndrome: Chest x-ray, sputum culture, blood culture, Swan–Ganz catheterization, arterial blood gasses (ABGs)

Agammaglobulinemia: Serum electrophoresis and immunoelectrophoresis, blood type, lymph node biopsy, B-lymphocyte and T-lymphocyte counts

Agranulocytosis, idiopathic: Complete blood count (CBC), bone marrow examination, spleen scan

AIDS: See Acquired Immunodeficiency Syndrome

Albright syndrome: X-ray of long bones, bone biopsy

Alcaptonuria: Urinary homogentisic acid, x-ray of spine

Alcoholism: Blood alcohol level, liver function tests, liver biopsy

Aldosteronism, primary: Electrolytes before and after spironolactone, plasma renin, 24-hr urine aldosterone, CT scan, exploratory laparotomy

Allergic rhinitis: Nasal smear for eosinophils, serum immunoglobulin E (IgE) antibody, radioallergosorbent test (RAST), skin test

Alveolar proteinosis: Luteinizing hormone (LH), sputum for periodic acid-Schiff–positive material (PSP), lung biopsy

Alzheimer disease: CT scan or MRI

Amebiasis: Stool for ova and parasites, rectal biopsy, hemagglutinin inhibition test

Amyloidosis: Congo red test, rectal biopsy, liver biopsy, gingival biopsy, subcutaneous fat aspiration and stain

Angina pectoris: Graded exercise tolerance test (GXT), thallium-201 scintigraphy, coronary angiogram, trial of nitroglycerin

Angioneurotic edema: C1 esterase inhibitor

Ankylosing spondylitis: Human leukocyte antigen (HLA) B27 tissue antigen

Anthrax: Smear and culture of lesion, skin biopsy, serologic test

Antitrypsin deficiency: Serum protein electrophoresis

Aortic aneurysm: Sonogram, CT scan, aortogram

Aortic valvular disease: Echocardiogram, CT scan, MRI, cardiac catheterization

Appendicitis: CBC, flat plate of abdomen, CT scan, ultrasonography

Aplastic anemia: Bone marrow, lymph node biopsy, immunoelectrophoresis

Ascaris lumbricoides: Cathartic stool for ova and parasites, eosinophil count

Asthma: Spirometry, sputum for eosinophils, serum IgE antibodies, RAST, skin test

Attention deficit disorder: Clinical diagnosis

Atrial arrhythmias: Free thyroxine, TSH, electrocardiogram (ECG), Holter monitoring, His bundle study

Atypical pneumonia, primary: See *Mycoplasma pneumoniae*

B

Bacillary dysentery: Stool smear (for leukocytes) and culture, febrile agglutinins

Balantidiasis: Stool for ova and parasites

Banti's syndrome: Liver function tests, liver–spleen scan, bone marrow examination, hepatic vein catheterization

Barbiturate poisoning: Blood or urine for barbiturates, electroencephalogram (EEG)

Basilar artery insufficiency: Four-vessel cerebral angiogram, magnetic resonance angiogram

Bell palsy: CT scan of mastoids and petrous bones, electromyogram (EMG)

Beriberi: Transketolase activity coefficient, urine thiamine afterload, therapeutic trial

Bilharziasis: Stool or urine sediment for eggs, rectal biopsy

Biliary cirrhosis: Liver function tests, mitochondrial antibodies, serum bile acids, endoscopic retrograde cholangiopancreatography (ERCP), liver biopsy

Blastomycosis: Potassium hydroxide (KOH) prep, culture, chest x-ray, skin test, serologic test

Boeck's sarcoid: Chest x-ray, transbronchial lung biopsy, lymph node biopsy, Kveim test, liver biopsy, angiotensin-converting enzyme, liver gallium scan

Botulism: Culture of food and stool, mouse assay of toxin

Brain tumor: CT scan, MRI

Brill–Symmers disease: Lymph node biopsy

Bromide poisoning: Blood bromide level

Bronchiectasis: Bronchogram, bronchoscopy, CT scan of lung

Bronchitis: Sputum culture, chest x-ray

Bronchopneumonia: Sputum smear and culture, chest x-ray, CBC, cold agglutinins

Brucellosis: Blood cultures, serologic tests, skin test

Bubonic plague: Culture of bubo, blood, or sputum; animal inoculation; serologic test

Buerger's disease: Phlebogram, arteriogram, biopsy of affected vessels, ultrasonography

C

Carbon monoxide poisoning: Carboxyhemoglobin determination

Carbon tetrachloride poisoning: Liver function tests, infrared spectrometry, liver biopsy, blood carbon tetrachloride

Carcinoid syndrome: Serum serotonin, urine 5-hydroxyindoleacetic acid (5-HIAA), exploratory laparotomy, bronchoscopy

Carcinoma of the breast: Mammogram, sonogram, fine-needle aspiration, biopsy

Carcinoma of the cervix: Papanicolaou (Pap) smears, cervical biopsy, colposcopy

Carcinoma of the colon: Stool for occult blood, sigmoidoscopy, barium enema, colonoscopy, carcinoembryonic antigen (CEA), CT scan

Carcinoma of endometrium: Pap smear, endometrial biopsy, dilatation and curettage (D & C)

Carcinoma of the esophagus: Barium swallow, esophagoscopy, biopsy

Carcinoma of the lung: Chest x-ray, CT scan, sputum Pap smears, bronchoscopy and biopsy, needle biopsy, open-lung biopsy, scalene node biopsy

Carcinoma of the pancreas: Sonogram, CT scan of abdomen, liver function tests, ERCP, exploratory laparotomy, cancer antigen (CA) 19-9

Carcinoma of the stomach: Gastrointestinal (GI) series, gastroscopy and biopsy, gastric cytology

Cardiac arrhythmias: ECG, Holter monitoring, echocardiogram, electrophysiologic study

Cardiomyopathy: See Myocarditis/Myocardiopathy

Carpal tunnel syndrome: Nerve conduction velocity (NCV) study, MRI

Cat-scratch disease: Skin test, lymph node biopsy

Celiac disease: D-xylose absorption, mucosal biopsy, urine 5-HIAA, small bowel series, tissue transglutaminase autoantibody titer by ELISA

Cellulitis: Smear and culture of wound exudates, antistreptolysin O (ASO) titer

Cerebellar ataxia: CT scan, MRI

Cerebral abscess: CT scan, MRI

Cerebral aneurysm: CT scan, MRI, MRA, arteriogram

Cerebral embolism: CT scan, blood culture, echocardiogram, carotid scan, four-vessel cerebral angiogram, ECG

Cerebral hemorrhage: CT scan, MRI

Cerebral thrombosis: CT scan, MRI, MRA, carotid scan, digital subtraction angiogram, four-vessel cerebral angiogram

Cervical spondylosis: X-ray of cervical spine, EMG, MRI, myelogram with simultaneous CT scan

Chagas disease: Blood smear and culture, cerebrospinal fluid (CSF) smear and culture, bone marrow or tissue biopsy, animal inoculation, serologic tests

Chancroid: Smear and culture of lesion, skin biopsy, serology tests

Child abuse: Skeletal survey, chest x-ray, vaginal smear and culture

Chlamydia pneumonia: Chest x-ray, serologic tests

Cholangioma: Liver function tests, transhepatic cholangiogram, ERCP, CT scan of abdomen, exploratory laparotomy

Cholangitis: Liver function tests, transhepatic cholangiogram, ERCP, exploratory laparotomy

Cholecystitis: Sonogram, cholecystogram, liver function tests, hepatobiliary iminodiacetic acid scan (HIDA) test

Choledocholithiasis: Liver function tests, duodenal drainage, ERCP, transhepatic cholangiogram, sonogram

Cholelithiasis: Sonogram, cholecystogram, liver function tests, ERCP

Cholera: Stool smear and culture, dark field microscopy

Choriocarcinoma: Plasma B-subunit hCG, urine chorionic gonadotropin, D & C

Cirrhosis: Liver function tests, liver scan, CT scan, liver biopsy

Coarctation of the aorta: Chest x-ray, clinical evaluation, aortograms rarely required

Coccidioidomycosis: Smear, animal inoculation, serology, skin test, chest x-ray

Concussion: CT scan, MRI, EEG, evoked potentials, psychometric tests

Congestive heart failure: ECG, chest x-rays, spirometry, circulation time, ABGs, echocardiogram, B-type natriuretic peptide (BNP)

Coronary insufficiency: See Angina pectoris

Costochondritis (Tietze syndrome): Lidocaine infiltration

Craniopharyngioma: Skull x-ray, CT scan, MRI

Cretinism: Free T_4, thyrotropin, radioactive iodine (RAI) uptake and scan, x-ray for bone age

Crigler–Najjar syndrome: See Gilbert disease

Cryoglobulinemia: Serum protein electrophoresis and immunoelectrophoresis, (SIA) water test, cold agglutinins, rheumatoid arthritis (RA) test, hepatitis C antibody titer

Cryptococcosis: Spinal fluid smear and culture, sputum or blood cultures, CSF cryptococcal antigen

Cushing syndrome: Twenty-four-hour urine free cortisol, plasma cortisol, single-dose overnight dexamethasone suppression test, CT scan of brain or abdomen

Cystic fibrosis: Quantitative pilocarpine iontophoresis, sweat test

Cysticercosis: Serologic test, CT scan of brain, MRI, biopsy of subcutaneous cysticerci

Cystinosis: Slit-lamp examination, liver biopsy

Cystinuria: Serum and urine cystine and arginine, cyanide–nitroprusside test, thin-layer chromatography

Cytomegalic inclusion disease: Blood smear for atypical lymphs, cytomegalovirus (CMV), IgM antibody titer, human fibroblastic cell culture inoculation, immunofluorescence technique for viral demonstration

D

Dehydration: Intake and output of fluid, electrolytes, blood urea nitrogen (BUN) to creatinine ratio, serum/urine osmolality

Dengue: Viral isolation from blood, serology test

Dermatomyositis: Antinuclear antibody (ANA), aspartate aminotransferase (AST), lactate dehydrogenase (LDH), creatine phosphokinase (CPK), aldolase, EMG, muscle biopsy

Diabetes insipidus: Hickey–Hare test, serum/urine osmolality intake and output before and after pitressin, CT scan, serum antidiuretic hormone (ADH)

Diabetes mellitus: Glucose tolerance test, cortisone glucose tolerance test, glycosylated hemoglobin (HbAlc)

Digitalis intoxication: Serum digoxin level, ECG

Di Guglielmo disease: Bone marrow, peripheral blood study

Diphtheria: Nose and throat culture

Diphyllobothrium latum: Stool for ova and parasites, serum B_{12} level

Dissecting aneurysm: Chest x-ray, ultrasonography, CT scan or MRI of aorta, aortogram

Disseminated intravascular coagulation (DIC): Decreased fibrinogen, increased fibrin degradation products, D-dimer assay

Diverticulosis: Sigmoidoscopy, barium enema, colonoscopy, CT scan of abdomen, gallium scan, sonogram, exploratory laparotomy

Down syndrome: Chromosome study, urinary B-aminoisobutyric acid

Dracunculiasis: Noting presence of worms in subcutaneous tissues, serum IgE, antifilarial antibody titer

Dubin–Johnson syndrome: Liver function tests, liver biopsy

Ductus arteriosus, patent: Cardiac catheterization, angiocardiogram, echocardiogram

Duodenal ulcer: See Peptic ulcer

Dwarfism: X-ray of bones; endocrine, renal and GI function tests

Dysfunctional uterine bleeding: D & C, endometrial biopsy, progesterone challenge

E

Eaton–Lambert syndrome: EMG, Tensilon test, muscle biopsy, chest x-ray

Echinococcosis: CT scan, x-ray of long bones, Casoni skin test, serologic tests, liver biopsy

Eclampsia: Uric acid, renal function tests, renal biopsy

Ectopic pregnancy: Serum β-hCG by immunoassay, sonogram, laparoscopy, culdocentesis, exploratory laparotomy, serum progesterone levels

Eczema: Serum IgE levels

Ehlers–Danlos syndrome: Capillary fragility test, bleeding time, skin biopsy

Emphysema: Pulmonary function tests, chest x-ray, ABGs, α-antitrypsin level, single breath diffusing capacity for carbon monoxide

Empyema: Chest x-ray, sputum cultures, gallium scan, thoracentesis

Encephalitis: Viral isolation from brain tissue and spinal fluid, MRI, serologic tests

Encephalomyelitis: Viral isolation from brain tissue and spinal fluid, MRI, serologic tests

Endocardial fibroelastosis: ECG, chest x-ray, echocardiogram, angiocardiogram

Endocarditis: See Subacute bacterial endocarditis

Epilepsy: Wake-and-sleep EEG, CT scan or MRI, positron emission tomography (PET) scan, ambulatory EEG monitoring

Erectile dysfunction: Penile blood pressure nocturnal tumescence testing, sonogram

Erythema multiforme: Skin biopsy, patch test

Erythroblastosis fetalis: Bilirubin, direct Coombs test, amniocentesis

Esophageal varices: Esophagoscopy, splenovenogram, ultrasonography

Esophagitis: Bernstein test, esophagoscopy and biopsy, esophageal manometry, ambulatory pH monitoring

Extradural hematoma: Skull x-ray, CT scan, MRI

Endometriosis: Sonogram, CA-125 levels

Epididymitis: Sonogram, radionuclide scan

F

Fanconi syndrome: X-ray (pelvis, scapula, femur, ribs), urinary amino acids, glucose, electrolytes, serum uric acid, alkaline phosphatase, renal biopsy

Filariasis: Blood smear for microfilariae, skin test, complement fixation test

Folic acid deficiency: Serum folic acid, therapeutic trial

Friedlander pneumonia: Sputum smear and culture, blood cultures, lung puncture, serial chest x-rays

Friedreich's ataxia: Clinical diagnosis

G

Galactosemia: Paigon assay of blood galactose, red blood cell (RBC) assay of (GAL-1-PUT) transferase

Gallstone: See Cholelithiasis

Gargoylism: Urinary chondroitin sulfuric acid, serum assay of α-L-iduronidase, tissue culture, enzyme assay

Gastric ulcer: See Peptic ulcer

Gastritis: Serology for *Helicobacter pylori*, gastroscopy, biopsy

Gastroenteritis: Stool for culture, smear, and ova and parasites

Gaucher's disease: Assay of leukocytes for β-glucosidase, bone marrow examination, x-ray of long bones

General paresis: Blood and spinal fluid fluorescent treponemal antibody absorption (FTA–ABS) test

Giardia lamblia: Cathartic stool for ova and parasites, duodenal analysis, giardia antigen, string test

Gigantism: CT scan or MRI of brain, serum growth hormone

Gilbert disease: Liver function tests, liver biopsy

Gilles de la Tourette syndrome: Urinary catecholamines

Glanders: Culture of skin lesion, skin test, serologic tests, animal inoculation

Glanzmann's disease: Platelet counts, clot retraction, prothrombin time, bleeding time, capillary fragility test; see also Thrombocythemia

Glaucoma: Tonometry, gonioscopy, visual fields

Glomerulonephritis: Serum complement, streptozyme test, ANA, renal biopsy

Glossitis: Culture, biopsy, therapeutic trial of vitamins and iron

Glycogen storage disease: Glucose tolerance test, epinephrine test, liver biopsy and analysis for glucose-6-phosphatase

Goiter: Free T₄, RAI uptake and scan, thyrotropin, serum antibodies

Gonorrhea: Urethral, rectal, vaginal, or throat smear and cultures; DNA probes and polymerase chain reaction (PCR)

Goodpasture's syndrome: Circulating antiglomerular antibodies, chest x-ray, renal biopsy

Gout: Serum uric acid, synovial fluid analysis, x-ray of bones and joints

Granuloma inguinale: Wright stain of scrapings from lesion and biopsy

Graves disease: See Hyperthyroidism

Guillain–Barré syndrome: EMG, spinal fluid analysis

Gumma: FTA–ABS

H

Haemophilus influenzae: Nose, throat, and sputum culture or spinal fluid smear and culture

Hamman–Rich syndrome: Chest x-ray, pulmonary function tests, lung biopsy

Hand–Schuller–Christian disease: X-ray of skull, bone biopsy, bone marrow examination

Hansen disease: See Leprosy

Hartnup disease: Urinary amino acid, indican, and indoleacetic acid; FT₄ index; thyrotropin

Hashimoto's disease: FT₄ index, thyrotropin, serum thyroglobulin antibodies

Haverhill fever: Agglutination titer, aspiration of affected joint or abscess for *Streptobacillus moniliformis*

Hay fever: See Allergic rhinitis

Heart failure: See Congestive heart failure

Helminth infections: Stool for ova and parasites, serologic tests, skin tests, liver function tests

Hemangioblastoma: CT scan or MRI

Hemochromatosis: Serum ferritin, serum iron and iron-binding capacity, liver or skin biopsy

Hemoglobin C disease: Blood smear for target cells, hemoglobin electrophoresis

Hemoglobinuria, paroxysmal cold: CBC, Coombs test, Donath–Landsteiner test, FTA–ABS, serum haptoglobins

Hemoglobinuria, paroxysmal nocturnal: CBC, Ham test, sucrose hemolysis test

Hemolytic anemia: Serum haptoglobins, radioactive chromium–tagged red cell survival, urine and fecal urobilinogen, Coombs test, blood smear

Hemophilia: Coagulation profile, thromboplastin generation test, assay of factors VIII, IX, XI

Hepatitis: Liver function test, hepatitis profile, IgM, anti–hepatitis A virus (HAV), hepatitis B surface antigen (HBsAG), liver biopsy, anti–hepatitis C virus (HCV)

Hepatitis, chronic active: HBsAG, liver function tests, ANA, liver biopsy, anti–smooth muscle antibody

Hepatolenticular degeneration: See Wilson's disease

Hepatoma: Ultrasonography, CT scan, α-fetoprotein, liver biopsy, arteriogram, MRI

Hernia, diaphragmatic: See Hiatal hernia

Herniated disc: EMG, MRI, CT scan, myelogram, discogram

Herpangina: Serologic tests, viral isolation

Herpes genitalis: Examination of skin scrapings, Tzanck test, culture, serologic tests

Herpes simplex: Serologic tests, viral isolation, Tzanck test

Herpes zoster: Tzanck test, serologic tests

Hiatal hernia: Bernstein test, esophogram, esophagoscopy and biopsy, esophageal manometry, therapeutic trial

Hirschsprung's disease: Rectal or colonic biopsy

Histamine cephalgia: Test trial of histamine subcutaneously, response to sumatriptan

Histoplasmosis: Sputum culture, bone marrow culture, animal inoculation, skin test, serologic tests, chest x-ray

HIV infections: See Acquired Immunodeficiency Syndrome

Hodgkin's lymphoma: Lymph node biopsy, bone marrow lymphangiogram, CT scan, liver–spleen scan, exploratory laparotomy

Huntington's chorea: Clinical diagnosis, genetic markers, CT scan

Hurler syndrome: See Gargoylism

Hydronephrosis: CT scan of abdomen Intravenous pyelogram (IVP), sonogram

Hyperaldosteronism: See Aldosteronism, primary

Hypercholesterolemia, familial: Lipoprotein electrophoresis, lipid profile

Hyperlipemia, idiopathic: Lipoprotein electrophoresis, ultracentrifugation

Hypernephroma: IVP or retrograde pyelogram, CT scan, angiogram

Hyperparathyroidism: Serum calcium, phosphorus, and alkaline phosphatase; urine calcium; serum parathyroid hormone (PTH); 1,25-(OH)2D; phosphate reabsorption test; exploratory surgery

Hyperprolactinemia: CT scan, MRI of brain serum prolactin

Hypersplenism: CBC, blood smear, red cell survival, spleen/liver ratio, bone marrow, epinephrine test, exploratory laparotomy

Hyperthyroidism: Thyroid-stimulating hormone (TSH), free T3, FT_4 index, free T4

Hypoparathyroidism: Serum calcium and phosphorus, 24-hr urine calcium, skull x-ray, phosphate reabsorption, therapeutic trial, PTH assay, urine cyclic adenosine monophosphate (AMP)

Hypopituitarism: Serum cortisol, serum thyroxine, serum growth hormone, serum corticotrophin, thyrotropin, follicle-stimulating hormone (FSH), LH, CT scan, MRI

Hypotension, idiopathic postural: Clinical observation, tilt table test, response to vasopressin injection (Pitressin), tests to rule out causes of secondary hypotension

Hypothermia: EKG [J waves (Osborn waves)]

Hypothyroidism: Free T_4, thyrotropin-sensitive assay, thyroid microsomal antibodies, therapeutic trial

I

Idiopathic hypertrophic subaortic stenosis: EKG, echocardiography

Ileitis: See Regional enteritis

Inappropriate ADH secretion: Plasma and urine osmolality, spot urinary sodium, serum ADH

Infectious mononucleosis: Monospot test, heterophile antibody titer, smear for atypical lymphocytes, liver function tests, repeat tests, Epstein–Barr virus (EBV) antibody titer

Influenza, viral: Culture of nasopharyngeal washing, complement fixation tests, rapid antigen test

Insulinoma: See Islet cell tumor

Interstitial cystitis: Cystoscopy and biopsy

Intestinal obstruction: Flat plate of the abdomen with lateral decubitus films, double enema, sonogram, CT scan, GI series with diatrizoate meglumine and diatrizoate sodium (Hypaque), exploratory laparotomy

Iron deficiency anemia: Serum ferritin, serum iron and iron-binding capacity, free erythrocyte protoporphyrins

(FEP), bone marrow, therapeutic trial

Irritable bowel syndrome: Clinical diagnosis

Islet cell tumor: Glucose tolerance test, 72-hr fast, plasma insulin, C-peptide, tolbutamide tolerance test, pancreatic arteriogram, exploratory laparotomy

K

Kala azar: Blood smear, bone marrow or splenic aspirate for parasites, culture, serologic tests (ELISA)

Kaposi sarcoma: Human herpesvirus 8 (HHV8) antibody titer, biopsy

Klinefelter's syndrome: Sex chromatin pattern, testicular biopsy, serum FSH and LH

Kwashiorkor: Serum albumin, CBC

L

Lactase deficiency: Lactose tolerance test, mucosal biopsy, hydrogen breath test

Laennec cirrhosis: See Cirrhosis

Larva migrans, visceral: Eosinophil count, serum globulin, skin testing, serologic tests, liver biopsy

Laryngeal carcinoma: Laryngoscopy

Laryngitis: Nose and throat culture, washings for viral studies, laryngoscopy

Lead intoxication: Serum and urine lead content, urine for γ-aminolevulinic acid (ALA), coproporphyria FEP, test dose of diaminoethanetetraacetic acid (EDTA), x-ray of long bones

Legionnaire disease: Sputum culture, serology, urinary Ag assay

Leishmaniasis: CBC, blood spleen and bone marrow smears for parasites, biopsy, serologic tests

Leprosy: Wade's scraped incision procedure, culture of lesion, biopsy of skin nerves, x-ray of hands and feet, histamine tests, lepromin skin test

Leptospirosis: See Weil disease

Letterer–Siwe disease: X-ray of bones, bone marrow, lymph node biopsy

Leukemia: Blood smear, bone marrow, uric acid, serum B_{12} concentration, iron-binding capacity, Philadelphia chromosome

Listeriosis: Blood or spinal fluid smear and spinal fluid agglutination titer, bone marrow biopsy

Liver abscess: Liver scan with technetium or gallium, liver aspiration and biopsy, CT scan, amebic hemagglutinin inhibition titer, cathartic stool for ova and parasites

Loeffler's syndrome: Eosinophil count, sputum for eosinophils, stool for ova and parasites

Lung abscess: Chest x-ray, tomogram, CT scan, sputum culture, bronchoscopy, sputum cytology, needle aspiration, biopsy, and culture

Lupoid hepatitis: See Hepatitis, chronic active

Lupus erythematosus: ANA, anti–double-stranded DNA antibody titer (not usually positive in drug-induced lupus), Coombs test, lupus erythematosus prep, coagulation profile, biopsy of skin, muscle, lymph node, or kidney

Lyme disease: Serologic tests

Lymphangitis: CBC, sedimentation rate

Lymphogranuloma inguinale: Lygranum test, Giemsa-stained smear, serologic tests, tissue or lymph node biopsy

Lymphogranuloma venereum: Serologic tests, lymph node biopsy, aspiration of bubo for culture

Lymphoma: See Hodgkin disease

Lymphosarcoma: CT scan, x-rays of chest and abdomen, lymphangiogram

M

Macroglobulinemia: Serum electrophoresis and immunoelectrophoresis, ultracentrifugation, Sia water test, bone marrow

Malabsorption syndrome: D-xylose absorption test, urine 5-HIAA, mucosal biopsy, small-bowel series

Malaria: Blood smear for parasites, bone marrow, serologic tests

Mallory–Weiss syndrome: Esophagoscopy

Marfan syndrome: X-ray of long bones and ribs, slit-lamp examination of eyes, IVP, urinary hydroxyproline, CT scan of aorta

Marie–Strumpell spondylitis: X-ray of lumbosacral spine, bone scan, HLA typing

Mastocytosis: Skin biopsy, Darier's sign, long-bone x-ray, bone marrow biopsy

Mastoiditis: X-ray of mastoid, CT scan

McArdle's syndrome: Liver biopsy, enzyme assay of muscle phosphorylase, muscle biopsy, urine myoglobin

Measles: Smear of nasal secretions for giant cells, serologic tests

Meckel's diverticulum: Technetium scan, sonogram, exploratory laparotomy

Mediastinitis: CT scan or MRI of chest, mediastinoscopy, exploratory surgery

Medullary sponge kidney: IVP, CT scan

Medulloblastoma: CT scan, MRI

Megaloblastic anemia: See Pernicious anemia

Meigs syndrome: Thoracentesis, culdoscopy, laparoscopy, exploratory laparotomy, sonogram

Melanoma: Serum or urinary melanin, biopsy

Ménière's disease: CT scan, audiogram, caloric tests, electronystagmography (ENG)

Meningioma: CT scan, MRI, x-ray of skull or spine, myelogram

Meningitis: Spinal fluid examination, smear and culture, serum for viral serologic studies, blood culture

Meningococcemia: Blood culture spinal fluid examination, smear and culture, Gram stain of punctured petechiae

Menopause syndrome: Serum LH, FSH, serum estradiol, vaginal smear for estrogen effects, therapeutic trial

Mental retardation: CT scan or MRI, EEG, psychometric testing, skull x-ray, phenylketonuria (PKU), FT_4 index, thyrotropin, urinary amino acids, chromosomal analysis

Methemoglobinemia: Erythrocyte methemoglobin, ABG, blood diaphorase I, spectrophotometry

Migraine: Nitroglycerin test, histamine test, sedimentation rate to rule out temporal arteritis

Mikulicz's disease: CBC, bone marrow, tuberculin test, biopsy of lesion, ANA, lymph node biopsy

Milk–alkali syndrome: Serum calcium, phosphorus, alkaline phosphatase, urinary calcium and phosphates

Milroy disease: Clinical diagnosis

Mitral insufficiency or stenosis: ECG, chest x-ray, echocardiogram, phonocardiogram, cardiac catheterization

Moniliasis: Vaginal smear or culture, skin scrapings with KOH prep, biopsy

Mononucleosis, infectious: See Infectious mononucleosis

Mucormycosis: Nose and throat culture, biopsy

Mucoviscoidosis: See Cystic fibrosis

Multiple myeloma: Serum protein electrophoresis, 24-hr urine electrophoresis, bone marrow, x-ray of skull and spine, MRI

Multiple sclerosis: Somatosensory evoked potentials, (SSEP), visual evoked potential (VEP), spinal fluid globulin (IgG), and myelin basic protein, MRI

Mumps: Skin test, serologic tests, viral isolation from throat washings

Muscular dystrophy: EMG, muscle biopsy, urine creatine, chromosome analysis, serum enzymes (creatine phosphokinase, and so forth)

Myasthenia gravis: EMG, Tensilon test, acetylcholine receptor antibody titer, CT scan of chest to rule out thymoma

Mycoplasma pneumoniae: Cold agglutinins, (MG) streptococcal agglutinins, culture

Mycosis fungoides: Skin biopsy

Myeloid metaplasia, agnogenic: Red cell morphology, CBC, bone marrow, leukocyte alkaline phosphatase, urine and serum erythropoietin

Myelophthisic anemia: CBC, bone marrow, bone scan, lymph node biopsy

Myocardial infarction: Serial enzymes [MB, creatine phosphokinase (CPK), and so forth], serial ECGs serum troponin-1, thallium-201 scintigraphy, pyrophosphate imaging, echocardiogram

Myocarditis/Myocardiopathy: Echocardiogram, endomyocardial biopsy, cardiac catheterization

Myotonia atrophica: EMG, urine creatinine and creatine, muscle biopsy

Myxoma, cardiac: Echocardiogram, angiocardiogram

N

Narcolepsy: Sleep study, EEG, HLA-DR2

Nematodes: Gastric analysis, muscle biopsy, eosinophil count, skin test, serologic tests, stools for ova and parasites, duodenal aspiration for ova and parasites, GI series, rectal swabs with Scotch tape

Nephritis: See Glomerulonephritis

Nephrocalcinosis: Serum PTH, serum calcium, phosphorus and alkaline phosphatase, IVP, CT scan of abdomen renal biopsy

Nephrotic syndrome: Urinalysis serum complement, sedimentation rate, serum protein electrophoresis, renal function tests, ANA, renal biopsy

Neurinoma, acoustic: See Acoustic neuroma

Neuritis, peripheral: See Neuropathy

Neuroblastoma: Urinary vanillylmandelic acid (VMA) and homovanillic acid (HVA), CT scan, bone marrow, exploratory laparotomy

Neurofibromatosis: Biopsy, skeletal survey, CT scan, spinal fluid analysis, myelogram

Neuropathy: Glucose tolerance test, blood lead level, urine porphobilinogen, blood and urine arsenic levels, urine N-methylnicotinamide, ANA, serum B_{12} and folic acid, spinal fluid examination, NCV, EMG, serum transketolase activity coefficient, nerve biopsy

Neurosyphilis: Blood and spinal fluid FTA ABS

Niacin deficiency: See Pellagra

Niemann–Pick disease: Demonstration of sphingomyelin in reticuloendothelial cells, bone marrow biopsy, tissue biopsy, skeletal survey, culture of skin fibroblasts

Nocardiosis: Sputum smear and culture, spinal fluid examination, smear and culture

Nonketotic hyperosmolar coma: Blood sugar, plasma osmolality

Normal pressure hydrocephalus: CT scan, nuclear flow study [radioactive iodinated albumin (RISA)]

Nutritional neuropathy: See Neuropathy

O

Ochronosis: Urinalysis (Benedict solution, isolation of homogentisic acid), x-ray of spine

Oppenheim's disease: EMG, muscle biopsy

Optic atrophy: CT scan of brain and orbits, visual fields, spinal tap, serum B_{12}, x-ray of skull and optic foramina

Optic neuritis: FTA–ABS antibody titer, visual fields, MRI of the brain

Osteitis deformans: Serum calcium, phosphorus, alkaline phosphatase, skeletal survey, bone scan, bone biopsy, urine hydroxyproline

Osteoarthritis: X-ray of spine and joints, exclusion of other forms of arthritis

Osteogenic sarcoma: Alkaline and acid phosphatase, x-ray of bone, bone scan, bone biopsy

Osteomalacia: Serum calcium phosphorus, alkaline phosphatase, x-ray of long bones, response to vitamin D and calcium, serum vitamin D levels

Osteomyelitis: Sedimentation rate, blood culture, culture of bone biopsy, x-ray of bone, bone scan, CT scan, teichoic acid antibody titer (TAAB)

Osteopetrosis: Bone marrow, x-ray of bones, bone biopsy

Osteoporosis: Serum, calcium, phosphorus, alkaline phosphatase, bone biopsy, x-ray of spine, quantitative computerized tomogram, bone mineral density (BMD), bone densitometry

Otitis media: Nasopharyngeal or aural smear and culture, CBC, sedimentation rate, tympanometry, audiogram

Otosclerosis: Audiometry

Ovarian cancer: Serum CA-125, pelvic sonogram, CT scan of abdomen and pelvis

P

Paget's disease: See Osteitis deformans

Pancreatic carcinoma: See Carcinoma of the pancreas

Pancreatitis, acute: Serum amylase and lipase, blood sugar, serum calcium, paracentesis, flat plate of abdomen, 2-hr urinary amylase

Pancreatitis, chronic: Serum and urinary amylase and lipase before and after secretin, glucose tolerance test, duodenal analysis for bicarbonate and enzyme concentration, CT scan, ERCP, fecal fat, triolein iodine 131 (^{131}I) uptake

Panniculitis: Bone marrow, skin and subcutaneous tissue biopsy

Paralysis agitans: Clinical diagnosis

Pediculosis: Woods lamp, microscopic examination of hair shafts

Pellagra: Urine *N*-methylnicotinamide, urine niacin after loading dose therapeutic trial

Pelvic inflammatory disease (PID): Laparoscopy, culture of cervical mucus, exploratory laparotomy

Pemphigus: Skin biopsy, Tzanck test, immunofluorescence studies

Penicillin allergy: Skin testing with penicilloyl polylysine

Peptic ulcer: Upper GI series, stool for occult blood, gastroscopy and duodenoscopy, gastric analysis, serology for *H. pylori*

Periarteritis nodosa: ANA; eosinophil count; CBC; urinalysis; muscle, skin, subcutaneous tissue, and testicular biopsy; nerve biopsy; angiography

Pericarditis: ECG, echocardiogram, chest x-ray, angiocardiogram, pericardial tap, CT scan or MRI

Periodic paralysis, familial: Serum potassium, ECG, EMG, response to glucose

Peritonitis: CBC, flat plate of abdomen, CT scan, sonogram, peritoneal tap, exploratory laparotomy

Pernicious anemia: CBC, blood smear, serum B_{12} and folic acid, Schilling test, gastric analysis with histamine, bone marrow

Pertussis: CBC, nasopharyngeal smear and culture

Petit mal: Sleep EEG, CT scan

Peutz–Jeghers syndrome: Small bowel series, exploratory laparotomy

Pharyngitis: Nose and throat culture, rapid agglutination test of throat swab (Abbott test pack strep A, Abbott Laboratories, Abbott Park, IL), streptozyme test

Phenylpyruvic oligophrenia: Urine for PKU and phenylalanine, Guthrie test, serum phenylalanine

Pheochromocytoma: Plasma and urine catecholamines, 24-hr urine VMA, CT scan, MRI

Phlebitis: See Thrombophlebitis

Phlebotomus fever: Serologic tests

Pickwickian syndrome: Pulmonary function tests, ABG, sleep study

Pinealoma: CT scan or MRI

Pinworms: Scotch tape swab of perianal area with microscopic examination for eggs

Pituitary adenoma: CT scan, MRI, serum thyrotropin, corticotrophin, LH and FSH, Free T_4, serum cortisol, growth hormone

Placenta previa: Ultrasonography

Plague: See Bubonic plague

Platyhelminthes: Stool for ova and parasites, serologic tests, skin test, urine sediment for eggs, eosinophil count

Pleurisy: Chest x-ray, thoracentesis, pleural biopsy, bronchoscopy, CT scan, ultrasonography

Pleurodynia, epidemic: Serologic tests, stool and throat cultures for Coxsackie B virus

Pneumococcal pneumonia: See Pneumonia

Pneumoconiosis: Chest x-ray, pulmonary function tests, ABG, sputum smear, lung biopsy, lung scan, scalene node biopsy

Pneumonia: Stat sputum smear, culture, blood cultures, chest x-ray

Pneumothorax: Chest x-ray, ABG, CT scan

Poliomyelitis: Viral isolation from stool, serologic tests, spinal fluid analysis

Polyarteritis: See Periarteritis nodosa

Polycystic kidney: Sonogram, CT scan

Polycystic ovary: See Stein–Leventhal syndrome

Polycythemia vera: CBC, platelet count, uric acid, ABG, pulmonary function tests, serum erythropoietin, bone marrow

Polymyalgia rheumatica: Sedimentation rate

Polyneuritis: See Neuropathy

Porphyria: Urine porphyrins and porphobilinogen

Portal cirrhosis: See Cirrhosis

Pott disease: X-ray of the spine, aspiration and culture of synovial fluid, synovial or bone biopsy, purified protein derivative (PPD) skin test

Preeclampsia: See Eclampsia

Pregnancy: Blood or urine test for pregnancy

Prostate carcinoma: Serum acid and alkaline phosphatase, prostate-specific antigen (PSA) skeletal survey, bone scan, biopsy of prostate

Prostatic hypertrophy: Sonogram, cystoscopy, IVP

Protein-losing enteropathy: ^{131}I polyvinylpyrrolidone test, serum protein electrophoresis

Pseudogout: Synovial analysis

Pseudomembranous colitis: *Clostridium difficile* toxin B

Pseudohypoparathyroidism: Serum calcium, phosphorus, alkaline phosphatase, urine calcium, Ellsworth–Howard test, PTH, parathyroid tissue biopsy

Pseudotumor cerebri: CT scan, MRI, spinal tap

Psittacosis: Chest x-ray, serologic test, virus isolation

Pulmonary embolism: See Pulmonary infarction

Pulmonary emphysema: See Emphysema

Pulmonary fibrosis: Diffusion capacity, bronchoscopy, lung biopsy, CT scan

Pulmonary hypertension, idiopathic: ABG, pulmonary function test, cardiac catheterization, pulmonary angiogram

Pulmonary infarction: ABG, V/Q lung scan, pulmonary angiogram, impedance plethysmogram, helical CT scan, rapid D-dimer assay

Pyelonephritis: Urine culture, colony count, IVP, cystoscopy, renal biopsy

Pyloric stenosis: GI series, gastroscopy, sonogram

Pyridoxine deficiency: Serum iron and iron-binding capacity, blood pyridoxine, urine pyridoxic acid

Q

Q fever: Serologic tests

R

Rabies: Observation or autopsy of infected animals, isolation of virus from saliva, serum and CSF antibody titer, fluorescent antibody stain of corneal or skin cells

Rat-bite fever: Dark field examination, culture of lesion, aspiration and culture of regional lymph node, animal inoculation, serologic tests

Raynaud's disease: ANA, lupus erythematosus prep, immunoelectrophoresis, cold agglutinins, cryoglobulins, skin or muscle biopsy, cold challenge

Reflux esophagitis: See Esophagitis

Regional enteritis: Sedimentation rate, small bowel series, sigmoidoscopy or colonoscopy and biopsy, CT scan of abdomen, surgical exploration

Reiter disease: HLA typing, bone scan, synovial analysis

Relapsing fever: Peripheral blood smear for Borrelia organisms, animal inoculation, serologic tests, total leukocytes, spinal tap

Renal calculus: IVP, noncontrast helical CT scan, cystoscopy, retrograde pyelogram, sonogram, stone analysis

Renal tubular acidosis: Serum electrolytes, calcium, phosphorus, alkaline phosphatase, urine calcium, phosphatase and bicarbonate, urine pH after ammonium chloride load

Respiratory distress syndrome: Ratio PaO_2 to FiO_2, pulmonary artery catheterization

Reticuloendotheliosis: X-ray, CBC, tissue cholesterol content, biopsy of skeletal lesion, bone marrow, or lymph nodes

Reticulum cell sarcoma: Alkaline phosphatase, lymph node biopsy, x-ray of chest, skeletal survey, GI series, IVP, cytologic examination of pleural or ascitic fluid

Rheumatic fever: Throat culture, streptozyme test, C-reactive protein (CRP), sedimentation rate, ECG, echocardiogram, serial ASO titer

Rheumatoid arthritis: RA test, sedimentation rate, ANA, x-ray of joints, synovial fluid analysis

Riboflavin deficiency: Activity coefficient of erythrocyte glutathione reductase

Rickets: Serum calcium, phosphorus, alkaline phosphatase, urine calcium, x-ray of bones, serum PTH, serum 25-OHD, bone biopsy

Rickettsialpox: Serologic tests

Rocky Mountain spotted fever: Specific serologic tests, Weil–Felix test, fluorescent antibody staining of skin lesions

Rubella: Viral isolation, latex agglutination card assay, other serologic tests

Rubeola: See Measles

S

Saddle embolus of aorta: Oscillometry, Doppler flow study, aortogram

Salicylate intoxication: Serum or urine salicylates, electrolytes

Salmonellosis: Stool culture, febrile agglutinins

Salpingitis: Vaginal smear and culture, sonogram, CT scan of pelvis, laparoscopy, exploratory surgery

Sarcoidosis: Chest x-ray, Kveim test, lymph node biopsy, elevated angiotensin-converting enzymes, gallium scan

Scabies: KOH prep

Scalenus anticus syndrome: X-ray of cervical spine, arteriogram

Scarlet fever: Nose and throat culture, streptozyme test, Schultz–Charlton reaction

Schilder's disease: EEG, CT scan, MRI, spinal tap, brain biopsy

Schistosomiasis: Stool or urine for ova, rectal biopsy, liver biopsy, serologic tests

Schönlein–Henoch purpura: Urinalysis, platelet count, coagulation profile, bleeding time, capillary fragility

Schuller–Christian disease: See Hand–Schuller–Christian disease

Scleroderma: ANA, RA test, anticentromere antibody titer, skin biopsy, esophagram, malabsorption workup

Scurvy: Serum ascorbic acid, capillary fragility, x-ray of bones, therapeutic trial

Seminoma: Urine hCG, sonogram, exploratory surgery, α-fetoprotein

Septicemia: Blood culture

Sexual precocity: Skull x-ray, CT scan, urine 17-ketosteroids and 17-hydroxysteroids, plasma cortisol, metyrapone test, exploratory surgery

Shigellosis: Stool examination for leukocytes, stool culture

Sickle cell anemia: CBC, blood smear, sickle cell preparation, hemoglobin electrophoresis

Silicosis: Chest x-ray, pulmonary function tests, ABG, lung biopsy, CT scan

Silo-filler's disease: Chest x-ray, clinical observations

Simmonds disease: See Hypopituitarism

Sinusitis: X-ray of sinuses, CT scan of sinuses, nose and throat culture, erythrocyte sedimentation rate (ESR), CRP

Sjogren's syndrome: Schirmer's test for tear production, ANA, RA titer, HLA typing, thyroglobulin antibody titer, anti-Sjogren's syndrome B (La) antibody titer

Smallpox: Smear of vesicular fluid for virus particles, viral isolation, serologic test

Spherocytosis, hereditary: CBC, blood smear, red cell fragility test, reticulocyte count, serum haptoglobins, bilirubin

Spinal cord tumor: X-ray of spine, CT scan of spine, MRI

Spinal stenosis: CT scan, MRI, myelogram

Sporotrichosis: Cultures of exudates from ulcer, serologic tests, skin tests, chest x-ray

Staphylococcal pneumonia: Sputum smear and culture, chest x-ray

Steatorrhea: See Celiac disease

Stein–Leventhal syndrome: Culdoscopy, laparoscopy, serum LH, urine 17-ketosteroids, sonogram, exploratory surgery, biopsy of ovaries

Stevens–Johnson syndrome: Streptozyme test, nose and throat culture

Still's disease: RA test, sedimentation rate, CRP, synovianalysis

Stokes–Adams syndrome: ECG, Holter monitoring, event monitoring, electrophysiologic testing

Streptococcal pharyngitis: See Pharyngitis

Strongyloidiasis: Stool or duodenal aspirate for ova and parasites

Sturge–Weber syndrome: Skull x-ray, CT scan, MRI

Subacute bacterial endocarditis: Blood culture, bone marrow cultures, echocardiogram, RA test, FTA–ABS, transesophageal echocardiography

Subarachnoid hemorrhage: CT scan of brain, spinal tap, arteriogram

Subdiaphragmatic abscess: Chest x-ray, gallium scan, indium scan, CT scan, needle aspiration, exploratory surgery

Subdural hematoma: CT scan, MRI, arteriogram

Subphrenic abscess: See Subdiaphragmatic abscess

Substance abuse: Blood alcohol level, urine drug screen, CAGE questionnaire

Sulfhemoglobinemia: Shaking of venous blood in test tube, spectroscopic examination of blood

Syphilis: Blood and spinal fluid venereal disease research laboratory (VDRL) test or FTA–ABS, dark field microscopy

Syringomyelia: CT scan, myelogram, MRI

T

Tabes dorsalis: Blood and spinal fluid, FTA–ABS

Takayasu's disease: CT scan of aorta, aortogram, serum protein electrophoresis

Tapeworm infections: Stool for ova and parasites, serology, sonogram, CT scan

Tay–Sachs disease: Cortical biopsy

Temporal arteritis: Sedimentation rate, biopsy of temporal artery

Tetanus: Clinical diagnosis, positive culture does not establish diagnosis

Thalassemia: CBC, blood smear, reticulocyte count, serum haptoglobin, hemoglobin electrophoresis

Thromboangiitis obliterans: See Buerger disease

Thrombocythemia (thrombasthenia): Platelet count, bleeding time, clotting time, clot retraction, capillary fragility

Thrombocytopenic purpura, idiopathic: Coagulation profile, platelet count, platelet antibody titer, bone marrow, liver–spleen scan, capillary fragility

Thrombophlebitis: Impedance plethysmography, compression ultrasonography, fibrinogen I-125 scan, venogram, thermogram, ultrasonography

Thymoma: Chest x-ray, CT scan of mediastinum, mediastinoscopy, exploratory thoracotomy

Thyroiditis, subacute: FT_4 index, RAI uptake and scan, sedimentation rate, antithyroid autoantibodies

Thyroid carcinoma: Serum calcitonin, RAI uptake and scan, CT scan of the neck

Thyroid nodule: RAI uptake and scan, fine-needle aspiration, biopsy, FT_4 index, sonogram, trial of thyroid suppression therapy

Tonsillitis: See Pharyngitis

Torsion of testicle: Ultrasonography, radionuclide scintigraphy

Tourette syndrome: Clinical diagnosis

Torulosis: See Cryptococcosis

Toxemia of pregnancy: See Eclampsia

Toxoplasmosis: Indirect fluorescent antibody (IFA) titer, passive hemagglutination test (PHA), skin test, animal inoculation

Trachoma: Smear of conjunctival scrapings, culture for *Chlamydia,* tears for microimmunofluorescent antibodies

Transfusion reaction: Serum hemoglobins and methemalbumin, Coombs test

Transient ischemic attack (TIA): Carotid scan, digital subtraction angiogram, CT scan, four-vessel cerebral angiogram, MRI

Trichinosis: Eosinophil count, skin test, serologic tests, muscle biopsy

Trypanosomiasis: Smears and culture of blood, CSF, lymph node aspirate for parasites, animal inoculation, serology

Tuberculosis: Smear and culture of sputum and gastric washings, Guinea pig inoculation, skin test, chest x-ray, CT scan

Tuberous sclerosis: Skull x-ray, CT scan, skin biopsy, cortical biopsy, EEG

Tularemia: Smear and culture of ulcer, lymph nodes, or nasopharynx; Foshay skin test; serologic tests

Turner syndrome: Buccal smear for chromatins (Barr bodies), chromosome analysis, FSH

Typhoid fever: Culture of stool, blood, or bone marrow; febrile agglutinins

Typhus, epidemic: Serologic tests, Weil–Felix reaction

Typhus scrub: Isolation from blood, serologic tests, Weil–Felix reaction

U

Ulcer: See Peptic ulcer

Ulcerative colitis: Barium enema, sigmoidoscopy or colonoscopy, biopsy

Urethritis: Urethral smear and culture, vaginal smear and culture, urine culture, *Chlamydia* culture, cystoscopy

Uterine fibroids: Sonogram, CT scan, MRI

Urticaria: RAST, allergic skin testing, elimination diet, C1 esterase inhibitor

Uveitis: Slit-lamp examination, ANA, HLA-B27 typing, VDRL, Lyme serology

V

Varicella: Serologic tests

Varicose veins: Phlebogram, thermogram

Variola: See Smallpox

Ventricular septal defects: ECG, echocardiogram, cardiac catheterization

Visceral larva migrans: Blood typing, serologic tests, biopsy

Vitamin A deficiency: Serum vitamin A or carotene, skin biopsy

Vitamin B deficiency: See Beriberi

Vitamin C deficiency: See Scurvy

Vitamin D deficiency: See Rickets

Vitamin K deficiency: Coagulation profile including prothrombin time

von Gierke disease: See Glycogen storage disease

von Willebrand disease: Coagulation profile, thromboplastin-generation test, factor VIII assay

W

Waterhouse–Friderichsen syndrome: Blood cultures, spinal fluid examination, nose and throat culture, plasma cortisol

Wegener's granulomatosis: X-ray or CT scans of nose, sinuses, and chest; urinalysis; renal biopsy; lung biopsy; nasal biopsy; antineutrophil cytoplasmic antigen (ANCA)

Weil's disease: Dark field examination of blood, Guinea pig inoculation, serologic tests, spinal tap

Wernicke's encephalopathy: Response to intravenous thiamine

Whipple's disease: Small-bowel series, lymph node biopsy, jejunal biopsy, malabsorption tests

Whooping cough: See Pertussis

Wilson's disease: Urine copper and amino acids, serum copper and ceruloplasmin, liver biopsy, slit-lamp examination of cornea, uric acid

Y

Yaws: Dark field examination, serologic tests

Yellow fever: Viral isolation, serologic tests, liver biopsy

Z

Zollinger–Ellison syndrome: Twelve-hour quantitative and basal gastric acid output (BAO) gastric analysis, serum gastrin, GI series, gastroscopy, exploratory laparotomy

Auricular fibrillation
  syncope, 468, 470
  tachycardia, 471, 472
Auricular flutter, 471, 472
Avascular necrosis
  hip pain, 232, 233
  joint pain, 289, 290
Axillary mass
  algorithm, 51
  diagnostic workup, 50
  questions to ask, 50
Azotemia, 494

B
Babinski's sign
  algorithm, 54
  diagnostic workup, 53
  questions to ask, 52–53
Back pain
  algorithm, 57
  case history, 55
  diagnostic workup, 55–56
  questions to ask, 55
Bacteremia, 28, 179
Bacteria, toxigenic, 117, 119
Bacterial endocarditis
  cardiomegaly, 75, 76
  chills, 83, 84
  clubbing of the fingers, 86, 87
  diaphoresis, 113, 114
  palpitations, 352, 353
  splenomegaly, acute or subacute, 452, 453
  subacute
    fatigue, 173, 175
    fever, acute, 177, 179
    fever, chronic, 180, 181
    hemiparesis/hemiplegia, 223, 224
    nail abnormalities, 325, 326
Baker's cyst, 381, 382
Balanitis
  enuresis, 149, 150
  penile sores, 366
Baldness, 21
Barbiturates
  blurred vision, 61, 62
  insomnia, 282
  intoxication
    dementia, 109, 110
    hypersomnia, 247
  memory loss, 309, 310
  restless leg syndrome, 427
  stupor, 465, 466
Bartholinitis
  dyspareunia, 134
  vulval or vaginal mass, 500
Bartholin's cyst, 50
Basal cell carcinoma, 414, 415
Basilar artery
  aneurysm, 343, 344
  insufficiency, 221, 222
    ataxia, 47, 48
    drop attacks, 128

    hyperactive reflexes, 238, 239
    nose, regurgitation of food through,
      341, 342
    ptosis, 396, 397
  meningitis
    hemianopsia, 221, 222
    nystagmus, 343, 344
  occlusion
    sensory loss, 436, 438
    tinnitus, 485, 486
    vertebral-basilar, 396, 397
  thrombosis
    Babinski's sign, 53, 54
    early basilar artery, 253, 254
    nystagmus, 343, 344
    pathologic reflexes, 361, 362
  vertebral basilar insufficiency
    hyperactive reflexes, 238, 239
    ptosis, 396, 397
  vertebral-basilar occlusion, 396, 397
Battered baby syndrome, 63, 64
Bee stings, 487
Bell's palsy
  epiphora, 151
  facial paralysis, 166, 167
  taste abnormalities, 473, 474
Benzodiazepines
  insomnia, 282
  nightmares, 339
  restless leg syndrome, 427
Beriberi
  edema, generalized, 144, 145
  foot ulceration, 189, 190
  memory loss, 309, 310
Bilateral ankle clonus, 30
Bilateral recurrent laryngeal palsy,
  463, 464
Bile ducts carcinoma
  hepatomegaly, 228, 229
  jaundice, 284, 286
Biliary cirrhosis
  hepatomegaly, 228, 229
  jaundice, 284, 286
Biliary colic, 331, 332
Biliary tree carcinoma, 32, 33
Birth control pills, 85
Bismuth, 473, 474
Bites
  black widow spider. *See* Black widow
    spider bites
  insect. *See* Insect bites
Biting nails, 325, 326
Black widow spider bites
  abdominal pain, acute, 1, 3
  abdominal rigidity, 7, 8
Bladder
  abdominal swelling, focal, 9, 11
  calculus
    abdominal pain, chronic recurrent,
      5, 6
    frequency of urination, 193, 194
    pain in the penis, 350, 351

type IV
  hypercholesterolemia, 241
  hypertriglyceridemia, 250, 252
  type V, 250, 252
Lip pain
  algorithm, 302
  diagnostic workup, 302
  questions to ask, 302
Lip swelling
  algorithm, 303
  diagnostic workup, 303
  question, 303
Lithium, 244
Little's area, irritation of, 152
Liver, cirrhosis of. *See* Cirrhosis, liver
Liver disease. *See also* Hepatic *entries*
  acid phosphatase elevation, 16
  aspartate aminotransferase elevation,
    45, 46
  chronic, 28, 29
  cirrhosis. *See* Liver, cirrhosis of
  lactic dehydrogenase elevation, 298
Localized edema. *See* Edema, localized
Lorain-Lévi syndrome, 129, 130
Lordosis, 304
Lower extremity pain
  algorithm, 157
  diagnostic workup, 156
  questions to ask, 156
Low sodium syndrome, 97, 98
LSD
  euphoria, 153, 154
  hallucinations, 207, 208
  memory loss, 309, 310
  stupor, 465, 466
Ludwig's angina
  neck swelling, 337, 338
  tongue mass or swelling, 487
Lues
  delirium, 106, 107
  stupor, 465, 466
Lumbar spondylosis
  back pain, 55, 57
  paresthesias of the lower extremity,
    356, 358
Lumbosacral sprain, 430, 431
Lung abscess. *See* Abscess, lung
Lung disease/disorders
  carcinoma
    gynecomastia, 203, 204
    hemoptysis, 225, 226
    hoarseness, 235, 236
    Horner's syndrome, 237
    lymphadenopathy, 305, 306
    nail abnormalities, 325, 326
    rales, 410, 411
    weight loss502, 504
  emphysema. *See* Emphysema
  insomnia, 282
  mycotic, 180, 181
  pulmonary fibrosis. *See* Pulmonary
    fibrosis

pulmonary infarction. *See* Infarct/
    infarction, pulmonary
taste abnormalities, 473, 474
tumors, 94, 95
Lupus
  discoid, 412, 413
  fever, chronic, 180, 181
  thrombocytopenia, 482
  vulval or vaginal ulcerations, 501
Lupus erythematosus, systemic. *See*
    Systemic lupus erythematosus
Lye poisoning, 135, 136
Lymphadenitis
  axillary mass, 50, 51
  inguinal swelling, 280
  neck swelling, 337, 338
  popliteal swelling, 381, 382
Lymphadenopathy
  algorithm, 306
  diagnostic workup, 305
  questions to ask, 305
Lymphangitis
  acute, 146
  extremity pain, lower extremity,
    156, 157
Lymphatic leukemia. *See* Leukemia,
    lymphatic
  acute, 452, 453
  leucocytosis, 300
Lymphedema
  localized, 146
  nail abnormalities, 325, 326
Lymph node, enlarged, 176
Lymphogranuloma venereum
  penile sores, 366
  vulval or vaginal ulcerations, 501
Lymphoma
  axillary mass, 50, 51
  diffuse, 487
  flank mass, 182, 183
  hepatomegaly, 228, 229
  Horner's syndrome, 237
  pruritus, generalized, 393, 394
  splenomegaly, acute or subacute,
    452, 453
  tongue mass or swelling, 487
  weight loss, 502, 504
Lymphosarcoma
  lymphadenopathy, 305, 306
  weight loss, 502, 504

M
Macroglobulinemia
  gangrene, 198, 199
  Raynaud's phenomenon, 416, 417
Maduromycosis, 189, 190
Major coagulation defect, 407, 408
Malabsorption
  abdominal swelling, generalized,
    12, 13
  alkaline phosphatase elevation,
    18, 19

Nitroglycerin, 262, 263
Nocturia
    algorithm, 340
    diagnostic workup, 340
    questions to ask, 340
Nodes, singer's, 235, 236
Nose
    deviated septum
        nasal obstruction, 329, 330
        snoring, 447
    nasal discharge
        algorithm, 328
        diagnostic workup, 327
        questions to ask, 327
    nasal gumma, 329, 330
    nasal obstruction
        algorithm, 330
        diagnostic workup, 329
        questions to ask, 329
    regurgitation of food through
        algorithm, 342
        diagnostic workup, 341
        questions to ask, 341
Nummular eczema
    rash—distribution, 412, 413
    rash—morphology, 414, 415
Nutrition. *See* Diet and nutrition;
        Malnutrition
Nystagmus
    algorithm, 344
    diagnostic workup, 343
    ocular, 343, 344
    questions to ask, 343

O
Obesity
    diaphoresis, 109, 110
    edema, generalized, 138, 139
    gynecomastia, 203, 204
    idiopathic
        sleep apnea, 444
        snoring, 447
    infertility, female, 277, 278
    pathologic
        algorithm, 346
        diagnostic workup, 345
        questions to ask, 345
Obstructions
    advanced intestinal
        abdominal swelling, generalized,
            12, 13
        meteorism, 315
    bladder intestinal, 12, 13
    bladder neck. *See* Bladder, neck
        obstructions
    chronic intestinal, 275, 276
    complete intestinal, 86, 87
    incomplete intestinal, 86, 87
    intestinal. *See* Intestinal obstructions
    nasolacrimal duct, congenital causes, 144
    present gastric outlet, 20
    pyloric. *See* Pyloric obstructions

Obturator hernia. *See* Hernia, obturator
Occipital lobe tumors, 432, 433
Occlusion
    anterior cerebral artery
        hemianopsia, 221, 222
        monoplegia, 318, 319
    anterior spinal artery
        Babinski's sign, 53, 54
        hyperactive reflexes, 238, 239
        paresthesias of the lower extremity,
            356, 358
        pathologic reflexes, 361, 362
        sensory loss, 436, 438
    basilar artery
        sensory loss, 436, 438
        tinnitus, 485, 486
        vertebral-basilar, 396, 397
    central retinal artery, 54, 55
    middle cerebral artery, 221, 222
    posterior cerebral artery
        blindness, 54, 55
        blurred vision, 56, 57
    posterior inferior cerebellar artery,
        436, 438
    vertebral-basilar, 396, 397
Oculomotor nerve palsy, 405, 406
Odontoma, 288
Odor
    algorithm, 347
    diagnostic workup, 347
    questions to ask, 347
Oliguria or anuria. *See* Anuria or oliguria
Omental hernia, 9, 11
Onychia, 325, 326
Opacities, corneal
    diplopia, 122, 123
    scotoma, 432, 433
Ophthalmoplegia, 396, 397
Opisthotonus
    algorithm, 348
    diagnostic workup, 348
    questions to ask, 348
Opium poisoning
    coma, 84, 85
    hypothermia, 264, 265
    respiration abnormalities, 426
Optic atrophy
    blindness, 54, 55
    blurred vision, 56, 57
    hereditary, 432, 433
Optic cortex tumors, 221, 222
Optic nerve
    injury, 54, 55
    lesions, 405, 406
Optic neuritis
    blindness, 59, 60
    eye pain, 153
    papilledema, 354, 355
Optic tract tumors, 221, 222
Oral contraceptives, 241
Oral tumors, 287
Orbital abscess, 122, 123

Shoulder pain
  algorithm, 442
  case history, 440
  bursitis. *See* Bursitis
  diagnostic workup, 440-441
  questions to ask, 440
Shunt, right-to-left, 266, 267
Shy-Drager syndrome, 444
SIADH, 261
Sickle cell disease, 28, 29
  abdominal pain, acute, 1, 2, 3
  hematuria, 208, 209
  joint pain, 289, 290
  priapism, 387, 388
  Raynaud's phenomenon, 416, 417
  thrombocytopenia, 482
Sick sinus syndrome
  bradycardia, 66, 67
  cardiac arrhythmia, 71, 72
  pulse irregularity, 401, 402
Silicosis, 94, 95
Simmonds' disease
  amenorrhea, 24, 25
  infertility, female, 277, 278
  weight loss, 502, 504
Sinus
  arrhythmia. *See* Arrythmia, sinus
  cavernous, 155
Sinusitis
  acute
    exophthalmos, 155
    face pain, 162, 163
    headache, 210, 211
    nasal discharge, 327, 328
    nasal obstruction, 329, 330
    periorbital edema, 368, 369
  allergic, 327, 328
  chronic
    anosmia or unusual odors, 34, 35
    face pain, 162, 163
    nasal discharge, 327, 328
  eye pain, 161
  facial swelling, 168, 169
  halitosis, 205, 206
  nasal discharge, 327, 328
  nasal obstruction, 329, 330
Sinus thrombosis, 83, 84
Skin thickening, 443
  diagnostic workup, 443
Skin tumors
  facial swelling, 168, 169
  rash—distribution, 412, 413
Skull fractures
  anosmia or unusual odors, 34, 35
  blindness, 59, 60
Sleep apnea
  algorithm, 444
  diagnostic workup, 444
  idiopathic, 444
  insomnia, 273
  questions to ask, 444
  snoring, 447

Sleepwalking, 445
Smallpox
  rash—distribution, 412, 413
  rash—morphology, 414, 415
Smoking
  cough, 90, 91
  heavy cigarette, 374, 375
Sneezing, 446
  diagnostic workup, 446
Snoring, 447
Sodium fluoride poisoning, 129, 130
Sore throat
  algorithm, 449
  diagnostic workup, 448
  questions to ask, 448
Space-occupying lesions. *See* Brain,
    spaceoccupying lesions
Spasm, diffuse esophageal, 129, 130
Spastic diplegia
  failure to thrive, 171, 172
  gait disturbances, 196, 197
Spasticity, 450
Speech abnormalities, 451
Spermatocele, 478, 479
Spherocytosis
  anemia, 25, 26
  hereditary
  splenomegaly, acute or subacute,
    452, 453
  splenomegaly, chronic, 454, 455
Spinal cord
  diseases, 188
  disks. *See* Spinal disks
  injury, 318, 319
    acute, 120, 121
  trauma
    incontinence of feces, 270, 271
    incontinence of urine, 264, 265
    meteorism, 315
    priapism, 387, 388
  tumors
    ankle clonus, 27, 28
    Babinski's sign, 49, 50
  back pain, 51, 52
  cervical cord, 238, 239
  extremity pain, upper extremity,
    158, 159
  gait disturbances, 196, 197
  girdle pain, 201
  high cord, 49, 50
  Horner's syndrome, 237
  hyperactive reflexes, 238, 239
  impotence, 268, 269
  incontinence of feces, 270, 271
  incontinence of urine, 272, 273
  monoplegia, 318, 319
  muscular atrophy, 321, 322
  neck pain, 333, 334
  paresthesias of the lower extremity,
    356, 358
  paresthesias of the upper extremity,
    359, 360

Thirst
　algorithm, 481
　diagnostic workup, 480
　questions to ask, 480
Thoracic outlet syndrome
　extremity pain, upper extremity, 158, 159
　Horner's syndrome, 237
　neck pain, 333, 334
　paresthesias of the upper extremity,
　　359, 360
　pulses, unequal, 403, 404
　shoulder pain, 440, 442
Thoracic spinal cord tumors, 238, 239
Thoracic sprain, 430, 431
Thrombocytopenia
　algorithm, 482
　bleeding gums, 58
　diagnostic workup, 482
　drug-induced, 407, 408
　purpura and abnormal bleeding, 407, 408
　questions to ask, 482
Thrombophlebitis
　edema, localized, 140
　extremity pain, lower extremity, 149, 150
　extremity pain, upper extremity, 158, 159
　superficial, 149, 150
Thrombosis
　anterior cerebral artery, 53, 54
　basilar artery
　　Babinski's sign, 53, 54
　　nystagmus, 343, 344
　　pathologic reflexes, 361, 362
　carotid artery
　　blindness, 59, 60
　　Horner's syndrome, 237
　　scotoma, 432, 433
　cavernous
　　diplopia, 122, 123
　　exophthalmos, 148
　　eye pain, 153
　　periorbital edema, 368, 369
　　ptosis, 396, 397
　cerebral
　　ankle clonus, 30, 31
　　hemiparesis/hemiplegia, 223, 224
　　pathologic reflexes, 361, 362
　deep vein, 149, 150
　dural sinus, 354, 355
　early basilar artery, 253, 254
　exophthalmos, 148
　extremity pain, lower extremity, 149, 150
　femoral artery, 299
　hemiparesis/hemiplegia, 223, 224
　hepatic vein
　　abdominal swelling, generalized, 12, 13
　　hepatomegaly, 228, 229
　　jaundice, 284, 286
　　mesenteric
　　abdominal pain, acute, 1, 2, 4
　　abdominal rigidity, 7, 8
　　abdominal swelling, generalized,
　　　12, 13

　melena, 307, 308
　meteorism, 315
　rectal bleeding, 418, 419
　middle cerebral artery, 53, 54
　portal vein
　　hematemesis, 206, 207
　　splenomegaly, acute or subacute,
　　　452, 453
　　splenomegaly, chronic, 454, 455
　posterior cerebral artery
　　hemianopsia, 221, 222
　　scotoma, 432, 433
　retinal vein, 54, 55
　sinus, 78, 79
　venous
　　gangrene, 198, 199
　　hemiparesis/hemiplegia, 223, 224
　　leg ulceration, 299
Thyroglossal cyst
　neck swelling, 338, 339
　thyroid enlargement, 483, 484
Thyroid carcinoma
　clubbing of the fingers, 82, 83
　enlargement, 483, 484
Thyroid enlargement
　algorithm, 484
　diagnostic workup, 483
　questions to ask, 483
Thyroiditis
　stridor, 463, 464
　subacute
　　fever, chronic, 180, 181
　　sore throat, 448, 449
　　thyroid enlargement, 483, 484
Thyroid storm, 471, 472
Thyrotoxicosis
　diaphoresis, 109, 110
　diarrhea, chronic, 113, 114
　gigantism, 200
　tachycardia, 471, 472
　thirst, 480, 481
Tic douloureux, 136, 137
Tietze's syndrome, 76, 77
Tinea capitis
　alopecia, 20
　rash—distribution, 412, 413
Tinea versicolor
　hyperpigmentation, 246
　rash—distribution, 412, 413
Tinnitus
　algorithm, 486
　diagnostic workup, 485
　questions to ask, 485
Tobacco
　blurred vision, 56, 57
　halitosis, 205, 206
　hoarseness, 235, 236
　poisoning, 432, 433
Toe and foot pain
　algorithm, 187
　diagnostic workup, 187
　questions to ask, 187

Toenail, ingrown, 187
Tongue, large, 444
Tongue mass or swelling
  algorithm, 487
  diagnostic workup, 487
  questions to ask, 487
Tongue pain, 488
  diagnostic workup, 488
Tongue ulcers, 489
Tonsillitis, 205, 206
Tonsils, hypertrophied, 447
Toothbrush, injury with, 58
Tooth or teeth
  abnormalities, 490
  abscessed
    face pain, 162, 163
    facial swelling, 168, 169
    insomnia, 273
  carious, 205, 206, 398, 399
  impacted wisdom, 287
  pain referred from, 302
Torticollis, idiopathic, 335, 336
Tourette's syndrome, 80, 81
Toxemia of pregnancy, proteinuria, 390, 391
Toxic encephalopathy
  delirium, 102, 103
  delusions, 104
Toxicity. See also Poisoning
  drug, 98, 99
  levodopa, 80, 81
  phenothiazine, 80, 81
    dysarthria, 131, 132
  prochlorperazine, 80, 81
  salicylate, 19
Toxic metabolic disease, 253, 254
Toxins in food, 275, 276
Toxoplasmosis, 305, 306
Trachea carcinoma, 463, 464
Trachoma, 396, 397
Transient ischemic attacks. See Ischemic
    attacks, transient
Transverse myelitis. See Myelitis,
    transverse
Trauma
  acoustic, 98, 99
  deafness, 98, 99
  joint pain, 289, 290
  joint swelling, 291, 292
  leucocytosis, 30
  lip pain, 302
  lip swelling, 303
  nail abnormalities, 325, 326
  nasal obstruction, 329, 330
  nose, regurgitation of food through,
    341, 342
  pathologic reflexes, 361, 362
  proteinuria, 390, 391
  pyuria, 409
  recent, 300
  spinal cord. See Spinal cord, trauma
  splenomegaly, acute or subacute, 452,
    453

thirst, 480, 481
  tongue mass or swelling, 487
Tremor
  algorithm, 492
  case history, 491
  diagnostic workup, 491
  familial, 491, 492
  questions to ask, 491
  senile, 491, 492
Trichinosis
  musculoskeletal pain, generalized,
    323, 324
  nail abnormalities, 325, 326
  periorbital edema, 368, 369
Tricuspid regurgitation
  cardiac murmurs, 68, 69
  cardiomegaly, 70, 71
Tricuspid stenosis, 68, 69
Trigeminal neuralgia, 371
  face pain, 154, 155
  jaw pain, 287
  lip pain, 302
Trismus, 493
Tuberculosis
  axillary mass, 46, 47
  bladder
    frequency of urination, 193, 194
    incontinence of urine, 272, 273
  chills, 78, 79
  clubbing of the fingers, 82, 83
  cough, 90, 91
  fatigue, 173, 175
  femoral mass or swelling, 176
  fever, chronic, 180, 181
  flank mass, 173, 174
  flank pain, 175
  halitosis, 205, 206
  hematuria, 208, 209
  hemoptysis, 225, 226
  hoarseness, 235, 236
  joint pain, 279, 280
  joint swelling, 291, 292
  knee swelling, 295, 296
  kyphosis, 297
  leg ulceration, 299
  lymphadenopathy, 305, 306
  miliary, 452, 453
  muscular atrophy, 321, 322
  neck stiffness, 335, 336
  nose, regurgitation of food through,
    341, 342
  proteinuria, 390, 391
  pyuria, 409
  rales, 410, 411
  respiration abnormalities, 426
  scoliosis, 430, 431
  spine, 335, 336
  splenomegaly, acute or subacute, 452,
    453
  strangury, 460
  testicular atrophy, 475, 476
  weight loss, 502, 504

diarrhea, chronic, 113, 114
rectal bleeding, 418, 419
Ulnar entrapment, 158, 159, 359, 360
Upper extremity pain
algorithm, 159
diagnostic workup, 158
questions to ask, 158
Upper respiratory infections, 31, 32
viral
cough, 90, 91
fever, acute, 177, 179
hoarseness, 235, 236
nasal discharge, 320, 321
nasal obstruction, 329, 330
sore throat, 448, 449
Uremia
algorithm, 494
cramps, muscular, 93, 94
diagnostic workup, 494
halitosis, 205, 206
hiccups, 230, 231
hypercalcemia, 331, 332
hypothermia, 264, 265
indigestion, 275, 276
insomnia, 282
memory loss, 309, 310
nausea and vomiting, 331, 332
odor, 347
opisthotonus, 348
pruritus, generalized, 393, 394
questions to ask, 494
respiration abnormalities, 426
stupor, 465, 466
tinnitus, 485, 486
weight loss, 502, 504
Uremic coma, 84, 85
Uremic neuropathy, 427
Urethral caruncle
diffculty urinating, 120, 121
dyspareunia, 128
vulvar or vaginal mass, 500
Urethral discharge, 495
Urethral stricture
difficulty urinating, 120, 121
pain in the penis, 344, 345
Urethral syndrome, 139, 140
Urethral tumors, 387, 388
Urethritis
difficulty urinating, 120, 121
dyspareunia, 128
dysuria, 139, 140
frequency of urination, 193, 194
infertility, male, 270
nocturia, 340
nonspecific, 139, 140
pain in the penis, 344, 345
perineum pain, 367
pyuria, 409
strangury, 460
Urinary incontinence. *See* Incontinence,
urine
Urinary tract infection, 390, 391

Urination difficulty
algorithm, 121
diagnostic workup, 120
questions to ask, 120
Urination frequency
algorithm, 194
diagnostic workup, 193
questions to ask, 193
Urine color changes, 496
Uropathy, obstructive, 494
Urticaria
allergic, 296
facial flushing, 156
hoarseness, 235, 236
lip swelling, 296
pigmentosa, 156
pruritus, generalized, 393, 394
Uterine bleeding, dysfunctional. *See*
Bleeding, dysfuctional
uterine
Uterine fibroids
abdominal swelling, focal, 9, 11
frequency of urination, 193, 194
menorrhagia, 311, 312
pelvic mass, 363
pelvic pain, 364, 365
strangury, 460
Uterine prolapse, 500
Uterus
pregnant
abdominal swelling, focal, 9, 11
pelvic mass, 363
retroverted
dysmenorrhea, 133
dyspareunia, 134
frequency of urination,
193, 194
infertility, female, 268, 269
pelvic, 195
rectal mass, 421, 422
UTI, 390, 391
Uveitis, 59, 60
Uvula, 447

V
Vagina, imperforate, 24, 25
Vaginal carcinoma
metrorrhagia, 316, 317
pruritus, vulvae, 395
Vaginal discharge
algorithm, 498
diagnostic workup, 497
questions to ask, 497
Vaginal or vulval mass
algorithm, 500
diagnostic workup, 500
questions to ask, 500
Vaginal or vulval ulcerations
algorithm, 501
diagnostic workup, 501
question, 501
Vaginismus, 195